Clinical Oncology
Basic Principles and Practice
Fifth Edition

Clinical Oncology
Basic Principles and Practice
Fifth Edition

Peter Hoskin MD FRCP FRCR
Professor in Clinical Oncology at the University of Manchester
and Consultant in Clinical Oncology at Mount Vernon Hospital
Northwood, Middlesex, United Kingdom

with additional contributions from:

Peter Ostler MBBS MRCP FRCR
Consultant in Clinical Oncology at Mount Vernon Hospital
Northwood, Middlesex, United Kingdom
and Chair of the Final FRCR (Part B) Examination Board
at the Royal College of Radiologists
London, United Kingdom

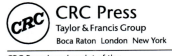

CRC Press is an imprint of the
Taylor & Francis Group, an **informa** business

CRC Press
Taylor & Francis Group
6000 Broken Sound Parkway NW, Suite 300
Boca Raton, FL 33487-2742

© 2020 by Taylor & Francis Group, LLC
CRC Press is an imprint of Taylor & Francis Group, an Informa business

No claim to original U.S. Government works

International Standard Book Number-13: 978-0-367-89696-6 (Hardback)
978-1-138-03555-3 (Paperback)

This book contains information obtained from authentic and highly regarded sources. While all reasonable efforts have been made to publish reliable data and information, neither the author[s] nor the publisher can accept any legal responsibility or liability for any errors or omissions that may be made. The publishers wish to make clear that any views or opinions expressed in this book by individual editors, authors or contributors are personal to them and do not necessarily reflect the views/opinions of the publishers. The information or guidance contained in this book is intended for use by medical, scientific or health-care professionals and is provided strictly as a supplement to the medical or other professional's own judgement, their knowledge of the patient's medical history, relevant manufacturer's instructions and the appropriate best practice guidelines. Because of the rapid advances in medical science, any information or advice on dosages, procedures or diagnoses should be independently verified. The reader is strongly urged to consult the relevant national drug formulary and the drug companies' and device or material manufacturers' printed instructions, and their websites, before administering or utilizing any of the drugs, devices or materials mentioned in this book. This book does not indicate whether a particular treatment is appropriate or suitable for a particular individual. Ultimately it is the sole responsibility of the medical professional to make his or her own professional judgements, so as to advise and treat patients appropriately. The authors and publishers have also attempted to trace the copyright holders of all material reproduced in this publication and apologize to copyright holders if permission to publish in this form has not been obtained. If any copyright material has not been acknowledged please write and let us know so we may rectify in any future reprint.

Except as permitted under U.S. Copyright Law, no part of this book may be reprinted, reproduced, transmitted, or utilized in any form by any electronic, mechanical, or other means, now known or hereafter invented, including photocopying, microfilming, and recording, or in any information storage or retrieval system, without written permission from the publishers.

For permission to photocopy or use material electronically from this work, please access www.copyright.com (http://www.copyright.com/) or contact the Copyright Clearance Center, Inc. (CCC), 222 Rosewood Drive, Danvers, MA 01923, 978-750-8400. CCC is a not-for-profit organization that provides licenses and registration for a variety of users. For organizations that have been granted a photocopy license by the CCC, a separate system of payment has been arranged.

Trademark Notice: Product or corporate names may be trademarks or registered trademarks, and are used only for identification and explanation without intent to infringe.

Visit the Taylor & Francis Web site at
http://www.taylorandfrancis.com

and the CRC Press Web site at
http://www.crcpress.com

Contents

List of abbreviations	ix
Preface	xiii
Acknowledgement	xv

1 Pathogenesis of cancer — 1
- Genetic factors — 1
- Chemical factors — 2
- Physical factors — 4
- Viral factors — 5
- Immune factors — 6
- Endocrine factors — 7

2 Principles of cancer diagnosis and staging — 9
- Securing a tissue diagnosis — 9
- Principles of cancer staging — 10
- The TNM staging system — 16

3 Decision-making and communication — 21
- Treatment options — 21
- Quality of life — 24
- Communication — 24
- Clinical evidence and clinical trials — 27

4 Principles of surgical oncology — 35
- Management of the primary tumour — 35
- Combined surgery and radiotherapy — 35
- Management of regional lymph nodes — 36
- Palliative surgery — 37

5 Principles of radiotherapy — 39
- Types of radiation — 39
- Biological actions of ionizing radiation — 39
- Radiotherapy equipment — 40
- Clinical use of radiotherapy — 42
- Side effects of radiotherapy — 46
- Radiation protection — 47

6 Principles of systemic treatment — 51
- Chemotherapy agents — 51
- Drug resistance — 55
- Administration of chemotherapy — 56

Contents

	Hormone therapy	60
	Biological therapy	62
	Immunotherapy	62
	Growth factors	63
	Experimental chemotherapy	63
7	**Lung cancer and mesothelioma**	**67**
	Lung cancer	67
	Mesothelioma	83
8	**Breast cancer**	**89**
	Epidemiology	89
	Aetiology	89
	Pathology	90
	Natural history	92
	Symptoms	93
	Signs	95
	Differential diagnosis	96
	Investigations	96
	Staging	98
	Treatment	98
	Prognosis	110
	Screening	112
	Prevention	113
9	**Gastrointestinal cancer**	**115**
	Carcinoma of the oesophagus	115
	Carcinoma of the stomach	121
	Carcinoma of the pancreas	126
	Hepatocellular cancer	131
	Cholangiocarcinoma	135
	Carcinoma of the gallbladder	138
	Carcinoma of the colon and rectum	138
	Carcinoma of the anus	146
	Tumours of the peritoneum	149
10	**Urological cancer**	**153**
	Renal cell carcinoma	153
	Prostate cancer	156
	Bladder cancer	165
	Cancer of the testis	170
	Cancer of the penis	174
11	**Gynaecological cancer**	**179**
	Cervical cancer	179
	Endometrial cancer	185
	Ovarian cancer	188
	Cancer of the vagina	192
	Cancer of the vulva	194
	Choriocarcinoma	196

Contents

12 CNS tumours — **201**
- Astrocytoma — 204
- Oligodendroglioma — 206
- Meningioma — 206
- Pituitary tumours — 207
- Craniopharyngioma — 208
- Pineal tumours — 209
- Germ cell tumours — 209
- Ependymomas — 210
- Medulloblastoma — 210
- Chordoma — 211
- Haemangioblastoma — 211
- Lymphoma — 211
- Metastases — 211
- Carcinomatous meningitis — 213

13 Head and neck cancer — **217**
- Carcinoma of the oral cavity — 217
- Carcinoma of the oropharynx — 223
- Carcinoma of the larynx — 223
- Carcinoma of the hypopharynx — 224
- Carcinoma of the nasopharynx — 225
- Carcinoma of the paranasal sinuses — 226
- Salivary gland tumours — 226
- Orbital tumours — 228

14 Endocrine tumours — **231**
- Thyroid cancer — 231
- Tumours of the parathyroid gland — 238
- Tumours of the adrenal glands — 238
- Carcinoid tumours — 240
- Multiple endocrine neoplasia (MEN) — 243

15 Sarcomas — **245**
- Soft-tissue sarcomas — 245
- Osteosarcoma — 250
- Ewing sarcoma — 254
- Other bone tumours — 256

16 Lymphoma — **259**
- Hodgkin lymphoma — 259
- Non-Hodgkin lymphoma (NHL) — 266

17 Haematological malignancy — **279**
- Leukaemia — 279
- Multiple myeloma — 290

18 Paediatric cancer — **301**
- Leukaemia — 301
- Central nervous system tumours — 301

	Bone and soft-tissue tumours	304
	Lymphoma	306
	Neuroblastoma	307
	Nephroblastoma (Wilms' tumour)	310
	Other tumours	312
19	**Skin cancer**	**317**
	Squamous and basal cell carcinoma	317
	Melanoma	323
	Metastases	328
	Rare tumours	328
20	**Carcinoma of unknown primary**	**331**
21	**Oncological emergencies**	**337**
	Hypercalcaemia	337
	Spinal cord and cauda equina compression	338
	Superior vena cava obstruction	340
	Neutropenic sepsis	342
	Tumour lysis syndrome	343
	Toxicities related to immunotherapy agents	343
22	**Palliative care**	**349**
	Pain control	349
	Other symptoms	355
	The dying patient	357

Appendix 1: Worldwide cancer burden – males and females	361
Appendix 2: Worldwide cancer burden – males	363
Appendix 3: Worldwide cancer burden – females	365
Appendix 4: Answers to self-assessment questions	367
Index	369

List of abbreviations

ABVD	chemotherapy schedule comprising Adriamycin, bleomycin, vinblastine and dacarbazine	CGL	chronic granulocytic leukaemia
AFP	α-fetoprotein	CHART	continuous, hyperfractionated, accelerated radiotherapy
AIDS	acquired immune deficiency syndrome	ChlVPP	chemotherapy schedule comprising chlorambucil, vinblastine, procarbazine and prednisolone
AIN	anal intraepithelial neoplasia	CHOP	chemotherapy schedule comprising cyclophosphamide, hydroxydaunorubicin (Adriamycin), oncovin and prednisolone
ALL	acute lymphoblastic leukaemia		
AML	acute myeloid/myeloblastic leukaemia		
AP	anteroposterior	CHRPE	congenital hypertrophy of the retinal pigment epithelium
APR	abdominoperineal resection		
APUD	amine precursor uptake and decarboxylation	CIN	cervical intraepithelial neoplasia
		CIS	cell carcinoma *in situ*
ATRA	all-trans-retinoic acid	CNS	central nervous system
AUC	area under the serum concentration vs. time curve	CRM	circumferential resection margin
		CRT	chemoradiotherapy
BBB	blood–brain barrier	CSF	colony-stimulating factors
BCC	basal cell carcinoma	CT	computed tomography
BEACOPP	chemotherapy schedule comprising bleomycin, etoposide, Adriamycin, cyclophosphamide, vincristine (Oncovin), procarbazine and prednisone	CVAD	chemotherapy schedule comprising cyclophosphamide, vincristine, doxorubicin (Adriamycin) and dexamethasone
BEAM	chemotherapy schedule comprising BCNU, etoposide, cytosine arabinoside and melphelan	DCIS	ductal carcinoma *in situ*
		DMC	data monitoring committee
		DNA	deoxyribonucleic acid
BEP	chemotherapy schedule comprising bleomycin, etoposide and cisplatin	DRE	digital rectal examination
		EBV	Epstein–Barr virus
BEV	beam's eye view	ECF	chemotherapy schedule comprising epirubicin, cisplatin and 5FU
BOPP	chemotherapy schedule comprising bleomycin, vincristine, cisplatin and prednisolone	ECX	chemotherapy schedule comprising epirubicin, cisplatin and capecitabine (xeloda)
BSE	breast self-examination	EDTA	ethylene diamine tetra-acetic acid
CAP	chemotherapy schedule comprising cyclophosphamide, Adriamycin, cisplatin	EGFR	epithelial growth factor receptor
		EMA-CO	chemotherapy schedule comprising etoposide, methotrexate, actinomycin D, cyclophosphamide and vincristine
CDT	chemotherapy schedule comprising cyclophosphamide, dexamethasone and thalidomide		
		EORTC	European Organisation for Research and Treatment of Cancer
CEA	carcinoembryonic antigen		

List of abbreviations

EPID	electronic portal imaging device	IVU	intravenous urography
ER	oestrogen receptor	KS	Kaposi's sarcoma
ERCP	endoscopic retrograde cholepancreaticogram	LCA	leucocyte common antigen
		LCIS	lobular carcinoma *in situ*
ESR	erythrocyte sedimentation rate	LD	latissimus dorsi
EUA	examination under anaesthetic	LDH	lactate dehydrogenase
FACT	Functional Assessment of Cancer Therapy questionnaire	LET	linear energy transfer
		LOPP	chemotherapy schedule comprising chlorambucil (Leukeran), vinblastine, procarbazine and prednisolone (same as ChlVPP)
FAD	chemotherapy comprising fludarabine in combination with Adriamycin and dexamethasone		
FDG	fluorodeoxyglucose	MAB	maximal androgen blockade
FDPs	fibrin degradation products	MAB	monoclonal antibody
FISH	fluoresence *in situ* hybridization	MALT	mucosal-associated lymphoid tissue
FMD	chemotherapy schedule comprising fludarabine in combination with mitoxantrone and dexamethasone	MDR	multidrug resistance
		MDT	chemotherapy schedule comprising melphalan, dexamethasone and thalidomide
FNA	fine-needle aspiration		
FOBT	faecal occult blood testing	MEN	multiple endocrine neoplasia
5FU	5-fluorouracil	mIBG	meta-iodobenzyl guanidine
GC	chemotherapy schedule comprising gemcitabine with cisplatin	MIP	maximum intensity projection
		MOPP	chemotherapy schedule comprising mustine, vincristine, procarbazine and prednisolone
G-CSF	granulocyte colony-stimulating factor		
GEP	gastroenteropancreatic		
GIST	gastrointestinal stromal tumour	MRA	magnetic resonance angiography
GnRH	gonadotrophin-releasing hormone	MRI	magnetic resonance imaging
GST	glutathione *S*-transferase	MTD	maximum tolerated dose
HAART	highly active antiretroviral therapy	MTIC	monomethyl triazenoimidazole carboxamide
HAD	Hospital Anxiety and Depression		
HCG	human chorionic gonadotrophin	MVAC	chemotherapy schedule comprising methotrexate, vinblastine and Adriamycin plus cisplatin
HHV	human herpes virus		
5-HIAA	5-hydroxyindoleacetic acid		
HIV	human immunodeficiency virus	MVC	chemotherapy schedule comprising methotrexate, vinblastine and cisplatin
HNPCC	hereditary non-polyposis colon or colorectal cancer		
HPOA	hypertrophic pulmonary osteoarthropathy	NAT2	*N*-acetyl transferase 2
		NHL	non-Hodgkin lymphoma
HPV	human papilloma virus	NLPHL	nodular lymphocyte-predominant Hodgkin lymphoma
HTLV-1	human T-cell lymphotropic virus type 1		
		NMDA	*N*-methyl-D-aspartate
HVA	homovanillylmandelic acid	NSAID	non-steroidal anti-inflammatory drug
IDL	indirect laryngoscopy	NSE	neurone-specific enolase
IJV	internal jugular vein	OAF	osteoclast-activating factor
IL	interleukin	OEPA	chemotherapy schedule comprising vincristine, etoposide, prednisolone and Adriamycin
IMRT	intensity-modulated radiotherapy		
INR	international normalized ratio		
IPI	International Prognostic Index		
IVC	inferior vena cava		

List of abbreviations

OPPA	chemotherapy schedule comprising vincristine, procarbazine, prednisolone and Adriamycin	RMI	Risk of Malignancy index
		RR	relative risk
		SCC	squamous cell carcinoma
PBPC	peripheral blood progenitor cell	SCLC	small-cell lung cancer
PCI	prophylactic cranial irradiation	SIADH	syndrome of inappropriate antidiuretic hormone secretion
PDGF	platelet-derived growth factor		
PDGFRB	platelet-derived growth factor receptor B	SRT	stereotactic radiotherapy
		STD	sexually transmitted disease
PET	positron emission tomography	SUV	glucose uptake rates (standardized uptake value)
PICC	peripherally inserted central catheter		
PIN	prostate intraepithelial neoplasia	SVC	superior vena cava
PLAP	placental alkaline phosphatase	SVCO	superior vena cava obstruction
PNET	primitive neuroectodermal tumour	TCT	transitional cell tumour
POMBACE	chemotherapy schedule comprising cisplatin, vincristine, methotrexate, bleomycin, actinomycin D, cyclophosphamide and etoposide	TME	total mesorectal excision
		TNM	tumour, nodes, metastases
		TP	thymidine phosphorylase
		TSH	thyroid stimulating hormone
		TURBT	transurethral resection of bladder tumour
PSA	prostate-specific antigen		
PTC	percutaneous transhepatic cholangiography	TURP	transurethral resection of the prostate
PUVA	psoralens and ultraviolet A	VAC	chemotherapy schedule comprising vincristine, actinomycin D and cyclophosphamide
PVI	protracted venous infusion		
RCHOP	chemotherapy schedule comprising rituximab, cyclophosphamide, hydroxydaunorubicin (Adriamycin), vincristine and prednisolone		
		VAIN	vaginal intraepithelial neoplasia
		VAS	visual analogue scale
		VDA	vascular disrupting agent
RCVP	chemotherapy schedule comprising rituximab, cyclophosphamide, vincristine and prednisolone	VEGF	vascular endothelial growth factor
		VHL	von Hippel–Lindau
		VMA	vanillylmandelic acid
REAL	Revised European American Lymphoma classification	Z-DEX	chemotherapy schedule comprising idarubicin and high-dose dexamethasone
RECIST	Response Evaluation Criteria in Solid Tumours		

Preface

Worldwide there were 17 million cases of cancer diagnosed in 2018, accounting for 9.6 million deaths. This is expected to increase to 27.5 million cases by 2040, with an increase in men greater than that for women. In Europe there were 4.2 million new cases and almost 2 million deaths. Over the past 20 years, in developed health-care systems the diagnosis of cancer at an earlier stage and advances in treatment and supportive care have led to an ongoing decline in age-standardized mortality. Over 12 million people were living with cancer in Europe in 2018.

Thus, the management of cancer patients forms a significant part of the daily practice of doctors in most clinical specialities and general practice. This concise textbook has been written to give an insight into the basic principles and practice of clinical oncology. With both general and site-specific chapters, it provides a readily available source of information on the epidemiology, aetiology, pathology, presentation, staging, management and prognosis of malignant disease. Recent advances and topical issues are covered. This book will be of interest and relevance to undergraduates in medicine, junior doctors, nurses with an interest in oncology and other health-care professionals who wish to acquire a core of basic knowledge in this field. Case studies and MCQs are used to reinforce key points. The text of this fifth edition has been fully revised to reflect recent advances and changes in practice in this field, the statistics updated and many new figures added to illustrate key points.

Peter Hoskin
2020

Acknowledgement

Clinical Oncology was first published in 1994 arising from an initiative by Anthony Neal when he was one of my trainees at the Royal London Hospital and to whom is the credit for driving the first edition to completion. I have valued his co-authorship for subsequent editions through to the fourth edition in 2007. He has chosen to leave the authorship for this edition but it is a tribute to him that much of this fifth edition retains the basic principles he established of a comprehensive textbook of oncology with carefully and consistently structured chapters across the various tumour sites.

I am also indebted to my colleague at Mount Vernon, Peter Ostler, who has made significant contributions to the chapters on the breast, lung, endocrine, sarcoma and oncological emergencies to ensure that they reflect the state-of-the-art practice in oncology at the time of publication.

Peter Hoskin
Northwood and Manchester, 2020

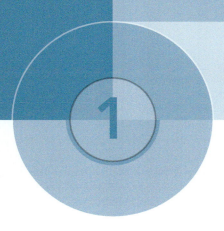

Pathogenesis of cancer

Pathogenesis is defined as 'the manner of development of a disease'. An understanding of the causes of a given cancer is an integral part of formulating strategies for successful treatment, screening and prevention. We owe much of our current understanding to epidemiologists who have discovered associations between different cancers and a number of genetic and environmental factors. The causative factors can be divided into genetic, chemical, physical and viral. Changes in the host genome are the final common pathway in the process of carcinogenesis whatever the initial trigger factors. However, for most patients with cancer it is still not possible to identify why that particular person developed cancer. Some of the examples cited are for historical interest only.

GENETIC FACTORS

Cell division, differentiation and cell loss are ultimately controlled by genetic signals within the cell. Changes in the genes responsible for these processes will lead to the development of malignant tumours characterized by the loss of the normal cellular mechanisms responsible for the control of proliferation, cell differentiation, programmed cell death (apoptosis), cellular organization and cellular adhesion. The uncoupling of the usual balance between cell loss and multiplication leads to the growth of tumour and its subsequent invasion both locally and at distant sites.

Genetic aberrations can be found in the majority of human cancers. The site of the responsible genes can be inferred by 'linkage studies' on individual members of families in which there is an inherited pattern of cancer incidence. The known positions of marker genes are used to deduce where the cancer gene lies along a given chromosome. The gene can then be sequenced, cloned and used to test patients thought to harbour the gene.

Factors suggesting a genetic predisposition to cancer include:

- Family clustering of a specific type(s) of cancer
- Cases occurring in very young individuals relative to the age distribution of that cancer within the rest of the population
- Associations noted between different tumour types
- Multiplicity of cancers, e.g. bilaterality

The genetic aberrations associated with cancer can be classified based on whether they are associated with activated oncogenes or tumour-suppressor genes.

UPREGULATED ONCOGENES

These are the genes which code for a protein that in some way is related to the proliferative cycle of cells or cell differentiation. These products may be growth factors, growth factor receptors on the cell surface or the chemicals that transmit the receptor signals from the cytoplasm to the nucleus. These oncogenes are well preserved throughout the evolutionary scale, remaining very similar right down to primitive organisms such as yeasts. Their overexpression or amplification leads to the uncoupling of usual cell loss/gain equilibrium in favour of cell multiplication, resulting in an increase in cell numbers

Pathogenesis of cancer

and ultimately a clinically apparent tumour. They are activated during the intense cell proliferation and differentiation of embryogenesis but, in the mature cells, are suppressed by regulating genes at other points along the chromosome. DNA strand breaks (e.g. from ionizing radiation or chemical carcinogens) with aberrant repair or translocations of genetic material might lead to the loss of the genes responsible for the regulation of a given oncogene. This may in turn lead to its activation.

The best characterized example is that of the Philadelphia chromosome of chronic myeloid leukaemia, which is confined to the malignant clone and can be identified in 95% of patients with the disease. There is a translocation of part of chromosome 9 to chromosome 22 and vice versa, placing the *abl* oncogene from chromosome 9 adjacent to the breakpoint cluster region (*bcr*) on chromosome 22. The fusion of these genes leads to the transcription of a protein with tyrosine kinase activity, which leads to leukaemic transformation by increasing lymphocyte proliferation.

TUMOUR-SUPPRESSOR GENES

Each cell has one of a pair of tumour-suppressor genes on each homologous chromosome, and both must be inactivated for the cancer to develop. This means that individuals from a 'cancer family' with only a single gene inherited owing to a 'germ line' mutation will have a normal phenotype, act as a carrier, but will develop cancer if the second gene is lost owing to a somatic mutation or other form of genetic miscoding. Normal individuals must lose both genes by a somatic mutation for a sporadic cancer to develop. Thus, tumour-suppressor genes cause cancer not by amplification or overexpression (as with oncogenes) but by the loss of their function.

The best known example of a tumour-suppressor gene is the *P53* gene, which has been called 'the guardian of the genome' and is found to be mutated in the majority of sporadic cancers. It is also mutated in Li–Fraumeni syndrome, characterized by cancers of the breast, adrenal glands, leukaemia, gliomas and soft-tissue sarcomas. This gene induces cell cycle arrest, which allows cells with DNA damage to repair these mutations before entering mitosis. The mutation of *P53* therefore makes the cell susceptible to carcinogenic mutations. Other examples include the retinoblastoma gene which is located on chromosome 13, breast cancer susceptibility genes *BRCA1* (chromosome 17) and *BRCA2* (chromosome 13), the Wilms' tumour gene on chromosome 11, and the familial polyposis coli gene on chromosome 5.

Some examples of the inherited diseases associated with the development of cancer are listed in Table 1.1.

The causes of genetic change may be classified as chemical, physical or viral.

CHEMICAL FACTORS

CIGARETTE SMOKING

Cigarette smoking is the single most important cause of preventable death. It accounts for around a quarter of all deaths from cancer, and 90% of deaths from lung cancer. Polycyclic aromatic hydrocarbons in the tar (e.g. benzpyrene) rather than the nicotine are carcinogenic. Smoking is strongly associated with carcinomas of the lung (squamous and small cell variants), oral cavity, larynx, bladder and pancreas.

ASBESTOS

A history of asbestos exposure is usually elicited from dockers, plumbers, builders and engineers, and is associated with the carcinoma of the lung, and mesotheliomas of the pleura and peritoneum. The blue variant is particularly carcinogenic.

PRODUCTS OF THE RUBBER AND ANILINE DYE INDUSTRY

Both β-naphthylamine and azo dyes are carcinogenic. These substances and their products are excreted in the urine, and cause cancers of the renal pelvis, ureter and bladder.

WOOD DUST

The inhalation of hardwood dusts has been associated with adenocarcinoma of the nasal sinuses, and has been first reported in workers in furniture factories.

Chemical factors

Table 1.1 Inherited diseases associated with the development of cancer

Disease	Type of cancer
Autosomal dominant	
Familial adenomatous polyposis	Adenoma/carcinoma of the colon/rectum
Peutz–Jeghers syndrome	Adenoma/carcinoma of the colon/rectum
Gardener's syndrome	Adenoma/carcinoma of the colon/rectum
Multiple endocrine neoplasia types 1 and 2 (see Chapter 14)	Endocrinologically active adenomata
von Recklinghausen disease	Neurofibromas, schwannoma, phaeochromocytoma
Palmar/plantar tylosis	Carcinoma of the oesophagus
Cowden's disease	Colorectal cancer, breast cancer
Gorlin's syndrome	Basal cell carcinoma of skin, medulloblastoma
Von Hippel–Lindau disease	Cerebellar haemangioblastoma, hypernephroma
Autosomal recessive	
Albinism	Melanoma, basal cell and squamous cell carcinomas of the skin
Xeroderma pigmentosum	Melanoma, basal cell and squamous cell carcinomas of the skin
Ataxia telangiectasia	Acute leukaemia
Fanconi anaemia	Acute leukaemia
Wiskott–Aldrich syndrome	Acute leukaemia
Bloom's syndrome	Acute leukaemia
Chromosomal disorders	
Down's syndrome (trisomy 21)	Acute leukaemia
Turner's syndrome (X0)	Dysgerminoma

SOOT

Before the advent of vacuum machines for cleaning chimneys, there was an increased risk of carcinoma of the scrotum in chimney sweeps from the trapping of soot in the rugosity of the scrotal skin and poor personal hygiene.

TAR/BITUMEN

As with cigarette smoke, polycyclic aromatic hydrocarbons may lead to cancer of exposed skin.

MINERAL OILS

An increased risk of skin cancer was noted in workers using spinning mules from the exposure to lubricating oils.

CHROMATES, NICKEL

These are associated with the development of lung cancer.

ARSENIC

Its use as a 'tonic' during the early 20th century led to multiple basal and squamous cell carcinomas of the skin. It has also been associated with lung cancer.

AFLATOXIN

This is a product of the fungus *Aspergillus flavus*, which is a contaminant of poorly stored cereals and nuts, and causes hepatocellular carcinoma.

NITROSAMINES

These are the products of the action of intestinal bacteria on nitrogenous compounds in ingested food and have been implicated in stomach cancer.

VINYL CHLORIDE MONOMER

Industrial exposure has led to angiosarcomas of the liver and cerebral gliomas.

ALKYLATING CHEMOTHERAPY AGENTS

The addition of alkyl groups to the DNA double helix drastically changes its configuration and causes errors when the cell undergoes mitosis or meiosis, ultimately leading to the loss and distortion of the genome. Prior use of these agents in the chemotherapy of lymphoma has led to an increased risk of acute myeloid leukaemia in long-term survivors.

PHYSICAL FACTORS

Physical factors can cause direct damage to the genome, such as DNA strand breaks or point mutations. This is a phenomenon of everyday life and the changes are either repaired by cellular protection mechanisms or are so severe that the cell perishes and does not multiply. However, if the effects are such that these mechanisms for repair are overloaded, the cell may divide and the genetic error expresses itself, possibly leading to a cell with a malignant phenotype. As the skin and mucosal surfaces are exposed to the external environment, it is these cells that are most prone to physical carcinogenic influences.

SOLAR RADIATION

Excessive ultraviolet exposure in normal individuals or minimal amounts in susceptible individuals (e.g. albinos, xeroderma pigmentosum) can lead to melanoma, basal cell carcinoma and squamous carcinoma (Figure 1.1).

IONIZING RADIATION

Several categories of exposure can be identified and implicated in carcinogenesis:

- *Excessive background radiation*: Radon gas is colourless and odourless, being a daughter product from the radioactive decay of uranium in the Earth's crust, particularly in granite-rich areas. It seeps into homes and reaches its highest level during winter when ventilation of dwellings is at its minimum. When inhaled,

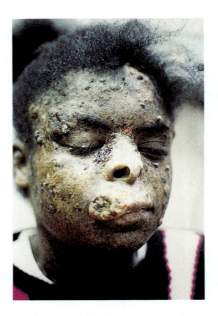

Figure 1.1 A young girl having xeroderma pigmentosum. She has developed multiple facial solar keratoses and both pigmented and non-pigmented skin cancers owing to exposure to ultraviolet radiation.

solid α particle-emitting daughter products can get deposited on the bronchial epithelium leading eventually to lung cancer. Uranium miners are at particular risk, and many have died of lung cancer in Eastern Europe and Germany. The distribution of radon varies with region and in the UK it is highest in Cornwall and parts of Scotland where levels may be 10 times that of low radon areas. Modern dwellings are built with radon membranes to protect occupants from undue exposure. The Japanese atomic bomb survivors have an increased incidence of a number of solid tumours, particularly breast cancer, and radioiodine exposure from atomic bomb test fallout has caused thyroid cancer.
- *Excessive diagnostic radiology exposure*: There was an increased risk of carcinoma of the breast in a cohort of women who had many chest fluoroscopies to monitor iatrogenic pneumothoraces once used as a treatment for tuberculosis. The use of thorotrast (containing thorium, which has properties similar to radium) as a contrast agent led to tumours

of the hepatobiliary tract and nasal sinuses. Exposure of utero is particularly harmful.
- *Therapeutic radiation*:
  - *Thyroid*: There is an increased incidence of papillary carcinoma of the thyroid after thyroid irradiation for benign disease.
  - *Sarcoma*: Soft-tissue sarcomas may arise at the edge of a previously irradiated area and skin carcinomas in previously irradiated skin.
  - *Breast*: Breast irradiation for postpartum mastitis has caused breast cancer.
  - *Ankylosing spondylitis*: A cohort of patients receiving radiation for ankylosing spondylitis have also been found to have an increased incidence of malignancies within the irradiated area.
  - *Hodgkin*: Patients receiving radiotherapy for the treatment of Hodgkin lymphoma during young adult life have an increased incidence of second malignancy, particularly breast cancer and lung cancer in smokers after irradiation of the mediastinum.

HEAT

Carcinomas of the skin have been described in chronic burn scars and the skin of Indians who wear heating lamps against their skin for warmth. Clay pipe smokers are at risk of carcinoma of the lip.

CHRONIC TRAUMA/INFLAMMATION

Carcinomas can arise at sites of chronic skin/mucosal damage (e.g. the tongue adjacent to sharp teeth or a syphilitic lesion), at the site of a sinus from chronic osteomyelitis or inflammatory bowel disease, chronic venous (Marjolin's) ulcer on the lower limb (Figure 1.2), or colonic carcinoma after chronic ulcerative colitis. Calculi and the associated infection may predispose to carcinomas of the urinary and hepatobiliary tracts. Skin cancers can arise in scarring from a previous burn (Figure 1.3), and lung scars from previous tuberculosis may lead to adenocarcinoma.

VIRAL FACTORS

Viruses reproduce by integrating their own genes with those of the infected host, and in doing so the gene sequence of host chromosomes is adjusted. This may in turn lead to the deregulation of oncogenes or the inactivation of tumour-suppressor genes, ultimately resulting in malignant transformation.

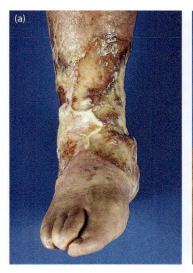
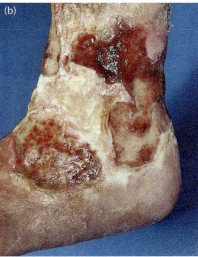

Figure 1.2 A large venous skin ulcer had been present for many years on the medial malleolus of the ankle. More recently it had enlarged and become irregular in shape with everted margins. Biopsy confirmed the clinical diagnosis of squamous carcinoma: (a) frontal view and (b) lateral view.

Pathogenesis of cancer

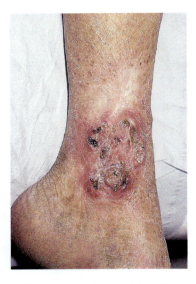

Figure 1.3 A woman who has sustained burns to the skin above the lateral malleolus of the ankle 10 years ago. She then developed nodularity and ulceration within the scar. Biopsy confirmed squamous carcinoma.

Evidences suggesting that a viral infection might have led to a tumour include:

- Geographical and community case clustering
- Serological evidence of infection
- Visualization of viral particles in the tumour cells, or
- Identification of viral genome in the tumour DNA

General observations include the following:

- The prevalence of infection is always much higher than the incidence of the associated tumour.
- Additional factors (e.g. genetic, immune) must be operative for malignant transformation.
- There is usually a long latent period between infection and presentation with cancer.

Some specific viruses related to cancer are as follows.

HEPATITIS B VIRUS

There is a high lifetime incidence (up to 100 times) of hepatoma in parts of Africa where hepatitis B is endemic and there are many chronic carriers of the virus.

EPSTEIN–BARR VIRUS

There is very strong evidence that Epstein–Barr virus is the causative agent of undifferentiated nasopharyngeal carcinoma in Southeast Asia, B-cell lymphomas in the immunosuppressed and Burkitt's lymphoma in Africa. There is also evidence linking it with Hodgkin disease.

HUMAN PAPILLOMA VIRUS

The potential for human papilloma virus (HPV) to cause cancer is most frequently expressed as the development of benign papillomas (warts) on the genitalia. It is generally considered to be sexually transmitted, infection risk being related to the number of sexual partners and sexual practices such as oral sex. HPV types 6 and 11 are considered low risk for malignant change. HPV types 16 and 18 are high-risk types and account for 70% of cervical cancers. HPV infection is also implicated in the genesis of cancers of the oral cavity, oropharynx, and cancers of the vulva and anal canal. The mechanism is related to viral production of two oncoproteins, E6 and E7, which inactivate the *P53* tumour-suppressor gene leading to cancer induction. Routine vaccination against HPV in girls is now available in many countries which is expected to reduce the incidence of such cancers in the future.

HUMAN T-CELL LYMPHOTROPIC VIRUS TYPE 1 (HTLV-1)

This is a retrovirus related to the human immunodeficiency virus (HIV, HTLV-3). It causes adult T-cell leukaemia–lymphoma in the endemic regions of Japan and the Caribbean where more than 95% of cases have positive viral serology.

HUMAN HERPES VIRUS TYPE 8

This is the causative agent in HIV-associated Kaposi sarcoma, primary effusion lymphoma and variants of multicentric Castleman disease.

IMMUNE FACTORS

The body's immunosurveillance system mediated by T cells is capable of mounting an immune response to tumour cells. This is manifest as a lymphocytic infiltrate in tumours such as seminoma and melanoma, which correlates with a favourable prognosis, the phenomenon of spontaneous regression in hypernephroma and melanoma, and the objective responses seen when the T-cell population is boosted by cytokines such as interleukin 2 and interferon. An increased susceptibility to malignant transformation is seen in heavily immunosuppressed individuals such as post-transplant patients. New therapeutic approaches to enhance the immune response targeting immune checkpoints such as PD-1, PDL-1 and CTLV4 show considerable promise.

ACQUIRED IMMUNE DEFICIENCY SYNDROME

Up to 40% of patients with acquired immune deficiency syndrome (AIDS) will ultimately develop some form of malignant disease (see Chapter 20).

DRUG-INDUCED IMMUNOSUPPRESSION

Transplant recipients receiving steroids and azathioprine or cyclosporin have an increased incidence of Kaposi's sarcoma, non-Hodgkin lymphoma and skin cancer.

ENDOCRINE FACTORS

Many cells have receptors for hormones on their surface, within their cytoplasm and nucleus. Overstimulation of these receptors by endogenous or exogenous hormones can lead to excessive cell proliferation, usually resulting in an adenomatous change but sometimes malignancy.

Excessive endogenous steroids (e.g. from a granulosa cell tumour of the ovary) or long-term exogenous oestrogens (e.g. high-dose oestrogen-only oral contraceptive or hormone replacement therapy) can predispose to hyperplasia of the endometrium, which may progress to a well-differentiated adenocarcinoma. Similarly, excess physiological secretion of hormones can lead to hyperplasia, adenomatous change and eventually malignant transformation.

For example, chronic severe iodine deficiency leads to a rise in thyroid-stimulating hormone (TSH), leading to goitre and in some cases follicular carcinoma.

UNDERSTANDING THE CAUSE OF CANCER: THE CONTRIBUTION TO PATIENT CARE

The identification of the aetiological agents responsible for cancers is vital for identifying individuals at high risk. Avoiding exposure of employees to industrial carcinogens either by providing protective clothing or restricted access to the area is a vital part of health and safety practice to prevent cancers. Similarly, screening of high-risk asymptomatic individuals might be indicated, e.g. regular urine cytology in rubber workers at risk of bladder cancer. The identification of cancer patients in whom industrial exposure to a carcinogen is implicated will entitle the patient to industrial injuries compensation.

Understanding the cause of cancer also forms the backbone of more general health education programmes aimed at reducing tobacco consumption and exposure to excessive ultraviolet irradiation.

Molecular biology has already given us a particularly valuable insight into the mechanisms of carcinogenesis. Specific applications include:

- Risk factor determination
- Genetic counselling
- Therapy
- Screening
- Prevention

The ultimate goal of such research must be to provide a greater understanding of cancer and ultimately facilitate more effective cancer therapies. The identification of precise genetic abnormalities may in turn make it possible to insert the appropriate genetic code into the genome (e.g. to replace a missing tumour-suppressor gene) or inactivate/downregulate an overexpressed oncogene, thereby reversing the cellular processes underlying the malignant phenotype.

Examples of such translational research include the development of monoclonal antibodies such as trastuzumab (Herceptin®), which is a very active treatment in women with breast cancer who

Pathogenesis of cancer

overexpress a receptor of the epidermal growth factor family, HER2 (see Chapter 8).

The antibody imatinib (Glivec®) is another example of rational drug design. It is highly active for blast-phase chronic myeloid leukaemia, as the tyrosine kinase protein it targets is BCR-ABL, produced by the Philadelphia chromosome (see section on 'Upregulated oncogenes'). Similarly, the recognition of gastrointestinal stromal tumours (GISTs) and their overexpression of *c-kit* have led to an effective therapeutic option with imatinib in a tumour that was previously unresponsive to conventional treatments (see Chapter 9).

FURTHER READING

Bunz F. *Principles of Cancer Genetics*. 2nd ed. Springer, New York, 2016.

Weinberg RA. *The Biology of Cancer*. 2nd ed. Taylor & Francis Group, New York, 2014.

SELF-ASSESSMENT QUESTIONS

1. Which three of the following suggest a familial cancer?
   a. Other affected first degree relatives
   b. Cancer of the female genital tract
   c. Young age at diagnosis
   d. Cytogenetic abnormalities in the tumour
   e. Follicular carcinoma of the thyroid
   f. Presentation with metastatic disease
   g. Bilaterality

2. Which one of the following statements is not true about tumour-suppressor genes?
   a. They prevent the development of cancer
   b. Mutations can be identified in most cases of cancer
   c. *P53* is a tumour-suppressor gene
   d. *BRCA1* is a tumour-suppressor gene
   e. Mutation analysis is clinically useful even if cancer has already developed

3. Which three of the following are cancers that can be caused by the exposure to ionizing radiation?
   a. Pancreatic cancer
   b. Breast cancer
   c. Gallbladder cancer
   d. Parathyroid cancer
   e. Papillary carcinoma of the thyroid
   f. Kidney cancer
   g. Lung cancer

4. Which one of the following is not a form of cancer associated with viral infection?
   a. Nasopharyngeal cancer
   b. Hepatocellular cancer
   c. Adult T-cell leukaemia–lymphoma
   d. Non-Hodgkin lymphoma
   e. Kidney cancer

Principles of cancer diagnosis and staging

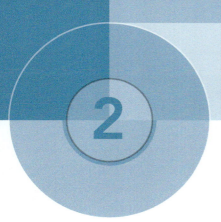

Diagnosis and staging are vital for determining the optimum management of a patient with cancer. Staging is essential not only for treating a specific patient but also to communicate treatment data and outcomes with other centres around the world.

SECURING A TISSUE DIAGNOSIS

Cancer treatment usually involves major procedures with significant toxicity and the diagnosis of cancer has profound psychological, social and physical consequences for the patient. It is therefore mandatory to be certain of the diagnosis before informing the patient or starting therapy. This may entail a simple biopsy or a more invasive procedure such as a laparotomy or a craniotomy. As a rule of thumb, the least invasive means of obtaining tissue should be employed. However, occasionally, several attempts at obtaining tissue from an ill-defined and poorly accessible tumour prove unsuccessful or the patient may be unfit to undergo an essential procedure by virtue of age or general condition. Under these circumstances, clinical judgement and common sense must prevail. Clearly, it would be inappropriate to investigate exhaustively an elderly and infirm person with an extensive asymptomatic brain tumour or widespread metastatic disease if no treatment or change in management would be considered. Specific methods of obtaining tumour tissue include the following techniques.

CYTOLOGY OF FLUIDS

A small specimen of body fluid (e.g. sputum, ascitic fluid, pleural fluid, urine, cerebrospinal fluid) may be spun down and the cells in it stained and examined under the microscope within minutes of its collection. An experienced cytologist can then give an immediate and accurate diagnosis. The false-positive rate is very low, although false negatives occur owing to errors in interpretation or sampling. This analysis has the advantage that the specimen can often be collected as an outpatient procedure with minimal discomfort and it gives a result quickly so that treatment can be started as soon as possible. Of course, the cellular material obtained may be insufficient for immunohistochemical analysis unless a centrifuge is used to produce a cellular pellet, which can be fixed in wax and sectioned/stained in the usual way.

CYTOLOGY OF TISSUE SCRAPINGS

Superficial cells are removed from a body surface (e.g. skin, vagina, cervix, bronchial mucosa, oesophageal mucosa) by scraping or brushing, before being stained and examined under the microscope. The advantages and limitations are the same as for fluid cytology.

FINE-NEEDLE ASPIRATION

This entails the passage of a fine-gauge hypodermic needle into a suspected tumour. Ultrasound or computed tomography (CT) guidance may be necessary for deep-seated tumours that cannot be palpated, such as those at the lung apex or retroperitoneum. Cells are aspirated, smeared onto a microscope slide and sent to a cytologist. This method can be useful for discriminating between reactive and malignant lymphadenopathy. The advantages and disadvantages are comparable to those previously cited for fluid cytology. If the needle washings are very cellular, a centrifuge can be used to produce a pellet for fixation, sectioning and staining as for a piece of tissue.

NEEDLE BIOPSY

This is now preferred wherever possible rather than fine-needle aspiration (FNA). A core of tissue is taken with a biopsy needle under local anaesthetic and the specimen is sectioned after mounting and fixing in wax, which means that the result will not be available for a few days after collection. The larger specimen makes a false-negative result less likely. Tumour grading and architectural subtyping are often possible. It is also possible to distinguish *in situ* malignant change from invasive. More extensive immunohistochemical analysis will be possible, and tissue is available for further molecular testing, the latter becoming increasingly essential in patient management.

INCISION BIOPSY

A small ellipse of tissue is taken from the edge of the tumour using a small scalpel under local anaesthetic. A punch biopsy instrument can be used instead of a scalpel to obtain a core of tissue, but this is more traumatic.

EXCISION BIOPSY

The tumour is excised in toto with a narrow margin of normal tissue. Unlike the other investigations, this has the advantage of removing the lesion, which may be curative for benign tumours and certain skin malignancies if the microscopic margins are clear. It can, however, make further management difficult if the original boundaries of the tumour are not apparent after excision.

PRINCIPLES OF CANCER STAGING

Once the diagnosis has been confirmed, the stage of the cancer, which defines the size and extent of the tumour, must be ascertained. Staging has several purposes:

- It defines the locoregional and distant extent of disease.
- It helps to determine the optimum treatment.
- It permits a baseline against which response to treatment can be assessed.
- It provides prognostic information.

Staging entails a detailed assessment as to the local extent of the tumour and whether there is evidence of spread elsewhere, e.g. regional lymphatics, distant metastases. This will in turn help the referring specialist and oncologist to decide on the most appropriate therapy. For example, a patient with distant metastases is unlikely to be a candidate for aggressive surgery to remove the primary tumour but may be a candidate for systemic treatment such as chemotherapy. Alternatively, the detection of lymph node metastases alone may indicate to the surgeon that excision of the primary tumour should be combined with a lymph node dissection and/or systemic adjuvant therapy. Detailed surgical staging is also valuable to the radiotherapist in deciding the volume of tissue to be irradiated.

Staging permits assessment of the response to treatment. A thorough assessment of the tumour dimensions prior to therapy will permit a critical evaluation of the response to treatment at a later date. Accurate measurements in two planes perpendicular to each other can be used as a crude measure of tumour size before, during and after therapy.

Staging provides a guide to the likely prognosis. In most cancers, the ultimate outcome and therefore life expectancy is related to the stage. Patients with metastatic disease at presentation will clearly fare worse than patients with disease localized to the site of origin. The only tumours that are potentially curable when distant metastases are present are seminoma, teratoma, choriocarcinoma, lymphoma and leukaemia.

Staging may be *clinical*, based on the clinician's history and examination; *non-clinical*, comprising blood tests and radiological studies; or *pathological*, based on the surgical specimen.

HISTORY

A thorough and systematic history can reveal symptoms that may suggest the need for specific staging investigations or a certain disease stage. For example, systemic symptoms such as weight loss, anorexia, malaise and fever raise the suspicion of metastatic disease. Specific symptoms at a site away from the primary tumour may also cause suspicion of distant metastases, e.g. skeletal pain, early morning headache, haemoptysis, hepatic pain.

EXAMINATION

A full physical examination should be performed in all cases. The primary tumour's size, shape, position and mobility should be recorded, preferably with a diagram. The regional lymph nodes should be carefully palpated – involved nodes are enlarged, usually non-tender and hard, and may be fixed to each other, the overlying skin or underlying tissues. The sclerae should be examined for jaundice and the abdomen palpated for hepatomegaly in which the liver is typically hard and knobbly. The chest is examined for signs of collapse, consolidation or effusion. The skin should be surveyed for any abnormal appearances, which may be biopsied if suspicious. A detailed neurological examination should be performed to exclude focal or global neurological deficit, and the fundi examined to exclude papilloedema. Tenderness over sites of bone pain is suspicious and should be followed up by appropriate x-rays.

INVESTIGATIONS

A knowledge of the patterns of spread of tumours will aid the selection of staging investigations. All patients should have a full blood count, liver function tests, calcium and alkaline phosphatase levels taken. The interpretation of deranged values is outlined in Table 2.1. Measurement of the erythrocyte sedimentation rate (ESR) is useful in lymphoma and myeloma. Although a chest x-ray may on occasion be adequate the most common staging examination is a CT scan. Other investigations may be indicated depending on site and nature of the malignant disease:

- Plain x-rays
- Liver ultrasound
- Isotope bone scan
- CT
- Magnetic resonance imaging (MRI)
- Positron emission tomography (PET)
- Other specialized investigations, e.g. bone marrow trephine, lumbar puncture
- Tumour marker assays

PLAIN X-RAYS

Plain x-rays of the skeleton should be taken at sites of any unexplained bone pain, particularly if it is affecting a long bone as it is prone to pathological fracture (Figure 2.1), which may be prevented if the metastasis is detected early. A skeletal survey comprising views of the skull, thoracic spine, lumbar spine and pelvis is indicated in suspected myeloma, as an isotope bone scan may be insensitive for this condition owing to the lack of an osteoblastic response in the involved and surrounding bone (see the section 'Isotope bone scan').

Table 2.1 Interpretation of abnormal screening blood tests

Test result	Interpretation
Normochromic normocytic anaemia	Suggests possibility of advanced cancer
Leucoerythroblastic anaemia	Suggests heavy bone marrow infiltration
Thrombocytopenia	Suggests heavy bone marrow infiltration or DIC
Elevated alkaline phosphatase with normal γ-glutamyltransferase	Suggests possible bone metastases ± elevated calcium
Elevated alkaline phosphatase and γ-glutamyltransferase ± elevated bilirubin	Suggests possible liver metastases

Principles of cancer diagnosis and staging

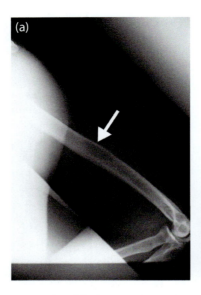 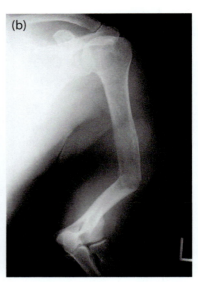

Figure 2.1 Plain radiographs of the humerus in a patient with lung cancer and a painful arm. (a) Lytic metastasis in the mid-shaft. This was noted by the radiologist but no prophylactic treatment was undertaken. (b) Subsequent pathological fracture at the same site.

ULTRASOUND

It is sensitive, specific, non-invasive and can be performed at short notice but is no substitute for high-quality cross-sectional imaging. It is to some extent subjective and the final hard copies can be difficult for the non-radiologist to interpret and utilize. Liver ultrasonography can be used for rapid staging of cancer, particularly gastrointestinal malignancies, as they preferentially metastasize to the liver via portal circulation. Transoesophageal ultrasonography can be of help in staging oesophageal cancers and tumours arising in the trachea and proximal bronchial tree. Transvaginal ultrasonography may be of value in staging malignancies of the lower female genital tract.

Endoscopic US is now the standard for assessing nodes of concern in the chest in lung cancer (EBUS—endobronchial ultrasound).

ISOTOPE BONE SCAN

This is a useful way of imaging the whole skeleton. It is routinely performed as part of the staging of prostate cancer and breast cancer, which have a propensity for early dissemination to the skeleton, but is otherwise reserved for patients with widespread skeletal symptoms or when plain x-rays are equivocal for metastatic disease. A metastasis leads to an osteoblastic response, which in turn leads to increased accumulation of the bone-seeking radioisotope and therefore a hot spot (Figure 2.2). Myeloma bone lesions are not particularly well visualized as they do not evoke a significant osteoblastic response. A very diffuse involvement of the skeleton may produce an intense uptake of isotope producing a 'superscan'. Benign disease such as degenerative changes in joints, vertebral collapse from osteoporosis or Paget disease of bone can also lead to abnormal isotope uptake. Bone scans can be unreliable in assessing response to therapy in the short term, as activity may be increased at the sites of metastatic disease with regression of the metastasis and subsequent bone healing (Figure 2.3). Isotope images can be linked to CT imaging (SPECT—single photon emission computed tomography).

COMPUTED TOMOGRAPHY

CT gives good soft tissue and bone contrast. A contrast-enhanced CT scan of the brain, thorax, abdomen and pelvis is indicated for potentially curable tumours with a propensity for widespread multiple

Principles of cancer staging

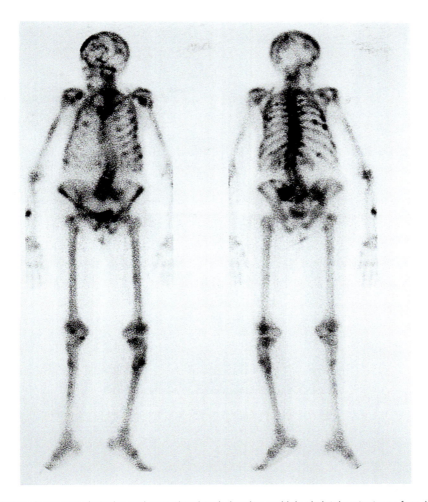

Figure 2.2 Isotope bone scan (anterior and posterior views) showing multiple skeletal metastases from breast cancer. Radioactive technetium has been injected and taken up by the skeleton, particularly in regions of increased bone metabolism. Metastases are seen in the skull, spine, pelvis and right proximal femur.

metastases, and in all patients with metastatic disease as a baseline for assessing response to therapy. Abnormal lymph nodes on CT are defined as >1 cm in diameter, although CT cannot detect abnormal lymph node architecture and therefore cannot distinguish between benign and malignant enlargement. Localized CT imaging may be used to position a needle for biopsy of a mass.

MAGNETIC RESONANCE IMAGING

This gives soft-tissue contrast superior to that of CT and superb anatomical definition in transverse, sagittal and coronal views (Figure 2.4). No ionizing irradiation is involved and it is therefore better for investigating young children and pregnant women. Contraindications include cardiac pacemakers, metallic intracranial vessel ligation clips, previous metallic intraocular foreign bodies and claustrophobia. It is particularly sensitive for imaging the brain and spinal cord. MRI is useful for patients with apparently solitary cerebral metastases on CT as a means of excluding multiplicity, which may be important in determining optimal management, and is the investigation of choice for patients with primary CNS (central nervous system) tumours. It also

Principles of cancer diagnosis and staging

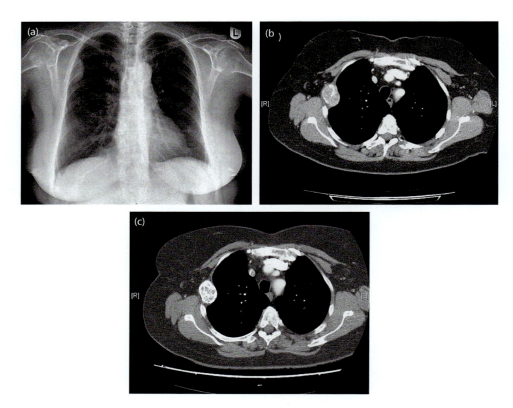

Figure 2.3 (a) Plain chest radiograph showing a peripheral opacity in the right upper zone. (b) Corresponding CT image showing a large, destructive, soft-tissue mass arising from a rib. (c) After appropriate systemic therapy, there has been a response showing as healing and sclerosis. Paradoxically, the isotope bone scan indicated increased isotope uptake at this site, which suggested disease progression.

has a role in the delineation of the local extent of soft-tissue sarcomas and primary liver tumours prior to definitive surgery where the tumour can be related to adjacent major blood vessels, and is the staging method of choice for pelvic tumours (e.g. carcinomas of the prostate, cervix, rectum).

MRI can be useful in determining the nature of persistent skeletal symptoms when both plain x-rays and isotope bone scans are normal (Figure 2.5). Functional MRI imaging allows the assessment of tumour activity and is playing an increasing role in assessing the nature of the primary tumour and the response of tumours to treatment.

POSITRON EMISSION TOMOGRAPHY

This entails the systemic administration of positron-emitting molecules, which form part of the everyday metabolic processes of the living cell, e.g. fluorodeoxyglucose (FDG). These tracers are preferentially taken up by fast metabolizing tissues (e.g. tumours) and can then be detected and their uptake spatially localized. Patients fast beforehand to maximize glucose uptake, and have to be warm and relaxed to avoid shivering and brown fat metabolism, which can lead to spurious glucose uptake. These studies provide functional information entirely different from the structural information obtained from CT and MRI, and can provide a whole body snapshot of the likely sites of disease activity. CT imaging is often undertaken in the scanner at the same time as the PET study to facilitate anatomical appreciation of the sites of tracer uptake. PET is of particular value in the assessment of residual soft-tissue masses after chemotherapy (e.g. lymph node masses in lymphoma and testicular tumours) where the presence

Principles of cancer staging

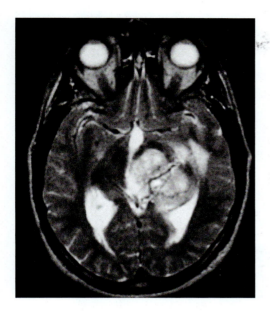

Figure 2.4 Brainstem glioma. MRI of the brain showing (a) transverse, (b) sagittal and (c) coronal views.

of viable tumour may be distinguished from fibrosis and/or necrosis. PET can also be used as part of a whole body staging procedure, particularly prior to radical surgery in diseases with an innately high risk of distant dissemination, e.g. lung cancer, pancreatic cancer (Figure 2.6). It can be of value in assessing the response to therapy (Figure 2.7). PET imaging is sensitive for detecting low-volume malignant lymphadenopathy (e.g. in the mediastinum, pelvis) that would otherwise be indeterminate by CT criteria (Figure 2.8). PET is, however, not a good imaging modality for surveying the brain as this is an area of very avid glucose uptake and the co-registered CT imaging is usually of low resolution and without contrast enhancement.

PET imaging using specific agents is proving useful, e.g. choline PET in prostate cancer.

OTHER SPECIALIZED INVESTIGATIONS

Bone marrow aspirate and trephine

This is a relatively non-invasive method for obtaining a sample of bone and bone marrow for microscopic examination. It is particularly useful in the diagnosis and staging of haematological malignancies (lymphoma, myeloma, leukaemia) and some solid tumours (small cell carcinoma of the lung, Ewing's tumour of bone).

Lumbar puncture

Some tumours have a particular propensity to spread to the central nervous system, particularly the meninges, and the CNS may act as a sanctuary allowing malignant cells to survive systemically administered chemotherapy. It is relatively easy to obtain a specimen of cerebrospinal fluid from the lumbar subarachnoid space, which can then be submitted for cytological examination. Lumbar puncture forms part of the routine staging of high-risk non-Hodgkin lymphomas (e.g. primary testicular lymphomas, those with bone marrow involvement, lymphomas affecting the paranasal sinuses).

TUMOUR MARKER ASSAYS

Tumour markers are usually proteins associated with the malignant process. Common methods of detection include:

- Immunohistochemistry
- Fluorescence *in situ* hybridization (FISH)

Tumour markers in the serum, urine or cellular material are useful in many aspects of cancer management, and testicular tumours provide a number of examples (Table 2.2). The following are examples of tumour markers used for other tumour types:

- CA15-3 (blood) in breast cancer
- Carcinoembryonic antigen (CEA – blood) in gastrointestinal cancer
- Prostate-specific antigen (PSA – blood) in prostate cancer
- CA125 (blood) in ovarian cancer
- CA19-9 (blood) in pancreatic cancer
- α-Fetoprotein (AFP – blood), β-human chorionic gonadotrophin (HCG – blood), placental alkaline phosphatase (PLAP – blood) and lactate dehydrogenase (LDH – blood) in testicular teratoma/seminoma
- Thyroglobulin (blood) in follicular carcinoma of the thyroid
- Calcitonin (blood) in medullary carcinoma of the thyroid

Principles of cancer diagnosis and staging

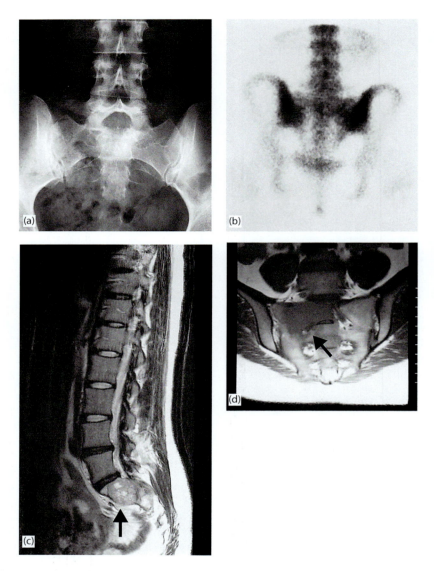

Figure 2.5 A woman with previously treated breast cancer presented with sciatica: (a) normal plain radiograph of lower lumbar spine and adjacent pelvis, (b) isotope bone scan of the same region showing normal, symmetrical uptake (c) sagittal MRI of the lumbar spine and sacrum showing a soft-tissue mass at S1 and (d) transverse MRI showing a large metastasis in the superior aspect of the sacrum impinging on the ipsilateral S1 nerve root.

- 24-hour urinary vanillylmandelic acid (VMA) in phaeochromocytoma
- 24-hour urinary 5-hydroxyindoleacetic acid (5-HIAA) in carcinoid tumours
- Urinary Bence–Jones protein, paraprotein/immunoglobulin levels (blood) and electrophoresis (blood) in myeloma

THE TNM STAGING SYSTEM

The origins of this staging system go back to the 1940s. Since then it has evolved into a comprehensive system covering all types and stages of cancer. It is accepted and contributed to by the most eminent

Use of pathological information

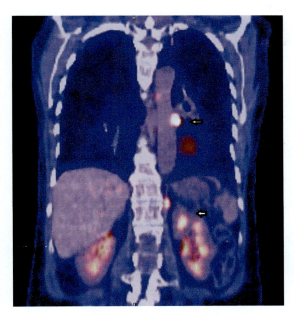

Figure 2.6 PET imaging for staging cancer. Coronal PET scan of the thorax and abdomen performed in a patient with lung cancer who was being considered for surgery. Although the staging CT scan was reported as normal, there is intense glucose metabolism in the left adrenal gland and a further focus just lateral to the thoracic aorta (arrows), both suggesting metastatic disease.

- Tis: carcinoma *in situ*
- T0: no evidence of primary
- Tx: primary cannot be assessed
- Nx: nodes cannot be assessed
- Mx: metastases cannot be assessed
- Gl: well differentiated
- G2: moderately differentiated
- G3: poorly differentiated
- G4: undifferentiated
- pT/N/M: pathological staging

The reader is referred to the site-specific chapters for more detailed staging descriptions.

USE OF PATHOLOGICAL INFORMATION

The pathologist plays a vital role in tumour diagnosis. The information on a pathology report is an integral part of the decision-making process for the clinician. Essential details include:

- Tumour size and macroscopic appearance
- Tissue of origin
- Benign versus malignant
- If malignant, primary versus secondary
- Tumour differentiation, i.e. grade
- Degree of local invasion (blood vessels, lymphatic vessels, nerve fibres, organ capsule)
- Number of regional lymph nodes retrieved and number involved
- Host immune response
- Tumour excised with an adequate margin of normal tissue
- Immunocytochemical markers, e.g. HER2 in breast cancer, EGFR (epidermal growth factor receptor) and ALK (anaplastic lymphoma kinase) in lung cancer

cancer research groups such as the World Health Organization, International Union Against Cancer and International Society of Paediatric Oncology. A formalized, universally applied staging scheme has several advantages. First, it aids the clinician in his or her appreciation of the extent of the cancer and gives a meaningful guide to likely prognosis. Second, it gives a consistency in the reporting of clinical trials and facilitates an exchange of meaningful information between clinicians without ambiguity; this staging method has been adopted around the world.

The system describes the anatomical extent of the disease by using three components:

- 'T' for the primary tumour
- 'N' for regional lymph nodes
- 'M' for distant metastases

Each of these categories is assigned a number according to the extent of disease, which will vary according to anatomical site and type of malignancy. Other categories include:

Much of this information is of prognostic value and may assist in determining the optimal treatment of the patient. The recent advances in immunocytochemistry have allowed pathologists to identify the tissue of origin in very poorly differentiated tumours (see Chapter 20) which has improved the management of this small group of patients. As with the radiologist, it is not only courteous but essential that

Principles of cancer diagnosis and staging

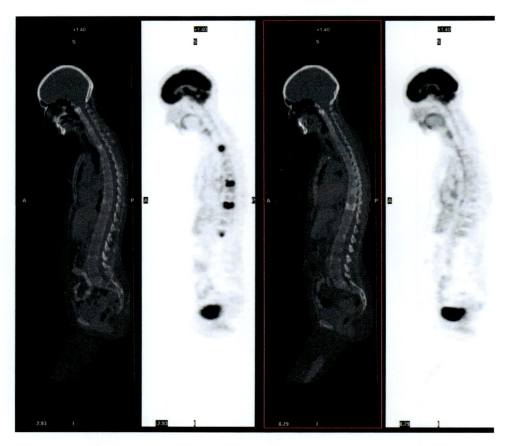

Figure 2.7 PET imaging to assess response to treatment. Sagittal whole body images of a patient with bone metastases. Left-hand panes represent the CT and PET images before treatment; the PET image shows four areas of intense glucose uptake in the thoracic spine. The right-hand panes are the corresponding images after successful systemic therapy showing a metabolic response. Note the area of sclerosis that has appeared in the lower thoracic region which suggests a healing area of osteoblastic activity.

Table 2.2 Role of serum tumour markers in the management of patients with testicular tumours

Role	Example
Diagnosis	Elevation of AFP suggests yolk sac teratoma elements, elevation of HCG suggests trophoblastic teratoma elements, while elevated LDH is associated with seminoma
Staging	Failure of AFP/HCG/LDH to return to normal after orchidectomy suggests residual disease elsewhere
Prognosis	Very high levels of AFP/HCG are associated with poor prognosis in testicular teratoma
Indicator of response	Failure of AFP/HCG/LDH to fall with chemotherapy suggests drug-resistant disease
Detection of relapse	Sudden elevation of AFP/HCG/LDH while in clinical remission suggests subclinical relapse

Self-assessment questions

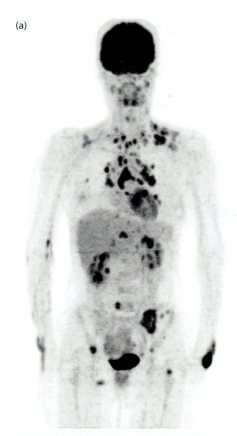

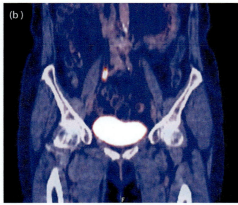

Figure 2.8 PET staging of cancer. (a) Coronal whole body PET image showing widespread metastatic disease. The mediastinal lymphadenopathy was not appreciated on an earlier CT scan. (b) Coronal PET image of the pelvis. Small but abnormal lymph node in the right iliac chain (arrow). Again, this had not been appreciated in an earlier CT scan.

as much relevant clinical information as possible is put onto any form submitted to the pathologist.

FURTHER READING

Greene FL, Compton CC. *AJCC Cancer Staging Atlas*. 8th ed. Springer, New York, 2016.

UICC. TNM Classification of Malignant Tumours. https://www.uicc.org/resources/tnm

Wittekind C, Asamura H, Sobin LH. *TNM Atlas*. 6th ed. Wiley-Liss, New York, 2014.

SELF-ASSESSMENT QUESTIONS

1. Which three of the following statements apply to cytology as a diagnostic tool?
   a. Can only be performed on specimens of body fluid
   b. Can provide a rapid diagnosis
   c. Allows precise characterization of the tumour
   d. Cannot distinguish *in situ* disease from invasive
   e. It has a low false-positive rate
   f. A negative result makes cancer very unlikely
   g. Very useful for immediate diagnosis of lymphoma

2. Which of the following is the least important objective of staging cancer?
   a. Provides baseline of current disease status for assessing response to treatment
   b. Allows optimization of treatment
   c. Informs both patient and clinician
   d. Allows time for patient to come to terms with diagnosis
   e. Gives insight into likely prognosis

3. Which three of the following statements apply to an isotope bone scan?
   a. Images all the skeleton except the ribs
   b. Complements plain radiographs of painful areas of the skeleton
   c. Relies on isotope being taken up in areas of osteoclastic activity
   d. It is not good at imaging myeloma bone lesions

Principles of cancer diagnosis and staging

    e. Increased isotope uptake always suggests disease progression
    f. Benign disease can produce a hot spot
    g. Contraindicated in hypercalcaemia

4. Which three of the following are contraindications to having a magnetic resonance scan?

    a. Previous hip replacement surgery
    b. Pregnancy
    c. Claustrophobia
    d. Raised intracranial pressure
    e. Cardiac pacemaker
    f. Spinal cord compression
    g. Intraocular metallic foreign body

Decision-making and communication

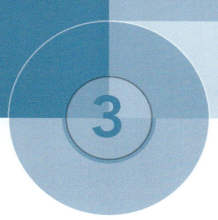

This chapter describes clear treatment policies for different types of malignant disease. These policies are based on the knowledge of the natural history of the disease and, as detailed in Chapter 2, details of its extent – the clinical or pathological stage of the tumour.

However, the practice of clinical oncology demands more than simple application of these instructions in an uncritical manner. The individualization of treatment for any given patient is influenced by sociological, economic and psychological factors as well as oncological principles. The three levels of decision-making used when formulating a treatment policy for an individual are as follows:

- The decision to treat or not to treat
- Treatment intent, whether radical or palliative
- Specific aspects of treatment policy regarding local, systemic and supportive therapy

Figure 3.1 illustrates various options for treatment.

TREATMENT OPTIONS

TO TREAT OR NOT TO TREAT

Not every patient in whom a diagnosis of cancer is made will benefit from active treatment of their disease. There is for example good evidence to show that active local treatment in the form of radiotherapy for inoperable carcinoma of the bronchus in poor performance status patients will have no impact whatsoever on the survival of a patient. It follows, therefore, that in asymptomatic patients diagnosed with this condition, treatment will only be meddlesome and indeed may detract from that patient's quality of life by invoking side effects for no positive outcome. In contrast, treatment with radiotherapy or chemotherapy in good performance status patients may result in a 2-month gain in survival; it is then a judgement as to whether for an individual asymptomatic patient this is an appropriate treatment. The actual decision to treat patients will be based not only on their clinical state but also on the availability of treatment facilities and the views of the patient and their relatives. It is often very difficult for patients to accept that, having been told they have cancer, no treatment is proposed other than symptomatic measures, even though specific cancer treatment may have no proven benefit.

A different scenario in which a no-treatment decision may be taken is when the prognosis is so good and the risk of relapse so small that treatment for all patients will result in overtreatment with consequent side effects for the majority. An example of this situation is the management of stage 1 testicular teratoma following orchidectomy where the probability of relapse is around 20% and the use of tumour markers and scans enables early diagnosis of relapse in a tumour readily cured on exposure to appropriate chemotherapy. This is a much easier scenario for patients who will easily accept that they are almost certainly cured and require no further treatment other than close follow-up for a finite period.

Treatment should always have a positive benefit for the patient but treatment outcome for any

Decision-making and communication

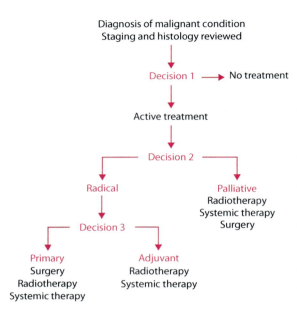

Figure 3.1 Treatment options.

individual is not predictable. The decision to treat or not to treat then becomes a matter of balancing the probability of improving a patient's condition, whether by symptom control with palliative treatment or by cure with radical treatment, against the toxicity and disturbance to lifestyle that treatment will entail. Thus, it is possible to justify an intensive course of chemotherapy with major side effects when there is a high probability of cure but more difficult to do so in a patient with limited life expectancy in whom only minor symptom improvement can be anticipated. Wherever possible, patients should be allowed to determine the level of input they wish to undergo; there is good evidence that, as a group, patients will often wish to undertake treatments with significant toxicity and very limited chances of possible benefit in contrast to the views of healthcare professionals.

RADICAL OR PALLIATIVE TREATMENT

- Radical treatment is that which is given with the intent of long-term control or cure for the patient.
- Palliative treatment is that which is given to improve the quality of life for a patient with no implied impact on their survival.

While this may seem to be a clear distinction, in practice it may be difficult to define treatment aims in these terms. For example, a patient presenting with small cell lung cancer may be offered a course of radical treatment comprising intensive chemotherapy and radiotherapy. However, it is recognized that, while this treatment may prolong survival, the likelihood of cure is less than 15%. Thus, the treatment intent, although radical, will result for most patients in only very limited benefit. Conversely, a patient with breast cancer relapsing with a single site of painful bone metastases may receive a low palliative dose of radiation for pain relief only, yet live, pain free, for several years.

In many cases the decision of treatment intent if not outcome will be clear. Those patients who present with localized tumours accessible to local therapy and those with metastatic disease from chemosensitive tumours, such as germ cell tumour or lymphoma, will be offered radical treatment. However, increasingly patients relapsing with local disease and those with up to three metastases (oligometastases) are treated with ablative procedures such as radical surgery or high-dose radiation in the hope that cure may be achieved. Those who present with a widespread metastatic disease from other tumours will, with few exceptions, fall into the palliative group.

Palliative oncological treatment has the aim of improving a patient's well-being usually through treatment for specific local symptoms such as pain, obstruction or haemorrhage. It follows therefore that patients in whom radical treatment is not appropriate and who have no symptoms do not require palliative treatment. The concept of prophylactic palliative treatment, in other words treatment to prevent symptoms emerging, is for most patients inappropriate and, in the asymptomatic patient, introduces treatment toxicity with little benefit. There may be occasional exceptions to this concept for example the prophylactic fixation of a bone damaged by extensive osteolytic metastases with impending pathological fracture. As always the probability of treatment benefit must be weighed against the natural history of the condition and probability of disease-related and treatment-related symptoms.

LOCAL, REGIONAL OR SYSTEMIC TREATMENT

As a general principle, a primary malignant tumour will require ablation with local treatment, which may be surgical excision and/or radiation treatment. Similarly, metastatic disease requires systemic treatment, which may be chemotherapy, hormone therapy or a biological agent.

Local treatment may involve simple excision of a tumour, removal of the entire organ or removal of the involved organ and regional tissues at risk of tumour involvement. In the past there have been advocates of extensive regional surgery around a tumour site in the hope of improving cure; however, such approaches are only rational where a tumour is known to spread in a predictable manner. In practice, most common tumours are thought to spread at an early stage in their evolution through blood and lymphatic dissemination of tumour cells. For this reason, the use of radical regional surgery is usually considered inappropriate. This is well illustrated in the case of breast cancer where it is clear that survival is largely independent of the type of local treatment for a given stage of the disease. Thus, radical mastectomy is no better at curing breast cancer than simple removal of the lump from the breast.

Although local control of a tumour is an important goal, most patients die from cancer because of metastatic disease. If a cancer has been detected prior to the establishment of metastases, then radical local treatment can result in cure. However, the natural history of many cancers is such that even relatively early tumours would be associated with distant micrometastases. In these cases improvements in survival are likely to come only from the use of adjuvant systemic treatment.

ADJUVANT TREATMENT

Adjuvant treatment is the prophylactic use of local or systemic treatment following primary treatment of a malignant tumour to prevent recurrence.

One of the most common adjuvant treatments given today is post-operative radiotherapy following the excision of a malignant tumour for example irradiation of the breast following local excision of an early carcinoma. Such adjuvant treatment may add significantly to patient morbidity and it is important therefore to consider the relative merits of treatment in these situations. For example, the risk of local relapse in the breast following simple excision with no radiotherapy is around 30%–50% depending on the tumour size. On this basis, if all patients are treated following lumpectomy, half may never have required treatment; the difficulty lies in predicting accurately who will relapse. A further consideration is the fact that local relapse following lumpectomy may be treated successfully in many women and would still occur in up to 5% even with radiotherapy. A small survival advantage with post-operative radiotherapy has also been shown. The decision to offer a woman breast radiotherapy following excision of a malignant breast lump therefore has to balance the potential benefits with the likely side effects for each individual patient. The substantial reduction in local relapse in the breast from 20% to 5% will be seen in most cases enough to justify a relatively simple, low morbidity treatment.

The use of adjuvant systemic therapy is also the one in which the decision to offer a particular treatment must be balanced against the possible acute toxicity which, with chemotherapy, may be significant. There are, in fact, few sites of cancer where the use of adjuvant systemic therapy is of proven value. The area where there has been the greatest endeavour and the most reliable information is once again breast cancer. There is good evidence that an overall survival benefit is achieved by offering women with early operable breast cancer some form of adjuvant systemic therapy. In postmenopausal women tamoxifen or anastrazole is recommended. This reduces the likelihood of dying from breast cancer by one-third and is a simple treatment involving the administration of a single tablet daily for a number of years with few, if any, associated side effects. Therefore, the decision in this case is reasonably straightforward. In contrast, there is a less reliable effect of anti-oestrogen treatment in premenopausal women with an oestrogen receptor-negative tumour, but there is proven advantage with chemotherapy for those with high-risk tumours defined by high tumour grade or positive regional lymph nodes. However, this treatment involves 6 months of intravenous chemotherapy with attendant side effects. The greatest efficacy is seen in patients with positive axillary lymph nodes, but

Decision-making and communication

even so the difference in survival at 10 years between women who receive chemotherapy and those who do not in prospective randomized trials is only 6%. Therefore, there is a much finer balance between toxicity and benefit in a premenopausal patient with negative lymph nodes in whom there may be only a small probability of survival gain.

It can be difficult to translate clinical trial and population-based data to the individual patient. Breast cancer is a common cancer and therefore even a very small treatment effect of, say, an improvement in survival of 5% over 10 years will result in many thousands of women worldwide living for longer after breast cancer. However, for an individual woman the odds that she will benefit from adjuvant treatment in that setting are small and it is possible that she will undergo a toxic treatment with no effect on her ultimate survival.

It is also difficult for those around the patient, be they family, friends or physicians, to evaluate and balance the risks of having a toxic treatment against the risk of relapse, particularly when there can never be a certainty of cure. There is evidence to suggest that patients have a much lower threshold for accepting treatment, even where there is significant associated toxicity, than would the nurses or doctors who look after them.

QUALITY OF LIFE

Whilst survival will always be the most important end point of cancer treatment, the quality of life experienced and the impact of different treatment regimens on this are important additional considerations. The measurement of quality of life has become increasingly sophisticated. Early attempts relied heavily on assessments by a physician on a broad scale measuring physical performance status as illustrated in Chapter 6 (see Table 6.2). A true measure of the quality of life for an individual can, however, be acquired only from that individual, and a number of formal patient questionnaire-based scales have now been developed. These include the Rotterdam symptom checklist, the Hospital Anxiety and Depression (HAD) score and the European Organisation for Research and Treatment of Cancer (EORTC) standardized quality of life questionnaire (EORTC QLQ-C30), consisting of a core questionnaire to which disease site-specific modules can be added. The importance of quality of life assessments in clinical trials is discussed later.

COMMUNICATION

Whilst the principles of communication in oncology should be no different than any other branch of medicine there are specific features that require consideration. In Western society the term 'cancer' remains one that is frequently surrounded by fear and dread for most of the population. In other cultures, it may not even be mentioned in open discussion. Many patients passing through an oncology unit will have an incurable and ultimately fatal disease. This requires special skills in communication and support, which will span the entire range of oncological practice. Radical treatment might require lengthy discussion to consider a choice between different treatment options; at the other extreme, specific skills are required in imparting the news that a cancer may be incurable and death imminent.

Patients are increasingly well informed and wish to discuss the details of their disease and options for treatment. The diagnosis of cancer is often associated with many emotional responses, which will colour the consultation including anger, frustration, guilt and despair. These may present considerable barriers to open discussion particularly where there is a perception that earlier medical care has been inadequate or delayed the diagnosis of cancer.

Communication with a patient is affected by many factors relating to both the patient and the healthcare professional including environment, culture and content.

ENVIRONMENT

Wherever possible important discussions relaying news of a diagnosis of cancer, discussions relating to treatment options and the 'bad news interview' relaying news that the condition may be incurable and terminal should be carried out in an environment comfortable for the patient. Privacy is important but often difficult to achieve in a busy ward and wherever possible a dedicated side room or communication room should be available. The patient should be adequately clothed and not given important information during the process of physical examination or while still undressed.

If possible and provided this is desired by the patient they should have a relative or friend accompanying them or alternatively a healthcare professional with whom they have empathy for example their ward or specialist nurse. Despite inevitable pressures on the time available for such interviews the patient should not be aware of time pressures that may hinder their willingness to interact and ask questions.

CULTURE

There will be cultural differences in the way a diagnosis of cancer, a potentially fatal illness, and death are approached. Increasingly in Western civilization a direct approach is preferred. The word 'cancer' should not be avoided or hidden behind euphemisms. A clear and simple explanation of the disease relevant to that particular patient and the treatment options should be given. Patients may be unfamiliar with surgical procedures and the processes of radiotherapy and chemotherapy; these will require additional explanation. It is unwise to assume that a patient has any background information unless confirmed. It is often helpful early in a consultation to ask the patient to give their understanding of their illness or the treatments being offered, a background against which further discussion can proceed. A particular pitfall to avoid relates to fellow healthcare professionals who may be disadvantaged by the assumption that they already are familiar with their condition and will have to decide on the treatment they wish to receive; usually this is far from the case and they will welcome putting aside any background knowledge they may have acquired for a full and simple explanation of their position.

CONTENT

Three common consultations can be identified in oncology that present specific challenges in communication; these are the choice between different radical or palliative treatments, the discussion of likely prognosis and discussion of matters related to the process of dying.

TREATMENT CHOICES

Where there is a choice of treatment, this should be laid out for the patient and in each case the possible advantages and disadvantages discussed. It may be difficult to give a balanced view of treatment options particularly for specialists outside their own area of interest; this is the advantage of multidisciplinary discussions. Realistic estimates of success should be given with a clear explanation of the expected end point, whether 'cure', by which the patient will interpret a complete return to normal life and normal life expectancy; 'control' of the disease, which may be only temporary; or simply control of symptoms without any impact perhaps on survival. Possible side effects of treatment should be discussed fully, in particular, those that may result in a long-term alteration in lifestyle for the patient. Again realistic estimates of their likelihood and the balance between side effects and positive benefit should be discussed.

It is well recognized that most patients do not retain information from their initial interview for long and a significant amount of the information will be forgotten or misinterpreted. It is therefore important that written information is given to the patient to support the facts imparted in the interview and that this is followed up by an opportunity for the patient to return for further discussion. A readily available point of contact should be given to the patient and often it is helpful for another healthcare professional such as a specialist nurse to be available for them to discuss matters further.

PROGNOSIS

The prediction of life expectancy is notoriously difficult and there is considerable evidence that estimates by healthcare professionals are often inaccurate. It may be difficult for patients and their relatives to accept that their medical advisers cannot give an accurate picture of the future. It is, however, usually possible to estimate survival in terms of days, weeks, months or years and, where lengthy survival is to be expected, a percentage likelihood of surviving, say, 5 years can be given. This should, however, be carefully interpreted since it is often difficult for patients to relate life-table curves giving a probability of survival at any point to their own individual survival.

The point at which patients wish to discuss such matters in detail will vary, some wishing to consider this in detail from the outset but many preferring to leave the matter unspoken for some time or even throughout their illness. This should be respected and the issue dealt with sensitively, giving patients the opportunity to 'set the pace', by asking specific details of their outlook, rather than giving bald and alarming statements of a short prognosis. Open questions such as 'Is there anything else you would like to ask?' may give them the lead to pursue specific areas of concern when they wish to do so.

DYING

The mention of death and dying is often avoided by both carers and patients perhaps in an attempt to avoid facing the inevitability of this event. Meaningful discussions with a patient who has advanced incurable cancer can, however, only progress once the notion of dying has been accepted, if only to subsequently agree not to mention it further. Patients and their relatives will often hide behind euphemisms such as 'the end' or 'when it's all over', whilst healthcare professionals may use terms such as 'very serious' or 'incurable' to introduce the idea that an illness is fatal. Realistic expectations are important for practical issues to be faced such as where and by whom the patient wishes to be cared for in his or her last days, clarification of practical and financial issues such as the transfer of assets and writing a will and where dependent children are involved, arrangements for their future care. Patients and their relatives are often concerned over the process of dying rather than the event itself, and it is important to explore these fears with appropriate reassurance over the availability and efficacy of symptom control and nursing care. Above all, it is important not to avoid the issue when faced with direct questions from the patient but to reply honestly and with sensitivity.

DIFFICULTIES IN COMMUNICATION

EXPECTATIONS VERSUS REALITY

For many patients and their carers the reality of a serious illness and the possibility of death are associated with unrealistic expectations from their treatment. This can be projected as anger and dissatisfaction when treatment failure is encountered. It is important that unrealistic expectations are not fuelled by unrealistic predictions of outcome from treatment and that such responses are met sympathetically but with clear and accurate information of realistic outcomes.

LACK OF KNOWLEDGE

Many patients may find it difficult to accept that their advisers do not understand all the details of their disease process and rarely can they attribute a cause to it. Patients often focus on events in their life and seek confirmation that this was the possible cause for their cancer, which it is often not possible to confirm or refute. Similarly, events may occur in their disease course that are unexpected and cannot necessarily be explained by previous experience. Healthcare professionals should not be reluctant to admit that they do not know or understand events and this is far better than fabrication of possible mechanisms which have no basis.

IDENTIFICATION

Patients who may be contemporaries of their carers and children are particularly likely to provoke strong emotional responses. This is a normal reaction to events and should be recognized as such but not be allowed to cloud objectivity. If this is found to be an overwhelming difficulty, healthcare professionals should have access to another colleague who can take their place or support them through difficult events.

CONFLICT WITHIN FAMILIES

The diagnosis of a life-threatening illness or impending death may unveil underlying conflicts between a patient and other family members. There is often guilt that the patient has not been given sufficient attention, symptoms have been missed and that more should have been done. This may be transferred to those looking after the patient as complaints relating to their diagnosis and care. Other more complex tensions may emerge with unmasking of relationship difficulties between partners or parents and children. There may be attempts to 'protect' the patient by asking professionals to withhold information, which relatives may see as distressing. Throughout the important principle is that the patient is pre-eminent and, while you must deal with relatives sympathetically, the patient's wishes should at all times be respected.

CONCLUSION

Decision-making in oncology is not as straightforward as a simple knowledge of the disease process may imply. Relating the large body of knowledge regarding disease outcome, treatment outcome and treatment-related morbidity to an individual patient can be difficult. The probability of benefit from any treatment can be interpreted differently by each patient so while one might accept a 90% probability of cure as very favourable, another will find a 10% probability of relapse unacceptable. Treatment decisions rely on an accurate and realistic presentation of the facts but individual interpretations might come to very different conclusions from the same facts.

CLINICAL EVIDENCE AND CLINICAL TRIALS

Ultimately treatment decisions rely upon interpretation of the available data for a given clinical situation. Different sources of data, however, have different levels of reliability when applying them to a patient population. Perhaps the least reliable, but often most memorable, is that of the anecdote recalling the course of a similar patient treated in the past. The most reliable data will come from the results of a large randomized trial addressing a specific question. Clinical evidence is graded according to its level of reliability as follows:

- *Level Ia*: Meta-analysis of randomized controlled trials
- *Level Ib*: Evidence from one or more randomized trial
- *Level IIa*: Evidence from a non-randomized trial
- *Level III*: Evidence from descriptive studies
- *Level IV*: Evidence from expert committee, reports or clinical experience

A particular clinical question, whether in cancer treatment or any other speciality, can be addressed in a number of ways. Types of trial include:

- Randomized controlled trials
- Case–control studies
- Cohort studies

A clearly defined path for new treatment development in the clinical setting is defined as follows:

- Phase 1
    - First exposure in man
    - Low doses initially based on animal data
    - Dose escalation to maximum tolerated dose (MTD)
    - Measurement of pharmacokinetics in man
    - Definition of significant and limiting toxicities
- Phase 2
    - Testing for activity in a range of tumours
    - Define response rates
- Phase 3
    - Randomized-controlled trial to compare with the best current treatment or placebo
- Phase 4
    - Post-marketing surveillance following successful phase 3 trial as use becomes widespread outside trial setting

RANDOMIZED-CONTROLLED TRIALS

These are statistically the most reliable way of comparing two or more different treatments in a population of patients. The characteristics of the population are defined and patients fulfilling these criteria are allocated to one of the treatment options by a random process akin to tossing a coin, but more usually derived from a computer-generated list of random numbers. In this way, fluctuations in the population that may affect the outcome of treatment are distributed evenly across the treatment groups allowing a true comparison of the treatment to be made.

END POINTS

It is important at the outset of a trial to *define* the end points by which the results will be judged. This will also guide the assessments that will be required during the trial to provide the necessary information to answer the main questions posed. End points are defined as primary, reflecting the main question addressed by the trial and on which its statistical power will be defined, and secondary, which will include other important outcomes such as side effects. Common end points are as follows:

- Survival
- Disease-free survival
- Response
- Toxicity
- Quality of life

Survival is the commonest end point for a large trial comparing two or more treatments for cancer. Whilst apparently straightforward in its definition time, cause of death may be difficult to trace, particularly in trials continuing for many years and where the condition has a long natural history for example patients in trials of prostate and breast cancer. It is important to define the cause of death. This will allow a comparison of not only overall survival but also disease-specific survival, i.e. counting only those patients dying from the disease under investigation. It is always important, however, to analyse all causes of death, since this may on occasions reveal an excess of deaths from the complications of the treatment. A typical example of this is the long-term analysis of the results of radiotherapy for breast cancer, where a reduction in breast cancer death rate is seen in patients receiving radiotherapy, but overall survival differences between those receiving radiotherapy and those who did not is less. The explanation for this apparent anomaly was explained by an excess of non-cancer deaths, predominantly cardiovascular disease in the radiotherapy group which partially negated the reduction in breast cancer deaths.

Disease-free survival is defined by the period during which a patient remains in remission, without detectable disease, following treatment. It may be further subdefined as 'local disease-free survival' taking into account only relapse within a specified site, typically the primary site of the cancer, after local treatment such as surgery or radiotherapy, which would not be expected to directly influence other distant sites. 'Distant disease-free survival' may also be used to assess a treatment for metastatic disease. Where this is used as an end point in a trial, it is important to account for the fact that relapse may only be defined by specific tests, which will be performed at specific time points. For example, if a patient is most likely to relapse with lung metastases detected on a chest CT scan, where the trial design defines a CT scan to be performed once a year, relapse can only be defined once a year, assuming that the patient does not become symptomatic and obtain a scan for their clinical management in the meantime. This would give only a very crude picture of the pattern of relapse, and a delay in the appearance of metastases by less than 12 months would not be detected; a design that called for a scan every 2–3 months during the period of risk might be more suitable in such a scenario. It is also important to realize that patients can only be compared by disease-free interval if they become disease free; for example it is a very common end point for trials after local treatment of early breast cancer where virtually all patients are 'disease free' after treatment, but of little value in trials of treatment for metastatic disease where only modest response rates might be anticipated.

In these patients a similar concept may, however, be applied using progression or symptom response rather than tumour response and measuring '*progression-free survival*' or '*symptom-free survival*'.

Response may be an important end point when testing new treatments to see whether they are effective. There are recognized formal definitions of response. The most commonly used criteria are the RECIST (response evaluation criteria in solid tumors) response criteria as follows:

- *Complete response (CR)*: Complete disappearance of all detectable disease for a period of at least 1 month
- *Partial response (PR)*: A 30% reduction in measurable disease for at least 1 month
- *Stable disease (SD)*: A reduction of <30% in measurable disease or no increase in size for at least 1 month
- *Progressive disease (PD)*: Any increase in the size of measurable disease during the assessment period

Response may be quoted as overall response rates (OR or RR), which usually include CR + PR, but it is important to check on precise definitions as some investigators include SD in this category.

Toxicity is a vital component in assessing the outcome of any clinical trial since ultimately any benefit will be balanced with side effects. Toxicity includes the immediate effects observed during the trial and may take the form of objective measures of organ function such as lung function tests, liver or renal function, and symptom scores for expected side effects of treatment. It is also important to consider later effects after treatment has been completed, and specific issues that might arise from cancer trials include the effects of treatment on fertility and the induction of second malignancies.

Quality of life measures give a global view of the impact of the intervention to be tested taking into account the response of the disease, side effects of treatment and also the more complex issues of the psychological and sociological consequences of the disease and its treatment.

Measurement of end points is a very important component of the design of any trial and requires a knowledge of the natural history of the disease being studied together with a knowledge of the effects of the treatment interventions available from the preceding use of the agents in phase 1 and 2 trials (see section 'Clinical Evidence and Clinical Trials'). Timing must be defined to give useful information but without burdening the patient or investigators with unnecessary measurements. In the early part of a trial, more measures are taken than later on, the most frequent being during treatment. However, as illustrated by the example of annual chest CT scans in a disease that may relapse within a few months, appropriate time points for assessment after treatment must also be incorporated. The nature of most cancer means that follow up will be most intensive during the first 2–3 years after treatment and then becomes less intrusive as the high-risk period for relapse passes.

Measurement may require a range of methods:

- *Death* is a clear end point but tracking patients after treatment to different centres and defining the cause of death can be more troublesome. In some countries cancer registries might be able to supply the information independently.
- *Clinical* measurement of a tumour mass may appear straightforward but clear parameters will need to be defined for example whether maximum diameter, minimum diameter or a calculated area or volume is to be used. Ideally measurements are made by independent observers or if made by the investigators, then they should be blind to the treatment received. Trials that do not include these safeguards are open to bias.
- *Radiological* measurements should similarly be carefully defined and ideally judged by an independent radiologist or preferably by a central panel convened for the trial. This allows any variation between observers to be ironed out and greater uniformity in the observations will be achieved.
- *Laboratory* measures are in general more objective but validation of the laboratory methods used is important. It is preferable to use a single reference laboratory distant from the treating centre with mechanisms in place to notify investigators of clinically relevant abnormal results.
- Measurement of *symptoms* is more complex. There are a number of accepted and validated measuring tools for common problems such as pain or vomiting and wherever possible these should be employed rather than individualized scales from a single trial or centre. These will typically take the form of categorical scales based on a none, mild, moderate, severe format or visual analogue scales, using a 10 cm scale, on which patients mark the severity of a symptom. Critical to achieving good data is careful explanation and continued support during the data collection. Wherever possible it is important to have data completed by the patient themselves rather than a surrogate.
- *Quality of life* instruments are detailed questionnaires relating to the patient's emotional and physical well-being. They can be general or have additional 'disease-specific modules' addressing issues that may be pertinent to a particular tumour site for example urinary and sexual function in carcinoma of the prostate. Common examples used in cancer trials are the FACT (Functional Assessment of Cancer Therapy) and EORTC QLQ-C30 (European Organisation for Research and Treatment of

Decision-making and communication

Cancer Core Quality of Life Questionnare C30) quality of life questionnaires.
- *Health economic* assessments are increasingly an integral component of randomized trials assessing new treatments as it becomes apparent that the resources allocated to health care in the developed world can no longer match the availability and demand for increasingly complex and expensive treatments. The demonstration of cost-effectiveness is therefore an important component of any clinical trial today evaluating new cancer treatments. The tools for evaluating this are also becoming more complex as it becomes clear that a simple balance sheet approach cannot address the issues that may arise. Attempts are made to relate the treatment effect with the length of time over which benefit may occur, resulting in concepts such as the Quality Adjusted Life Year (QALY) to measure treatment outcome.

PLACEBO-CONTROLLED TRIALS

Placebo-controlled trials will be appropriate when a new treatment is being tested in a situation where there is no recognized standard treatment with which to compare it. Although it may be possible to compare the new treatment with no treatment there is always the possibility that simply the process of delivering a treatment, whether a drug or other intervention, will have an unexpected beneficial or harmful effect. The use of a placebo, which will be made to resemble the active treatment as closely as possible, reduces this possibility. Placebos are most effective in trials that are blinded. This refers to a situation in which either the investigator or subject do not know the difference between the placebo and active drug (single-blind design). The optimum design is a double-blind trial in which neither the investigator nor the subject is aware whether a placebo or active drug is being used.

Where there is already a recognized treatment against which the new treatment is to be tested then placebo-controlled trials are inappropriate and the control arm will be the best available standard treatment. Alternatively, particularly in testing new treatments in advanced cancer, the control arm could be best supportive care. This is optimized symptomatic supportive care distinct from the use of 'anticancer' treatment and permits the test of a new treatment in the setting of symptomatic, advanced malignancy to evaluate the addition of an anticancer therapy where standard treatment is symptomatic care only.

RANDOMIZATION

Randomization describes the method by which subjects in a trial are distributed into different treatment groups. Most trials have two 'arms': the standard arm, which should be the recognized best available treatment or, if there is none, then this will be a 'no treatment' or placebo arm and the experimental arm in which the new treatment will be tested. In most trials there will be balanced randomization, i.e. the trial will comprise equal numbers in each of the arms of the trial. Occasionally, however, a design can be used in which there is a weighted randomization for example a 2:1 distribution of subjects, usually in favour of the experimental arm, i.e. twice as many subjects in the experimental arm as the control. Randomization should take place through an independent trials office totally separate from the facilities in which the trial will be undertaken; usually this involves computer-generated blocks of random numbers, which then allocate subjects to their arm of the trial. This may be accessed by researchers through a telephone call, fax or a voice-activated computer program.

STRATIFICATION

Stratification can be built into the design of a trial. This is to ensure that subgroups within the trial population, which may have different prognoses, are equally distributed. In oncology this might mean that trials are stratified by tumour stage or performance status. At randomization each tumour stage or performance status group will be independently randomized ensuring an equal distribution of stages or performance status across the arms of the trial. This precaution also aids later analysis using the stage or performance status subgroups without prejudice. Multicentre trials usually stratify by treatment centre also.

TRIAL STATISTICS

The major drawback of a randomized trial is that for a statistically robust result a large number of patients are required. The total number of patients required is defined beforehand by a trial statistician who predicts the number of subjects needed to give a defined level of statistical certainty for a given change in response rate from a known baseline. For example, if a standard treatment has a known response rate of 70% and a 5-year survival rate of 45%, the trial investigators must decide what improvement upon this they would expect, or wish to detect, in their trial. This should be based on the difference that would be expected to alter clinical practice. They will then need to define the power of the trial, i.e. how certain they wish to be of their result at the end. For example, if a particular treatment has a survival rate of 50%, in order to reliably detect an absolute improvement of 10%–60% from a new treatment, approximately 400 patients will be required to enter a randomized trial comparing the two. The precise number of patients will be affected by the degree of error in the trial results that will be accepted by those designing the trial. Two types of errors have been recognized:

- Type I(α) error in which a difference may be observed which does not really exist; and
- Type II(β) error in which a true difference may be missed.

These will commonly be set at an α error of 0.05 and a β error of 0.2 (often referred to as 80% power). This means that there is a 5% chance of the result observed being false. As a general principle, the more strict the statistical constraints are, i.e. the smaller the α and β errors accepted and the smaller the difference to be detected between the arms of the trials, the larger the number of patients required. For example, for a trial in a condition where, with standard treatment, a 5-year survival rate is 50%, to detect a 10% increase in survival with a new treatment in a two-arm randomized trial accepting an α error of 0.05 and β error of 0.2, a total of 760 patients will be required. Trials designed to show equivalence, i.e. no difference between the treatment arms, require the highest number of patients.

The 'p' value is often quoted alongside results of a clinical trial. This essentially relates to the α error accepted in the result. The conventional value required before a result is considered statistically significant is $p = 0.05$, which relates to an α error of 0.05 and means that there is a 5% chance of the results not being a true reflection of the comparison in the trial, or in other words there can be a 95% certainty that the result is a true result.

TRIAL INFRASTRUCTURE

Clinical trials demand an extensive infrastructure within a dedicated central clinical trials unit that will coordinate the trial and provide a central point for randomization, data collection and analysis. It should be independent of the investigators entering and treating patients in the trial who are usually based in many different centres all accruing relatively small numbers of patients. A randomized clinical trial may take several years before it is completed and analysed to give reliable results that will be translated into clinical practice. It is important during the running of such a trial that any new information from other trials that may affect the relevance of the outcome is considered and that any unexpected toxicity or difference in response is evaluated within the trial. For this reason, most large trials will have associated with them a data monitoring committee (DMC) usually comprising a statistician and two or three clinicians or scientists who are not involved in that particular trial. They will review the results of the trial at defined time points perhaps annually or after accrual of a predetermined number of subjects, e.g. after every 100 patients entered. They may recommend early closure of a trial if a large number of unexpected toxicities are found in one arm, or if a sufficiently large difference emerges between the arms of the trial early on which was unexpected and unlikely to be reversed by larger numbers. The data seen by the DMC must at all times remain confidential from the investigators involved in running the trial. In practice, early closure is rare in a well-designed clinical trial but the DMC is an important component to ensure that patients are not given inappropriate treatment.

ETHICS OF CLINICAL TRIALS

It is a fundamental principle in designing and partaking in a clinical trial comparing two treatments

Decision-making and communication

that the patient should not be disadvantaged compared with other patients not taking part in the trial. For this to be satisfied the investigators must be confident that there is no proven advantage for the new treatment over the existing management and equally that there is no evidence of any greater toxicity that would disadvantage the patient. This will be based on information gained from earlier phase I and phase II trials. In fact, it has been shown that patients taking part in clinical trials generally have a better outcome than those who do not, possibly because of the adherence to a rigid protocol and the greater clinical input that inevitably accompanies trial participation.

META-ANALYSIS

A meta-analysis is a means of overcoming the problem of patient numbers. This arises because most innovations in treatment have only a modest impact on outcome; an improvement in survival of more than 10% from any new intervention is very unusual. Other new treatments might not even be expected to improve survival but aimed at reducing toxicity or improving quality of life. Any clinical observation is inherently unreliable in statistical terms and will carry a range around which a repeat observation may be expected to fall – this is often quoted as the 95% confidence interval within which 95% of repeated observations might be expected. The smaller the number of observations the wider will be the confidence interval. To be certain that the observations in two groups of patients are truly different, there must be no overlap of the confidence intervals. Where there is a big difference, even relatively wide confidence limits will not overlap, but for a small true difference the confidence interval needs to be as small as possible to demonstrate the difference, and this will only be achieved with a large number of patients.

A meta-analysis therefore attempts to include as many patients as possible who have entered trials addressing a particular question. This approach has been used in several tumour sites of which breast cancer provides an excellent example. For some years a series of individual clinical trials across the world have addressed the question as to whether adding hormone therapy or chemotherapy to the primary treatment can prolong survival. The results of individual trials failed to give a clear answer, some showing benefit and others no benefit. A meta-analysis has therefore been performed combining the results of all known trials in this area and demonstrated that in 30,000 women adjuvant tamoxifen conveys a 6.2% survival advantage after 10 years and in 10,000 women polychemotherapy carries a 6.3% survival advantage after 10 years. These figures illustrate the very small overall survival effect seen and explain why series of small trials gave conflicting results. With large number of patients in the meta-analysis, small differences can be found with a high level of statistical reliability as demonstrated by the very low 'p' value associated with these data; the tamoxifen result above has a p value of <0.00001, i.e. only a 1 in 10,000 chance that the observation is not real.

CASE–CONTROL STUDIES

In many situations, particularly in rare tumours where it is not possible to study large number of patients, randomized trials are not practical. The next best type of trial is the case–control trial in which a new treatment is given to a series of patients and then compared with patients previously treated for that condition. It is important in such a comparison to exclude any factors that might affect the result other than the treatment being tested. This is achieved by selecting matched controls, i.e. patients with otherwise identical characteristics to one of the new treatment group with whom they are matched. Parameters important to match for include age, sex, tumour stage and histological type, together with any other known prognostic factors. The comparison may be refined by selecting two matched controls for each patient receiving the new treatment.

The difference between the two groups is often quoted as an *odds ratio* comparing the probability of an event (e.g. death or tumour recurrence) occurring in the control group with that in the new treatment group.

COHORT STUDIES

Cohort studies are not usually of value in comparing two different treatments but are used in particular to investigate aetiological factors. As their name suggests they are observational studies in which a group of patients (a cohort) is monitored over a period of time for a particular outcome, e.g. development of or death from cancer. This type of study is usually reported in terms of relative risk, comparing the incidence in the cohort with that of a control cohort. The value of this type of study is in defining the natural history of a particular tumour type and evaluating the impact of potential aetiological agents.

CONCLUSION

Different tumour types, their aetiology, natural history and various treatment options have been described in subsequent chapters. The accuracy of this depends critically on the data from which this information has been derived. It can be seen that there are many pitfalls in obtaining and interpreting the results of clinical data sets. Any advances in cancer management depend critically on rigorous evaluation with close attention to the design and interpretation of clinical trials to ensure that reliable outcome data are acquired to further advance knowledge. It also demands that clinicians and patients of the future are sufficiently informed to understand and partake in clinical trials.

FURTHER READING

Brody T. *Clinical Trials*. 2nd ed. Academic Press, San Diego, 2016.

Girling DJ, Parmar MKB, Stenning SP, Stephens RJ and Stewart LA. *Clinical Trials in Cancer: Principles and Practice*. Oxford University Press, Oxford, 2003.

Principles of surgical oncology

Surgery is the most effective treatment for localized cancers either alone or in combination with regional radiotherapy or adjuvant systemic chemotherapy. Over 50% of cures achieved in cancer patients are attributable to radical resection of localized cancer. Surgical input into multidisciplinary teams is essential to enable close liaison between surgeon and oncologist to optimize the use of each modality.

MANAGEMENT OF THE PRIMARY TUMOUR

Surgery may contribute to the management of a patient with cancer in several ways:

- Tissue biopsy to establish the diagnosis.
- Sampling of regional lymph nodes to confirm staging.
- Removal of malignant disease with a clear margin of normal tissue.
- Repair, reconstruction and restoration of function. This may vary according to the extent of resection and anatomical site, from simple primary wound closure to major reconstruction of bone and soft tissue with vascularized grafts and prostheses.

The type of surgery required will be determined by the type of tumour and the anatomical site, and may include:

- Wide local excision of the tumour mass, e.g. local excision of a breast lump
- Removal of part of an organ and surrounding tissue, e.g. partial glossectomy and neck dissection for a carcinoma of the tongue
- Removal of an entire organ, e.g. laryngectomy, cystectomy or hysterectomy.

En bloc removal of the immediate lymphatic drainage areas is usually an integral part of any cancer surgery, e.g. hysterectomy for cervical cancer includes pelvic lymphadenectomy.

Radiotherapy will give equivalent local control rates to surgery for small tumours (<5 cm) in many anatomical sites and has the potential advantage in certain sites of being able to preserve anatomical structure and function, e.g. in the treatment of laryngeal cancer where radical radiotherapy can result in tumour eradication with voice preservation in contrast to the surgical alternative, which is total laryngectomy. However, against this must be balanced the need for close post-radiotherapy surveillance and the potential need for later surgical salvage if recurrence is found. This may occur in around 20% of patients having organ-preserving treatment depending on the primary tumour and stage. Surgery following radiotherapy can be technically more difficult and have a higher complication rate.

COMBINED SURGERY AND RADIOTHERAPY

The combination of surgery with radiotherapy has two potential advantages and applications:

Principles of surgical oncology

Table 4.1 Relative merits of pre- and post-operative radiotherapy

Pre-operative RT	Post-operative RT
Early radiotherapy	No delay to surgery
Enables pre-operative preparation for planned surgery	True pathological staging may be masked by pre-operative RT
Surgery may be easier if tumour shrinks pre-operatively	Pathology of surgical specimen may guide later RT
	Lower dose of RT needed for microscopic disease

- It enables the extent of surgery to be limited by treating sites of microscopic disease immediately adjacent to the primary site with radiotherapy, e.g. the use of local excision and radiotherapy in place of mastectomy for breast cancer.
- For large tumours (>5 cm) local control rates are often better for combined therapy than either modality alone.

Radiotherapy may be given pre-operatively or post-operatively. The relative merits of each approach are illustrated in Table 4.1.

MANAGEMENT OF REGIONAL LYMPH NODES

The common epithelial tumours, such as those of the lung, breast, head and neck region and pelvis, metastasize through two routes: the lymphatic system and the blood circulation. Clinically involved lymph nodes and those at high risk of microscopic involvement require active treatment.

Surgery is indicated for the immediate draining of nodes around a primary tumour. Radical dissection of the involved node chain should be considered, and may involve:

- Axillary dissection for breast cancer
- Radical neck dissection for head and neck sites
- Inguinal node dissection for vulval, anal or penile cancers

A more conservative approach, sentinel lymph node mapping, is now the standard of care for breast cancer and melanoma. This entails the identification of the 'sentinel' lymph node. This is the node that is first to receive lymph from the tumour-bearing tissue. A vital blue dye and radiolabelled colloid microspheres are injected pre-operatively to allow perioperative identification of the lymph node(s) to be removed. If they are found to be involved by frozen section analysis or on definitive histological examination, a full lymph node dissection is mandatory. If this is negative, it is highly unlikely that other lymph nodes in that group will harbour cancer cells, and the patient may be spared the additional morbidity of the larger operation. The technique allows the identification of unusual patterns of lymphatic spread, e.g. to the internal mammary lymph nodes in breast cancer, or the axilla in truncal melanoma.

Radical excision of nodes is *not* indicated for:

- Lymphomas (Hodgkin disease or non-Hodgkin lymphoma) or leukaemias
- Those with metastatic involvement at visceral sites where there may be little or no quality of life gain by removing enlarged lymph nodes

SURGICALLY INOPERABLE NODES

Radiotherapy is indicated for lymph nodes which cannot be removed by surgery. This may be because they are too large, fixed to underlying structures or close to vital structures such as major blood vessels or nerves.

Pre-operative radiotherapy can succeed in rendering inoperable lymph nodes operable.

Post-operative radiotherapy following surgical dissection is recommended for patients with multiple node involvement and extension of tumour beyond the capsule of the gland (extracapsular extension).

CHEMOTHERAPY

Chemotherapy is indicated for enlarged lymph nodes from germ cell tumour and lymphoma. It may also play a role in the management of other chemosensitive tumours such as metastatic breast cancer, colorectal cancer or small cell lung cancer.

PALLIATIVE SURGERY

Even when cure is no longer a realistic aim, surgery can have an important role in the palliation of local symptoms. Specific examples where surgery should be considered include:

- Palliation of obstructive symptoms
- Control of haemorrhage
- Palliation of tumour fungation
- Fracture reduction and fixation

PALLIATION OF OBSTRUCTIVE SYMPTOMS

- Palliative resection of a bowel tumour or a simple bypass procedure such as a gastrojejunostomy will avoid symptoms of intestinal obstruction.
- Laser or cryotherapy resection of an obstructing tumour mass will restore the lumen of an obstructed bronchus or oesophagus.
- Intubation of the oesophagus with a rigid tube or flexible stent provides rapid and effective relief of dysphagia.
- Nephrostomy or passage of ureteric catheters will relieve obstructive hydronephrosis.
- Biliary stents or choledochojejunostomy will relieve obstructive jaundice owing to extrahepatic bile duct obstruction as in carcinoma of the pancreas.
- Gastroenterostomy will relieve gastric outflow obstruction.
- Rectal stents will overcome obstruction from a rectal cancer.
- Ventriculoperitoneal shunting of hydrocephalus may result in dramatic improvement in headache and neurological deficits even though the underlying tumour may be incurable.

CONTROL OF HAEMORRHAGE

- Diathermy at bronchoscopy or cystoscopy will control haemoptysis or haematuria, respectively.
- Bleeding tumours in the oesophagus, stomach or large bowel can be controlled by using diathermy or laser coagulation at endoscopy.

PALLIATION OF TUMOUR FUNGATION

Local resection, even if not complete, may be of value for a locally advanced tumour mass that is necrotic and breaking down. 'Toilet' mastectomy for a progressive breast cancer is perhaps the most common example of this.

FRACTURE REDUCTION AND FIXATION

- Pathological fracture of a weight-bearing bone is best dealt with by internal fixation, as shown in Figure 4.1, followed by post-operative radiotherapy.
- In certain circumstances prophylactic fixation may also be indicated; specific indications for this include diffuse lytic bone disease in a weight-bearing area and destruction of more than 50% of the cortex by a lytic deposit.
- Radiotherapy is often given following surgical fixation for patients with a prognosis of more than 3 months to reduce further tumour growth in the bone and maximize healing, without which subsequent progression of the underlying cancer will result in progressive bone damage around the fixation (Figure 4.2).

FURTHER READING

de Jolinière JB, Major A, Khomsi F, Ali NB, Guillou L, Feki A. *The sentinel lymph node in breast cancer: Problems posed by examination during surgery. A review of current literature and management. Front Surg.*, 2018.| https://doi.org/10.3389/fsurg.2018.00056

Sabel MS, Sondak VK, Sussman JJ. *Essentials of Surgical Oncology*. Mosby, London, 2007.

Silberman H, Silberman AW. *Principles and Practice of Surgical Oncology*. Lipincott, Williams and Wilkins, Philadelphia, 2010.

Principles of surgical oncology

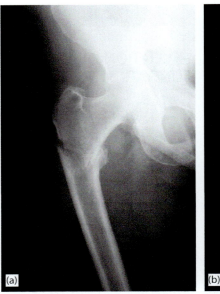
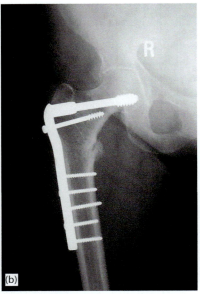

Figure 4.1 Pathological fracture of the right neck of femur: (a) before and (b) after internal fixation.

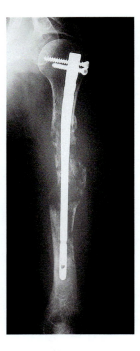

Figure 4.2 Uncontrolled bone metastases. This woman had internal fixation for a pathological fracture of the mid-shaft of the humerus. This was not followed by radiotherapy. She has now developed significant bone lysis compromising the mechanical integrity of the bone.

SELF-ASSESSMENT QUESTIONS

1. Which three of the following are indications for the surgical treatment of cancer?
   a. Long waiting time for radiotherapy
   b. Fracture of a weight-bearing bone
   c. Acute intestinal obstruction
   d. Hypercalcaemia
   e. Anaemia
   f. Hypoproteinaemia
   g. Intestinal perforation

2. Which one of the following is the most important feature of pre-operative radiotherapy?
   a. Allows treatment of regional lymph nodes
   b. Downstages disease to facilitate surgical resection
   c. Removes need for radiotherapy after surgery
   d. Lessens morbidity from radiotherapy
   e. Cost-effective

Principles of radiotherapy

Radiotherapy is the use of ionizing radiation to treat disease. The radiation used is either produced by specialist equipment designed for treating patients or by using a specific radioisotope that decays in a set manner to produce radiation.

TYPES OF RADIATION

Alpha (α): A heavy charged particle that has classically been difficult to harness in the treatment of patients. Radium 223 is an alpha emitter used in the treatment of metastatic prostate cancer.

Beta (β): An electron produced by the decay of certain radioisotopes or by specialist radiotherapy equipment. Electrons are an important part of therapeutic radiation treatment.

Gamma (γ): A beam of radiation, part of the electromagnetic spectrum. Gamma rays (or x-rays) are produced by the decay of certain radioisotopes and from specialist radiation equipment. Gamma radiation is the main type of radiation used to treat cancer patients (and in diagnostic CT units).

Proton: Protons are available in an increasing number of centres around the world and the first centre in the UK became operational in 2018. Their advantage is the production of a highly localized, high-energy peak of energy deposition (*Bragg peak*), which, by manipulation of the beam energy and by the use of absorbing materials, can be focused to a defined position in a patient. Biologically they are similar in action to x-rays. They have been used particularly for tumours in inaccessible sites such as the back of the eye, base of the skull and childhood brain and spinal tumours. Research is ongoing to see if they have any advantage for other disease sites.

Neutron: Neutrons have been evaluated extensively in a number of centres across Europe and the United States. Their advantages are that they have less dependence on oxygen for cell killing, have a recognized limitation for x-rays and cause more direct damage to the cellular DNA. While there is little doubt that they are more effective at achieving cell kill, they are not selective for cancer cells and their use has been accompanied by unacceptably high levels of normal tissue damage and severe late side effects. They are therefore not in routine clinical use.

Heavy ion particles: These are rarely used but in principle may overcome some of the issues in relation to oxygenation.

BIOLOGICAL ACTIONS OF IONIZING RADIATION

Ionizing radiation causes damage to cellular DNA by two mechanisms:

- *Direct damage* caused by the passage of the photon through the nucleic acid structure.
- *Indirect damage* owing to the production of toxic-free hydroxyl radicals from the interaction of radiation with water within the cell. This results in single- and double-strand breaks

in the DNA, which, unless repair occurs, will accumulate, resulting in the reproductive death of the cell.

Other factors important in the response to radiation are as follows:

- *Oxygenation*: Hypoxic tissues are considered relatively radioresistant. The delivery of radiotherapy in multiple fractions allows reoxygenation to occur between each treatment as the tumour shrinks and blood flow improves.
- *Repopulation*: Both tumour tissue and normal tissues continue to divide during a course of radiotherapy and there is even some evidence to suggest that repopulation may increase during this time as cells are lost. Gaps within a radiotherapy schedule should therefore be avoided wherever possible to avoid significant repopulation undoing any effects from irradiation in the previous days.
- *Repair*: Much of the damage produced by x-rays and gamma rays is not sufficient to kill the cell immediately (sublethal damage). The repair of such damage will mean that the cell retains its viability. This capacity is better developed in normal tissues than in many malignant tumours, which accounts for much of the differential cell kill between tumour and normal cells.
- *Redistribution*: Radiosensitivity varies as cells progress through cell cycle, being maximum during the periods of active DNA synthesis in late G1 and S phases and least during G2 and early M phases.

There is a spectrum of radiosensitivity for both tumour and normal cell types. Few, if any, tumours are truly radioresistant, although some may require a larger dose of radiation than others to achieve the same effect. There is also a wide spectrum of sensitivity in normal tissues. Particular care is required with certain normal tissues when irradiation is delivered:

- CNS tissue has a relatively low threshold for damage and has little or no capacity for repair. Radiation damage to the CNS is therefore often irreversible and can result in catastrophic morbidity if, for example, necrosis of the spinal cord or brainstem results.
- The small bowel is also relatively sensitive, and doses well below those required to sterilize an epithelial tumour will cause serious damage.
- The lens of the eye develops cataract after exposure to small doses and must therefore be carefully shielded whenever possible.
- Bladder and rectum are often dose-limiting tissues when pelvic tumours are treated.
- Lung damage occurs at around half the dose required to treat a lung cancer; damage to a large volume of lung will result in respiratory distress and even death from respiratory failure.

The balance between causing serious normal tissue damage and curing a malignant tumour is termed the 'therapeutic ratio'. Compromise of radiation dose to avoid excessive toxicity is the major limitation in successfully achieving local cure of malignant tumours with radiotherapy.

In certain circumstances, the effect of radiotherapy may be enhanced by the concurrent use of chemotherapy or agents that affect tumour oxygenation. An example is the radical radiotherapy of bladder cancer where radiotherapy is either given with chemotherapy or with the oxygenation enhancers carbogen and nicotinamide.

RADIOTHERAPY EQUIPMENT

EXTERNAL BEAM RADIOTHERAPY

External beam radiotherapy is the most common form of treatment in clinical use. A range of x-ray beams is available, varying according to their energy.

SUPERFICIAL VOLTAGE

These x-ray beams are of energy 50–150 kV and are, as their name implies, suitable for the treatment of superficial lesions in the skin; their useful treatment energy penetrates no more than 1 cm beneath the surface. For example, they could be used to treat a patient with a superficial skin cancer, e.g. basal cell carcinoma.

ORTHOVOLTAGE MACHINES

These machines produce x-rays of energy 200–300 kV and penetrate to a depth of approximately 3 cm. These are therefore useful for treating structures such as ribs, scapula or sacrum but are not sufficiently powerful to reach deeper internal organs. This is mostly used to deliver palliative radiotherapy. Many radiotherapy centres now provide such treatment using megavoltage equipment.

MEGAVOLTAGE MACHINES

Linear accelerators (LAs) produce high-energy x-ray beams of 4–20 MV and are the mainstay of most radiotherapy treatments. LAs have largely replaced machines such as cobalt machines which contain a radioisotope cobalt-60, which decays spontaneously to nickel-60 releasing gamma rays of 1.2 and 1.3 MV, respectively. A modern linear accelerator is shown in Figure 5.1.

Electron beams are also produced by linear accelerators and have the advantage that, as particulate radiation beams, they have a defined range in tissue with a sharp cut-off at the point where they deliver their energy. This is of value where a tumour is superficial and particularly when it is overlying a radiosensitive structure such as the spinal cord. In many centres, electron beam treatment has replaced older superficial and orthovoltage x-ray machines, providing a wide range of beams with varying effective treatment depths from the linear accelerator.

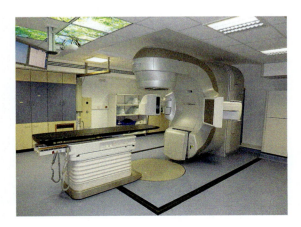

Figure 5.1 A modern linear accelerator.

BRACHYTHERAPY

Brachytherapy is a method where radioactive sources are placed either on or within the site involving the tumour. The great advantage of this form of treatment is the rapid fall-off of dose at a short distance from the source (obeying the inverse square law – double the distance will quarter the radiation dose).

There are three types of brachytherapy used:

- *Mould treatment*: In this therapy, radioactive sources are placed directly over a superficial tumour of the skin fixed in a plastic mounting (the mould).
- *Intracavitary treatment*: In this technique, radioactive sources are placed within a body cavity. Intrauterine tubes and vaginal sources in the treatment of gynaecological tumours are the common applicators of this technique.
- *Interstitial treatment*: In this therapy, radioactive sources, which may be in the form of needles or wires, are inserted directly into the area of interest. This technique is used for the treatment of cancer of the tongue, floor of the mouth and breast.

The first isotope to be employed was radium. It is no longer used because it constitutes a major radiation hazard as it has a long half-life (1620 years) and decays to a radioactive gas (radon). It has been superseded initially by cobalt sources and currently by caesium and iridium as the principal isotopes for brachytherapy.

LIVE SOURCE IMPLANTS

Direct handling of live sources is most commonly carried out today when iodine or palladium seeds are used for prostate implants. While the radiation from iodine-125 is short range and poses no major radiation hazard, that from iridium implants used in the past is more penetrating and its use has major disadvantages like exposure of staff and patients within the hospital to radiation from the time of insertion to the time of removal, which may be several days. This means that careful monitoring is required and that there are limits to the time that individuals can spend caring for the patient. It also means that friends and family are not permitted to be with the patient.

MANUAL AFTERLOADING

In this method, inactive source carriers are used initially to enable accurate siting of the treatment so that the patient can be moved within the hospital from theatre or the x-ray department without radioactive sources in place. The active isotope is introduced manually once the inactive carrier is correctly placed. This enables more accurate placement not constrained by the need for rapid placement and long-handled instruments required when a live source is used. Loading can be done in the operating theatre or once the patient has returned to a protected room and post-operative recovery is complete. An example although no longer in regular use, is iridium wire hairpins for tongue and floor-of-mouth implants.

REMOTE AFTERLOADING

Following placement of the source carriers, the radiation sources are introduced by remote control via pneumatic pipes or a cable connected to the source carriers within the patient. This system minimizes exposure to staff and in practice means that only the patient is exposed to radiation. It is also possible to interrupt the treatment so that the patient can receive attention without further exposing hospital personnel and there are no time limits on their stay. A modern afterloading machine is shown in Figure 5.2.

All such treatments require the patient to be isolated in a protected room with thickened or shielded walls, floors and ceilings while the source is in position in the patient.

Remote afterloading can deliver radiation at different dose rates; most centres now use high-dose rate machines, which deliver the dose in only a few minutes. This has substantial advantages in radiation protection and means that the patient no longer needs prolonged periods of isolation to receive brachytherapy.

INTERNAL ISOTOPE THERAPY

Internal isotope treatment involves the administration of a radioactive isotope systemically, which is then concentrated within the body at certain sites. Specific examples of this form of treatment are the use of radioiodine (^{131}I) for thyroid cancer and also neuroblastoma when conjugated in meta-iodobenzyl guanidine (mIBG), phosphorus (^{32}P) for polycythaemia rubra vera, strontium (^{89}Sr) for bone metastases and Ra223 for bone metastases in prostate cancer.

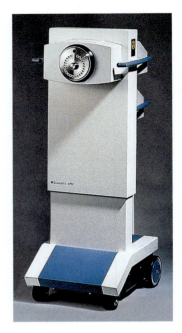

Figure 5.2 A modern brachytherapy afterloading machine, which uses a small iridium source located in the head of the machine that passes out a radiation source through a series of channels sequentially which are connected to applicators within a tumour volume. (Courtesy of Varian Medical Systems.)

CLINICAL USE OF RADIOTHERAPY

The patient attending radiotherapy treatment will pass through a series of steps to ensure that treatment is given as accurately and safely as possible; these include:

- Patient positioning and immobilization
- Tumour and normal tissue localization and definition
- Treatment planning
- Verification
- Treatment

Clinical use of radiotherapy

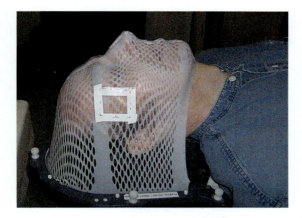

Figure 5.3 Patient in position for treatment to the orbit demonstrating immobilization mask.

POSITIONING OF A PATIENT

This is very important in order to enable an x-ray beam to reach a certain site. It is particularly the case in the head and neck region where small changes in the position of the neck or chin can greatly affect the tissues included in an x-ray beam.

In order to reproduce a particular position accurately, some form of immobilization may be designed, such as a plastic head shell to hold the head in a fixed position as shown in Figure 5.3.

TUMOUR AND NORMAL TISSUE LOCALIZATION AND DEFINITION

Localization can be achieved by simple clinical examination as in the case of skin tumour or plain x-rays as in bone metastases. It may also require more sophisticated imaging, e.g. CT scan, MRI scan or PET/CT scan for tumours in the thorax, abdomen or pelvis. Alongside this, it is important to identify the normal tissues and structures to which dose constraints apply – these will depend on the site being treated, e.g. normal lung tissue, heart and spinal cord when treating a patient with lung cancer.

The International Commission on Radition Units (ICRU) has defined target volumes to be used in radiotherapy:

- GTV = gross tumour volume.
- CTV = clinical tumour volume. The GTV with an expansion to take into account possible microscopic spread and movement of the target volume.
- PTV = planning target volume. The CTV with an expansion to take into account possible set-up errors on the actual treatment machine. These expansions are the disease site and machine type, and they are department specific.
- OAR = organs at risk. The normal tissues that must be defined and the radiation dose to these is kept within pre-defined limits that are known to be safe.

TREATMENT PLANNING

This defines the optimal arrangement of x-ray beams to cover the treatment area as evenly as possible while avoiding structures around it. At its simplest level this may be a single direct electron beam for a skin tumour; for internal tumours a more complex arrangement is required and radiotherapy techniques have advanced greatly with developments in computer planning. The following terms are used to describe different radiotherapy planning and delivery techniques:

Conformal radiotherapy using external x-ray beams shapes the high-dose treatment area as closely as possible to that of the tumour volume, even where this may have a highly irregular shape, while avoiding adjacent sensitive normal structures. This requires accurate three-dimensional reconstruction of the volume to be treated and irregular beam shaping using lead blocks, or more commonly a multi-leaf collimator shaping the beam typically by 80 or 120 interleaved projections into the beam, which can be adjusted as required. An example is shown in Figure 5.4.

Intensity-modulated radiotherapy (IMRT) is a further development, which varies the dose delivered within a tumour volume. This means that a central high-dose region can be defined surrounded by a low-dose region, minimizing inclusion of normal tissues, all within the same treatment volume.

Stereotactic radiotherapy is a means of treating a small volume with a very high dose of radiation. This can be achieved using a standard linear accelerator with a modified beam producing a small focused field, which builds up the high-dose volume using a series of rotating arc movements. Some equipment

Principles of radiotherapy

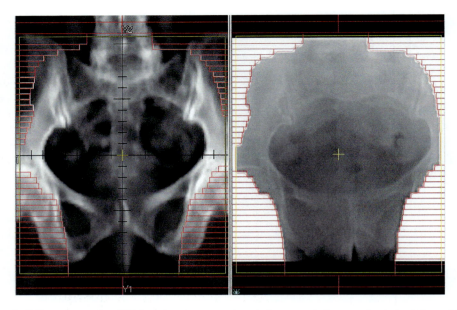

Figure 5.4 (Left) Beam's eye view (BEV) of planning scan pictures from a radiotherapy plan to treat the pelvis, demonstrating position of the beam and shaping using the multileaf collimator. (Right) An electronic portal image (EPI) has been taken using the high-energy linear accelerator beam prior to a treatment exposure to verify the beam size, shape and position. Note the loss of definition between bone and soft tissue characteristic of high-energy (megavoltage) x-rays.

is designed specially to deliver stereotactic radiotherapy, e.g. 'cyberknife', which incorporates a megavoltage x-ray beam into a gantry capable of multiple non-coplanar arcs controlled by software that enables variable beam profiles during the arc to build up a complex localized dose distribution. Gammaknife® is a machine containing multiple cobalt sources, each with its independent shield which can be opened to focus on the treatment volume in a spherical pattern (able to treat the head only).

VERIFICATION

Verification entails ensuring that the treatment plan can be translated back to the patient in the defined treatment position. Traditionally, this was performed on a machine called a treatment simulator, which reproduces precisely the movements of the treatment machine and produces diagnostic x-ray beams so that an x-ray picture of the proposed treatment beam can be taken.

Verification is essential during treatment and the ability to perform this is now a standard part of the design of modern radiotherapy equipment with megavoltage, kilovoltage or both imaging modalities being used. Verification protocols will depend on the disease site and equipment being used. The term image-guided radiotherapy (IGRT) is used when the actual patient and target volumes are checked against those planned directly before treatment. IGRT is usually performed by monitoring the position of tiny metal markers (fidcuial markers) which are inserted into or close to the target prior to the radiotherapy planning process as shown in Figure 5.5, or by taking a set of CT images on the treatment LA and comparing these with the initial planning CT scan. Complex techniques can be offered when it is important to take account of respiratory motion, e.g. gating in lung cancer, deep inspiratory breath hold for left-sided breast cancer.

TREATMENT DURATION

There is considerable variation in the dose and duration of radiotherapy treatment given to patients, which can appear confusing. Neither the total number of treatments nor the total dose given is necessarily a guide to the biological dose of radiation

Clinical use of radiotherapy

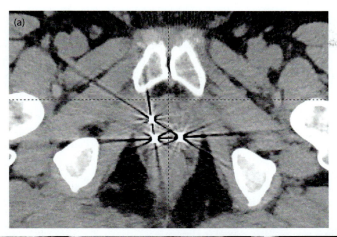

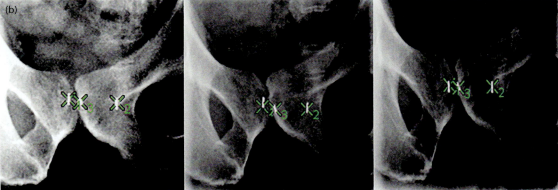

Figure 5.5 CT image showing markers placed in the prostate gland to ensure accurate delivery of radiotherapy (a) and cone beam CT images from the linear accelerator taken on three consecutive days showing consistency of position of markers during treatment delivery (b).

delivered. There are three components to biological radiation dose:

- Total dose
- Number of treatments (fractions) of a given dose
- Overall time of treatment

Formulae have been developed by radiobiologists to help compare different radiotherapy schedules. Linear quadratic equation is currently used. The following general principles can be applied:

- The same total dose given in a short time or fewer fractions has greater effect than the same dose given over a longer time in many fractions.

- Fraction size is an important determinant of normal tissue damage: small fractions minimize normal tissue effects. However, it follows from the previous point that, if used, small fractions demand a longer course of treatment with a higher total dose to have the same effect.
- Overall treatment time is important in achieving tumour control. Delays and interruptions in a course of treatment should be avoided as should an overall treatment time of greater than 7 weeks.

The unit of radiation dose used is the Gray, which is a measure of absorbed energy (1 Gy = 1 Joule/kg). This has replaced the rad but the conversion is simple: 1 Gy = 100 rads.

45

Principles of radiotherapy

Precise radiation schedules can vary from centre to centre and country to country but there are many radiotherapy schedules that are now standard around the world. A fundamental difference lies between palliative and radical doses.

Radical treatments require high doses of radiation to eliminate tumour but are divided into smaller fractions to minimize side effects and remain within the tolerance of normal tissues. Research developments have looked at the optimal schedules in relation to both dose and time. The delivery of a larger dose of radiotherapy per fraction with an overall shorter total duration of treatment is termed hypofractionation.

An example of the changes in radical radiotherapy fractionation can be seen in the total dose and fractionation used in the treatment of prostate cancer:

> 74 Gy 37 #s 7.5 weeks   =   60 Gy 20 #s 4 weeks
> conventional   moderate
> fractionation   hypofractionation
> (evidence from UK CHHIP trial in prostate cancer)
>
> 60 Gy 20 #s 4 weeks   =   35.75 Gy 5 #s 1 week
> moderate   severe
> hypofractionation   hypofractionation
> (ongoing clinical trial in early prostate cancer-UK PACE trial)

Palliative treatments require short schedules with few acute side effects. The ideal palliative treatment is a single dose and this is applicable in many cases; however, in some cases a short course of radiotherapy may be more appropriate. Examples include:

- 8–10 Gy in a single dose
- 20 Gy in five daily fractions over 1 week or 30 Gy in 10 daily fractions over 2 weeks

SIDE EFFECTS OF RADIOTHERAPY

The toxicity of radiotherapy is divided into two distinct groups: the early effects, which occur during treatment, and the late effects, which come about months or years following treatment and may be permanent.

EARLY EFFECTS

These effects develop during treatment usually in the second or third week of a course of radical irradiation. They may be divided as follows:

- *Non-specific effects*: Many patients feel tired and lack energy during treatment. There may be many factors in addition to radiation exposure to account for this, including depression, anxiety, daily travel for treatment and concomitant medication.
- *Specific local effects related to the area being treated*: It is important to note that areas outside the irradiation field do not exhibit acute toxicity. Examples are presented in Table 5.1 together with suggested treatment. As a general principle, these are all self-limiting effects, which resolve spontaneously after treatment, their pathogenesis being related to temporary loss of cell division at an epithelial surface.

LATE EFFECTS

These effects are potentially the most serious effects of treatment since, unlike the acute effects, they are

Table 5.1 Acute effects after radical radiotherapy

Site	Effect	Treatment
Skin	Erythema leading, if severe, to desquamation	Minimal; avoid irritants, trauma Aqueous or weak hydrocortisone cream
Bowel	Diarrhoea/colic	Low residue diet Codeine or loperamide
Bladder	Frequency/dysuria	Exclude infection
Scalp	Hair loss	Order wig in advance; hair will re-grow after palliative but not radical doses
Mouth/pharynx	Mucositis	Avoid irritants and alcohol; treat candidiasis; topical chlorhexidine or benzydamine

Radiation protection

Table 5.2 Late effects after radical radiotherapy

Site	Effect	Treatment
Skin	Fibrosis; telangiectasia; rarely necrosis	Usually none
Bowel	Stricture; perforation; bleeding fistulae	If severe, resection of affected segment
Bladder	Fibrosis causing frequency; haematuria; fistulae	If severe, surgical resection
CNS	Myelitis causing paraplegia; cerebral necrosis	None
Lung	Fibrosis	None

Table 5.3 Examples of second malignancies after therapeutic radiation exposure

Disease	What irradiated	Effect radiotherapy	Action as a result
Hodgkin disease	Chest (breast tissue)	Increase risk of breast cancer	1. Breast cancer screening in such patients 2. Reduced use of radiation and more use of chemo
Seminoma	Para aortic nodes	Increase risk of bowel cancer	1. Reduced use of radiation and more use of chemo 2. Low threshold for bowel screening

not self-limiting and indeed tend to be progressive and irreversible. They arise owing to the loss of stem cell recovery potential and progressive damage to small blood vessels resulting in their occlusion (endarteritis obliterans).

Fortunately, in practice they are rare but any radical treatment dose will carry a risk of late damage. Patients are consented to these risks similar to a patient being consented to the risks of surgery or chemotherapy. These side effects are not usually seen before 6 months after treatment but there is an ongoing risk, which is never entirely lost. Examples of late effects are provided in Table 5.2.

Finally, the risk of inducing second malignancy should be considered. In practice, this is exceedingly rare and invariably outweighed by the risk from the established malignancy for which radiation is given. A clear pattern is recognized with leukaemia and lymphoma seen in the first few years after exposure, reaching a peak incidence around 3 years and not seen after 10 years. In contrast, solid tumours have an increasing risk with time, are rarely seen before 10 years and may occur 30 years or more after exposure.

The greatest risk may be associated with low-dose exposure and there are many historical examples of treatment of benign diseases such as tinea capitis, goitre and ankylosing spondylitis. After therapeutic radiation the risk is small but there is some evidence that this may increase in patients who receive combined modality treatment with the addition of chemotherapy (Table 5.3).

RADIATION PROTECTION

Indiscriminate use of radiation is dangerous. There are strict regulations regarding its use for medical purposes to ensure that exposure to staff, visitors and patients is kept to an absolute minimum. This is achieved by physical separation and protection from the sources of radiation and subsequent monitoring of exposure in those at particular risk.

SEPARATION AND PROTECTION

Radiotherapy machines are localized in one area or even in a separate hospital. Their design incorporates shielding of scattered radiation to produce a defined beam, the penetration and qualities of which are carefully measured and maintained. They are housed within a room designed to contain the radiation, using lead barriers within the walls for low-energy beams and thick high-density concrete walls for high-energy beams (the linear accelerator is housed in such a building often called the radiotherapy bunker).

Similarly, radioisotopes are stored under carefully controlled conditions in a radiation-safe environment and administered to the patient in a designated area, again designed to contain any radiation exposure. Patients having implants or high doses of radioiodine will be isolated in single rooms that have additional shielding to prevent radiation reaching other areas of the ward. Staff are given strict time limits to be spent with the patient. Visitors are usually not permitted while there are high levels of radioactivity present. Patients given certain radioactive treatments will be given clear instructions on what they can and cannot do and for what period of time these restrictions apply, e.g. after the treatment of thyroid cancer with I131.

RADIATION MONITORING

All staff involved in the direct care of patients receiving radiation treatment will be designated as workers who require regular monitoring for radiation exposure. The mainstay of monitoring is the film badge worn by these staff, which, when processed, would detect those who may have been inadvertently exposed to radiation. There are clearly defined exposure limits for adults within which all personnel must remain. All departments must have local rules regarding the handling and use of radiation sources and staff must be fully acquainted with these.

It is important to keep the dangers of radiation as used under controlled medical conditions in context, while not relaxing the rules governing its use. There is no evidence that hospital workers are at greater risk than the general population of malignant disease. The entire population is exposed to levels of background radiation and many other common daily activities carry a greater risk than low-level exposure. For example, it has been estimated that all of the following activities carry a one in a million risk of death:

- Driving for 65 miles
- Flying in civil aircraft for 400 miles
- Smoking less than one cigarette
- Drinking half a bottle of wine

FURTHER READING

Hoskin P (ed.). *Radiotherapy in Practice: External Beam Therapy*. 3rd ed. Oxford University Press, Oxford, 2019.

Hoskin P, Coyle C (eds.). *Radiotherapy in Practice: Brachytherapy*. 2nd ed. Oxford University Press, Oxford, 2011.

Joiner M, van der Kogel A. *Basic Clinical Radiobiology*. 5th ed. Arnold, London, 2019.

SELF-ASSESSMENT QUESTIONS

1. Which of the following best describes radiotherapy?
   a. It uses non-ionizing radiation
   b. It is a useful systemic treatment for cancer
   c. It can use beams of ionizing particles
   d. Toxicity is usually limited to acute effects during treatment
   e. It is suitable for tumours at any site

2. Which of the following applies to megavoltage x-ray machines?
   a. They are useful for diagnostic x-ray production
   b. They are usually portable
   c. They can be used to produce neutrons for superficial radiotherapy
   d. A linear accelerator can produce both electrons and photons to treat patients
   e. They are commonly used for brachytherapy

3. Which three of the following are important in modifying the response of radiotherapy in the cell?
   a. White cell count during irradiation
   b. Oxygen levels during irradiation
   c. RNA repair after irradiation
   d. Cell repopulation after irradiation
   e. Phase of cell cycle during irradiation
   f. Water content of the cell during irradiation
   g. Interstitial pressure during irradiation

4. Which of the following statements is correct regarding radiation dose?
   a. Total dose alone will indicate the biological effect
   b. The same dose given over a longer time is more effective
   c. A dose is most effective given in multiple small doses (fractions)
   d. Large doses per fraction are more effective than smaller fractions
   e. The overall time is more important than the dose per fraction

Self-assessment questions

5. When the clinical use of radiotherapy is considered, which of the following is correct?
    a. Palliative treatments will require high total doses
    b. Radical treatments are best given in large daily fractions
    c. A typical radical dose would be 30 Gy in 10 daily fractions
    d. Single doses are the best palliative treatment for painful bone metastases
    e. Radical doses work best when delivered slowly over a long time

6. Which three of the following are recognized acute effects of radiotherapy?
    a. Constipation
    b. Peripheral neuropathy
    c. Skin erythema
    d. Cataract
    e. Dysphagia
    f. Dysuria
    g. Lymphoedema

7. Which three of the following are recognized late effects of radiotherapy?
    a. Peripheral neuropathy
    b. Skin fibrosis
    c. Cataract
    d. Constipation
    e. Dysuria
    f. Lymphoedema
    g. Fatigue

8. With regard to radiation protection, which of the following is correct?
    a. There is no significant risk from doses used in clinical practice
    b. High-energy beams are shielded behind lead screens
    c. Patients receiving radioisotope therapy can be visited regularly
    d. Hospital workers have higher rates of exposure than the public
    e. The entire population is exposed to radiation

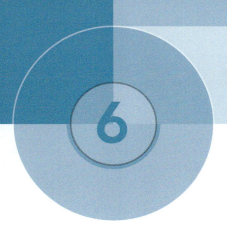

Principles of systemic treatment

Cancer chemotherapy is the treatment of malignant disease with drugs rather than radiation or surgical removal. The drugs used are often highly toxic since they are rarely totally selective for cancer cells. They should therefore be given within an oncology unit by those experienced in their use.

Systemic therapy can be used alone or, more commonly, in combination with surgery or radiotherapy as an adjuvant to enhance local control and to attack potential sites of metastases.

CHEMOTHERAPY AGENTS

Cancer chemotherapy agents act upon cell division, interfering with normal cell replication. They can be broadly classified as follows:

- Drugs acting on the structure of DNA
  - Antimetabolites
  - Alkylating agents
  - Intercalating agents
  - Topoisomerase inhibitors
- Drugs acting on mitosis
- Signal transduction inhibitors
- Drugs inducing apoptosis
- Drugs targeting tumour vasculature
  - Antiangiogenesis
  - Vascular disrupting agents (VDAs)

DRUGS ACTING ON THE STRUCTURE OF DNA

ANTIMETABOLITES

These drugs function at the level of DNA synthesis, interfering with the incorporation of nucleic acid bases (cytosine, thymine, adenine and guanine). They can be classified into two groups:

- Drugs based on chemical modification of a nucleic acid so that the drug rather than the true nucleic acid is incorporated into the DNA, thereby preventing accurate replication of the complementary base sequence. 5-Fluorouracil (5FU) is the classic example now available as an oral prodrug capecitabine. Others include gemcitabine, cytosine arabinoside and fludarabine. These drugs may also have additional modes of inhibiting DNA synthesis, e.g. the inhibition of thymidine synthetase by 5FU and of ribonucleotide reductase by gemcitabine.
- Drugs which inhibit the reduction of folic acid (essential for the transfer of methyl groups in DNA synthesis) from its inactive dihydrofolate form to the active tetrahydrofolate, e.g. methotrexate.

ALKYLATING AGENTS

These agents directly interfere with the DNA double strand of base pairs by chemically reacting with the structure, forming methyl cross-bridges. They then prevent the two DNA strands coming apart in mitosis to form daughter DNA fragments, and division therefore fails. Drugs in this group include cyclophosphamide, chlorambucil, melphalan, mitomycin C and the nitrosoureas BCNU (bischloroethyl nitrosoureas) and CCNU (1-(2-chloroethyl)-3-cyclohexyl-1-nitrosourea).

INTERCALATING AGENTS

They act in a similar way as the alkylating agents but, rather than directly forming cross-strands in the DNA molecule, they bind between the base pair molecules, i.e. bind adenine to thymine and cytosine to guanine. This again prevents the DNA double strand from dividing in order to replicate, thus preventing cell division. Platinum compounds (cisplatin, oxaliplatin and carboplatin) act by binding specifically to guanosine, forming DNA adducts that cross-link either within one DNA strand or across strands. Other compounds, active through DNA intercalation, are the anthracycline group of drugs (Adriamycin, epirubicin and idarubicin).

Bleomycin is not a true intercalating agent but does partially intercalate with DNA and produces direct DNA damage through forming a complex with iron, resulting in the production of reactive toxic products.

TOPOISOMERASES INHIBITORS

Topoisomerases are enzymes that control the tertiary coiling of DNA molecules. Two main classes are recognized: topoisomerase I and II. The camptothecin group of drugs including topotecan and irinotecan are topoisomerase I inhibitors, and the podophyllotoxins, etoposide and teniposide, are topoisomerase II inhibitors.

DRUGS ACTING ON MITOSIS

Mitosis requires spindle formation essential in the sorting and moving of chromosomes following replication at the end of mitosis. Spindle formation is affected through two mechanisms:

- *Spindle poisons*: The vinca alkaloids (vincristine, vinblastine and vindesine).
- Tubulin polymerization resulting in abnormal spindle formation, thereby leading to cell death. The taxane group of drugs (paclitaxel and docetaxel) are cytotoxic through this mechanism.

Microtubule formation is also affected by podophyllin, so etoposide and teniposide both inhibit spindle formation in addition to their effects through topoisomerase.

SIGNAL TRANSDUCTION INHIBITORS

Communication within and between cells is mediated by extensive biochemical interactions triggered by cell surface receptors. Tyrosine kinases are frequent components of these cascades, particularly those related to the epidermal growth control receptor (EGFR) and angiogenesis (VEGF [vascular endothelial growth factor] and PDGF [platelet-derived growth factor]). Drugs which act primarily through the inhibition of tyrosine kinases include imatinib, gefitinib, sorafenib and sunitinib.

DRUGS INDUCING APOPTOSIS

Proteosome inhibitors enhance apoptosis in a population of tumour cells. Proteosomes are large protein complexes within the cell, which regulate the degradation and removal of proteins. The inhibitors of proteosomes have been shown to enhance apoptosis by disrupting the ordered degradation of proteins controlling the cell cycle. The most successful agent in this group is bortezomib which is used in multiple myeloma.

DRUGS TARGETING TUMOUR VASCULATURE

New blood vessel formation is an essential prerequisite for a tumour to become established and remain viable. VEGF is an important component in this process. Tumour blood vessels differ from normal vasculature forming a random chaotic network with little structure and variable flow controlled primarily by fluctuations in interstitial pressure. Both the formation of blood vessels (angiogenesis) through VEGF and the new blood vessels themselves are therefore potential targets to inhibit tumour growth.

Antiangiogenic drugs include bevacizumab, which is a monoclonal antibody to the VEGF receptor, and sorafenib, which inhibits signalling from the VEGF receptor through tyrosine kinase inhibition. Thalidomide and lenalidomide, both used in multiple myeloma, also have antiangiogenic activity, although their main mode of action may relate to the inhibition of IL-6 and immunomodulatory effects.

The VDAs target the structure of the blood vessels and prevent their proliferation. This approach has had limited success to date and drugs such as combretastatin-4 phosphate and its analogues remain experimental.

CHEMOTHERAPY AND THE CELL CYCLE

Because of their mode of action, certain drugs require cells to be in specific phases of the cell cycle to have any effect. For example, those acting on the synthesis of DNA will act only on cells actively synthesizing at the time they are exposed to the drug. Cytotoxic drugs are therefore further classified into:

- *Phase-specific drugs*: These drugs act only in a specific phase of the cell cycle, e.g. antimetabolites during S phase and vinca alkaloids in M phase.
- *Cycle-specific drugs*: These drugs act on cells that are only dividing and passing through the cell cycle rather than being in the resting G0 phase. These include the alkylating agents and intercalating agents.

EFFICACY AND TOXICITY OF CHEMOTHERAPY

Although in principle all cycling cells should be sensitive to drugs that act on the cell cycle, in practice, chemotherapy for most cancers is only modestly effective. This is for a variety of reasons related to drug delivery to the cell and activation or deactivation within the target cells. Precise indications for the use of chemotherapy are detailed in the following chapters but in general the common malignant diseases can be broadly classified into three groups:

- Those extremely sensitive to chemotherapy where this is the treatment of choice
- Those with modest sensitivity where chemotherapy may play a part in their management but usually in combination with other treatment as an adjuvant or for recurrent disease
- Those where chemotherapy is only of limited value in the palliation of advanced disease

Examples of this classification are illustrated in Table 6.1.

Table 6.1 Classification of common malignant diseases according to their sensitivity to chemotherapy

Group 1: High sensitivity	Group 2: Modest sensitivity	Group 3: Low sensitivity
Leukaemias	Breast	Prostate
Lymphomas	Colorectal	Kidney
Germ cell tumours	Bladder	Primary brain tumours
Small cell lung cancer	Ovary	Adult sarcomas
Myeloma	Cervix	Melanoma
Neuroblastoma		
Wilms' tumour		
Embryonal rhabdomyosarcoma		

RESPONSE AND SURVIVAL

In describing the efficacy of chemotherapeutic agents, there are internationally accepted response criteria, the RECIST (Response Evaluation Criteria in Solid Tumours) criteria (see Chapter 3, Section 'Clinical evidence and clinical trials'), defined as follows:

- *Complete response (CR)*: Complete resolution of all clinically detectable disease
- *Partial response (PR)*: A reduction in the longest diameter of a tumour by at least 30%

- *Stable disease (SD)*: Small changes with a response less than a PR or a progression less than a 20% increase in measurable disease during the period of observation
- *Progressive disease (PD)*: An increase in measurable disease of at least 20% during the period of observation, or the development of any new lesions

It is important to interpret with care response data derived from clinical trials. Unless an agent or drug combination achieves a CR in a significant proportion of patients, it is unlikely to have any impact on overall survival when used to treat that disease in the general population. PRs may be of value in delaying progression of a disease, but as they represent only a very small decrement in total cancer cell burden, significant effects on overall survival are unlikely. An exception to this principle may be applied to immunotherapy where stabilization and slow disease regression is seen in responders.

With this in mind, performance status and quality of life measures are important measures of the efficacy of cancer treatment. Numerous scales of performance status have been devised, usually based on a 4- or 5-point scale ranging from normal to moribund. Common examples are the Karnofsky and the WHO performance scale illustrated in Table 6.2.

Quality of life measures are more complex; they should be completed by the patient and will involve a structured questionnaire often divided into domains, evaluating different aspects of the patient activities, e.g. physical activity, pain and specific symptoms, emotional response, social interaction and financial impact. The most widely used quality of life questionnaires are the EORTC QLQ-C30 and the FACT (Functional Assessment of Cancer Therapy).

Table 6.2 Scales for performance status

Score	Status
Karnofsky	
100	Normal; no complaints; no evidence of disease
90	Able to carry on normal activities; minor signs or symptoms
80	Normal activity with effort, some signs or symptoms of disease
70	Cares for self; unable to carry on normal activity or do active work
60	Requires occasional assistance but able to care for most needs
50	Requires considerable assistance and frequent medical care
40	Disabled; requires special care and assistance
30	Severely disabled; hospitalization indicated although death not imminent
20	Very sick; hospitalization necessary; active supportive treatment necessary
10	Moribund; fatal processes progressing rapidly
0	Dead
WHO	
0	All normal activity without restriction
1	Restricted in physically strenuous activity but ambulatory and able to do light work
2	Ambulatory and capable of all self-care but unable to carry out any work. Up and about >50% of waking hours
3	Capable of only limited self-care, confined to bed or chair >50% of waking hours
4	Completely disabled. Cannot carry on any self-care. Totally confined to bed or chair

CLINICAL USE OF CHEMOTHERAPY

Cytotoxic drugs can be given as single agents but are more usually given as multiple drug combinations. The major limitation in using these agents is toxicity to normal tissues. Because the majority are non-specific in their action, both malignant and normal cells are damaged when exposed to a cytotoxic drug. When the drugs are used within their defined dose limits, the normal cells will recover, and it is the need for this window of recovery that results in the typical intermittent scheduling of these agents, most being given at 3–4 weekly intervals.

Common limiting toxicities are bone marrow suppression, bowel toxicity and renal and neurological damage. The major limiting factors for specific drugs are illustrated in Table 6.3.

Table 6.3 Major toxicities for chemotherapeutic agents

Tissue affected	Toxic agents
Bone marrow[a]	All drugs, in particular vinblastine, etoposide, carboplatin, cyclophosphamide, melphalan, ifosfamide, paclitaxel
Bowel	Melphalan, cisplatin, 5FU, irinotecan, methotrexate
Renal	Methotrexate, cisplatin, ifosfamide
Neurological	Cisplatin, vincristine, ifosfamide, paclitaxel
Cardiac	Adriamycin, 5FU
Bladder	Cyclophosphamide

[a] In practice, bone marrow toxicity is becoming less important as a limiting toxicity as techniques for bone marrow support, such as autologous marrow or peripheral stem cell transplantation, become available.

COMBINATION CHEMOTHERAPY

For most malignancies, combinations of drugs are more effective than single agents. These are designed by adding together modestly active agents to give greater overall activity and choosing agents with different dose-limiting toxicities so that the antitumour effect but not the toxic effect is additive or synergistic. Combinations also aim to incorporate drugs from different classes thereby attacking cells with both phase- and cycle-specific agents with the intent of targeting as many cells in the population as possible. An example of spreading limiting toxicities is presented in Table 6.4 with R-CHOP used for non-Hodgkin lymphoma.

Combination therapy can also involve the use of a non-chemotherapy agent with a cytotoxic drug to enhance its activity. The most common example of this in clinical use is the addition of folinic acid to 5FU, which approximately doubles its response rates in the treatment of colorectal cancer. This works because the administered folinic acid increases the intracellular concentrations of folate, which is an essential cofactor in the incorporation of 5FU into RNA and also its action in inhibiting thymidylate synthetase, an important enzyme in DNA synthesis.

DRUG RESISTANCE

The resistance to chemotherapy drugs can be an intrinsic property of a malignant cell but can also be acquired after exposure to individual drugs. Mechanisms of resistance include:

- Altered biochemical pathways to avoid specific pathway blocks, e.g. modified folate is used to avoid dihydrofolate reductase block with methotrexate
- Altered cell transport mechanisms to prevent drug concentration in cancer cell by either reduced uptake or enhanced efflux
- Altered drug metabolism to increase clearance or reduce drug activation and
- Impaired mechanisms of apoptosis (programmed cell death)

It is often found that resistance to a number of drugs develops together, a phenomenon called 'multidrug resistance' (MDR). This is thought to result from common molecular mechanisms related to specific DNA sequences. The identification of one particular genetic change in drug resistance has led to the isolation of *MDR1* gene and the protein for which it codes, a transmembrane glycoprotein important in cell transport. As mechanisms of resistance are

Table 6.4 Drugs in R-CHOP

Drug	Action	Main toxicity
Rituximab	Complement activation	Allergy, anaphylaxis
Cyclophosphamide	Alkylating agent	Bone marrow, bladder
Adriamycin	Intercalating	Bone marrow, cardiac
Vincristine	Spindle poison	Neurological (peripheral neuropathy)
Prednisolone	Unknown	Fluid retention and weight gain, gastric irritation, hyperglycaemia

Principles of systemic treatment

elucidated, strategies to overcome them are emerging. For example, transmembrane transport can be modified by drugs such as verapamil and cyclosporin by inhibiting the efflux of drugs away from the cell.

ADMINISTRATION OF CHEMOTHERAPY

Chemotherapy should be administered only in specialized units with the experience and support to do so safely. Most of the agents used can be harmful if there is continuous contact with the skin and even more so if accidentally ingested through contamination of hands and work surfaces. Agents should therefore be prepared by a specialized chemotherapy pharmacist under strictly controlled conditions, and gloves should be worn by the clinical staff when they are administering these drugs.

Prior to the administration of drugs, all patients should have a full blood count measured. In varying circumstances and with different drugs the criteria for safe administration will vary but a general guide is that chemotherapy should only be given if the following parameters are met:

- *Haemoglobin >10 g/dL*: Although this is rarely a limiting factor, it is acceptable to proceed at lower levels and transfuse if necessary
- Total white count $>3.0 \times 10^9/L$ and total neutrophil count $>1.0–1.5$
- Platelets $>50–80 \times 10^9/L$

For certain drugs renal function must also be carefully checked prior to the administration of drugs. It is not usually sufficient to rely on serum urea or creatinine, and a measure of creatinine clearance should be performed. This applies in particular to the following:

- Cisplatin
- Carboplatin
- Ifosfamide
- Methotrexate (high dose)

Because of the close relationship between serum levels and creatinine clearance, the dose of carboplatin is usually defined by a formula (the *Calvert formula*), which relates the predicted area under the serum concentration versus time curve (AUC) to the clearance. This enables the drug to be given relatively safely, even where renal function is impaired, with a predictable AUC after administration.

Chemotherapy drugs can be given orally, by intravenous or intramuscular bolus injection or by intravenous infusion. Examples of these are presented in Table 6.5.

Many chemotherapy drugs are severe irritants when injected outside a vein and extreme care must be taken during intravenous injections. This should be performed ideally by experienced staff working in a dedicated chemotherapy administration unit. Large visible veins should be chosen as far as possible and it is safe to administer drugs into a running intravenous drip.

Table 6.5 Routes of administration

Oral	IV injection	Infusion	Intrathecal
Chlorambucil	Cyclophosphamide	Cisplatin	Methotrexate
Busulphan	Methotrexate	Carboplatin	Cytosine arabinoside
Melphalan (l.d.)	5FU	Mitozantrone	
Procarbazine	Adriamycin	Ifosfamide	
Etoposide	Vincristine	Methotrexate (h.d.)	
Capecitabine	Vinblastine	Melphalan (h.d.)	
Temozolamide	Vinorelbine	Paclitaxel	
		Gemcitabine	
		Oxaliplatin	
		5FU	

Key: l.d., low dose; h.d., high dose.

Administration of chemotherapy

Where venous access is difficult an indwelling central venous catheter has many advantages. For example:

- For schedules requiring lengthy infusions
- When continuous infusion pumps are to be used
- In procedures likely to require the administration of many intravenous drugs
- In transfusions such as bone marrow transplantation or high-dose chemotherapy

A common type is the Hickman catheter as shown in Figure 6.1. It can be inserted under radiological control with local anaesthetic and remain *in situ* for many months. Regular flushing with heparinized saline at least weekly is required, and some doctors also recommend continuous low-dose warfarin 1 mg daily while the line remains to prevent thrombotic complications. More sophisticated devices place a reservoir under the skin of the chest wall rather than an external line; this enables multiple access with less potential risk of infection, and is more convenient for an active patient.

An alternative type of central line, which may be less robust but simple to insert, is a line such as a PICC line, which is inserted through the antecubital vein and then directed through the brachial and subclavian veins into the vena cava; an example is shown in Figure 6.2.

The major complication from central lines in chemotherapy patients is infection, and infected lines or subcutaneous tracts require immediate removal of the catheter together with high-dose antibiotic cover.

Subclavian vein thrombosis may also occur, particularly around the infected line.

If extravasation of chemotherapy does occur then there should be clear guidelines for its management. Table 6.6 details the drugs for which this is an important issue.

The following principles apply:

- The chemotherapy injection or infusion must be stopped immediately.
- The cannula is left *in situ*, residual drug is aspirated and the area flushed with saline.
- Ice packs may be applied and some recommend administration of local steroids or hyaluronidase, except for vincristine and oxaliplatin, when gentle warming of the area is recommended.

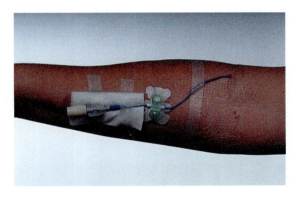

Figure 6.2 A PICC line *in situ* entering an antecubital vein.

(a)

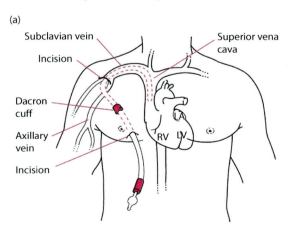

(b)

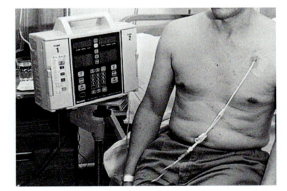

Figure 6.1 Central Hickman line shown (a) diagrammatically and (b) *in situ* in a patient.

Principles of systemic treatment

Table 6.6 Vesicant properties of common cytotoxic drugs

Vesicants	Exfoliants	Irritants	Inflammatory agents	Neutral
Causing pain, inflammation and blistering, leading to tissue death and necrosis	*Causing inflammation and shedding of skin*	*Causing inflammation and irritation*	*Causing mild to moderate inflammation and flare in local tissues*	*Causing no inflammation or damage*
Carmustine	Cisplatin	Carboplatin	Fluorouracil	Aspariginase
Dacarbazine	Docetaxel	Etoposide	Methotrexate	Bleomycin
Dactinomycin	Mitozantrone	Irinotecan		Cyclophosphamide
Daunorubicin	Oxaliplatin			Cytarabine
Doxorubicin	Topotecan			Fludarabine
Epirubicin				Gemcitabine
Idarubicin				Ifosfamide
Mitomycin				Melphalan
Mustine				
Paclitaxel				
Vinblastine				
Vincristine				
Vindesine				
Vinorelbine				

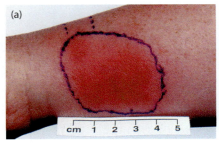 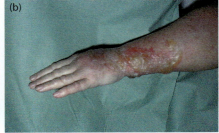

Figure 6.3 (a) Erythema following minor extravasation of epirubicin and (b) more severe soft-tissue damage following extravasation of chemotherapy given intravenously at the back of the hand.

In severe cases with irritant drugs such as Adriamycin or epirubicin, there may be extensive soft-tissue damage as shown in Figure 6.3, particularly if the problem is not identified immediately and action taken. Liaison with a plastic surgery unit for such eventualities is of great value. Occasionally damage may be such as to require surgical repair.

AVOIDING SIDE EFFECTS

As a general rule side effects are best anticipated and prevented. Chemotherapy agents vary in their emetic potential but all may cause nausea and some severe vomiting. Anti-emetics should therefore be considered for all but the most gentle of agents. A three-stage anti-emetic policy based on emetic potential will work for most patients.

EMETIC POTENTIAL OF COMMON CHEMOTHERAPY AGENTS

Chlorambucil and vincristine/vinblastine, used as single agents, rarely cause significant nausea and either anti-emetics are not required or simple oral agents are sufficient. Other drugs or combinations fall into the groups illustrated in Table 6.7.

Table 6.7 Classification of chemotherapy drugs according to their potential to provoke emesis

Low (<10%)	Moderate (10%–30%)	High (31%–90%)	Very high (>90%)
Vincristine	Cyclophosphamide	Adriamycin	Cisplatin
Vinblastine	Methotrexate	Epirubicin	Dacarbazine
Bleomycin	Mitomycin	Ifosfamide	Carmustine
Fludarabine	Mitozantrone	Carboplatin	Mustine
Rituximab	Etoposide	Oxaliplatin	Cyclophosphamide (>1.5 g/m^2)
Bevacizumab	5FU	Irinotecan	
	Paclitaxel		
	Gemcitabine		
	Cetuximab		
	Transtuzumab		

The use of specific anti-emetic drugs varies but a simple anti-emetic protocol is as follows:

- Low potential schedules
  - Metoclopramide 10 mg orally or prochlorperazine 25 mg rectally preceding chemotherapy
- Moderately emetogenic schedules
  - Dexamethasone 8 mg and metoclopramide 10 mg intravenously preceding chemotherapy followed by dexamethasone 2 mg three times daily orally for 2–3 days with metoclopramide 10 mg three times daily orally
- Highly emetogenic schedules
  - Dexamethasone 8 mg and ondansetron 8 mg orally or intravenously preceding chemotherapy followed by dexamethasone 4 mg twice daily and ondansetron 8 mg twice daily orally for 2–3 days

Anticipatory nausea and vomiting may be a particular problem for some patients. This occurs when they experience symptoms with any visit to the hospital, often on arrival, without exposure to the drugs. Lorazepam may be helpful in these instances. It is also often easier for inpatients to receive chemotherapy in the evening when they can receive added sedation and sleep through the administration.

Other side effects must also be anticipated and steps taken to prevent them; for example:

- Diarrhoea (e.g. from cisplatin, 5FU or irinotecan) – prescribe loperamide or codeine phosphate
- Mucositis (e.g. from 5FU, methotrexate) – use regular chlorhexidine and benzydamine mouthwashes
- Alopecia (e.g. from Adriamycin) – use of scalp cooling and provision of wig

SCHEDULING

Chemotherapy schedules vary from simple single oral drugs to complex multiple drug regimens. The design of drug schedules is based on a consideration of the effects on both normal tissues and tumour cells as discussed previously.

Normal tissues are inevitably damaged by chemotherapy agents. Particularly sensitive are the dividing cells of the bone marrow and mucosal epithelial cells lining the oropharynx, gut and bladder. The general principle of scheduling chemotherapy is that each successive course should be given only when damage from the previous drug exposure has been repaired. Fortunately, both bone marrow and epithelial lining cells have a large capacity for tolerating and recovering from damage and usually do so within 2–3 weeks. On this basis, most chemotherapy is given at 3–4 weekly intervals.

Damage to tumour cells may depend on both the absolute levels of drug that can be achieved within them and the duration of exposure. In order to achieve the maximum levels possible, a fine line may be drawn between serious side effects and maximizing tumour cell kill. In some circumstances where there is evidence that very high doses of drugs beyond normal tolerance will achieve more, e.g. in acute leukaemia, bone marrow, or usually bone marrow stem cells, can be removed prior to chemotherapy and stored to be used as an autograft once high-dose therapy has been given.

In order to achieve maximum levels for a suitable duration, a knowledge of the pharmacokinetics of the drug is important. Drugs with short half-lives, such as 5FU, may have a greater effect when given by infusion or in divided doses.

The design of chemotherapy drug schedules is often a combination of elegant hypothesis, serendipity and pragmatism. However, when the results of chemotherapy trials are assessed and translated into general oncological practice, careful attention to the drug dosing and scheduling is important. There is some evidence that patients who fail to receive full doses of drugs at the designated minimum intervals have a reduced benefit from the treatment, and this is a strong argument for chemotherapy being managed only in experienced units familiar with the complications and tolerance for each schedule.

HORMONE THERAPY

A small number of tumours are influenced by therapeutic changes in their hormone environment. In practice, hormone therapy is of value for breast and prostate cancer and to a lesser extent for endometrial cancer. The response to breast cancer is based primarily on the influence of oestrogen, and that to prostate cancer is based on the influence of androgens.

Occasional responses with other tumour types have been reported, particularly to the drug tamoxifen, but their basis remains uncertain.

BREAST CANCER

Oestrogen exerts its effect by binding to a receptor within the cell nucleus called the 'oestrogen receptor'. This process is thought to be fundamental to the way in which oestrogen can influence the development of breast cancer. Drugs that alter the balance of activity at the oestrogen receptor are therefore often of value in the treatment of breast cancer. Such drugs may act directly by binding to the receptor, thereby blocking its activity as typified by tamoxifen, or indirectly on the production and peripheral activation of oestriol and oestrone to oestradiol by inhibiting the enzyme aromatase; commonly used aromatase inhibitor drugs include anastrozole and letrozole.

The presence of oestrogen receptors can be demonstrated histologically using immunohistochemistry and the demonstration of oestrogen receptors (ER) in an individual tumour is important in predicting the likelihood of response to hormonal treatment. Overall, around 50% of patients with breast cancer respond to hormone therapy, but this figure reflects a response rate of up to 80% when oestrogen receptors are positive compared with around 10% where they are negative.

The observation that some patients who have no demonstrable receptors respond may be explained by the presence of receptors in these cancer cells that have a slightly different structure not detected by the routine methods of assay.

Characteristically, hormone responses have a finite duration and it would seem that all breast cancers eventually become resistant to the first hormone treatment to which they are exposed. This may, however, be followed by second, third and even fourth successive responses to further hormone manipulations.

The basis for hormone resistance development is thought to be the changes in the characteristics of the oestrogen receptor, varying from complete loss of receptor to alterations in its binding sites or in its transcriptional properties within the nucleus. In other cases access to the receptor may be denied because of alterations of transport mechanisms and metabolism within the cell. The exposure to an alternative hormone therapy may in many cases achieve a second response, which is observed in up to 45% of patients after an initial exposure.

Progestogens and androgens can also be effective as second- and third-line treatments in breast cancer. Drugs such as megestrol and medroxyprogesterone do indirectly affect activity at the oestrogen receptor causing downregulation (i.e. making them less sensitive to stimulation by oestrogen), but in addition specific progestogen receptors have been identified in breast cancers and found to correlate with response to treatment.

Hormone therapy

Table 6.8 Hormone therapy in breast cancer

Drug	Mode of action	Other actions and common side effects
Tamoxifen	Anti-oestrogen	Hot flushes, fluid retention, vaginal dryness/discharge, uterine bleeding, deep-vein thrombosis
Faslodex		
Exemestane	Aromatase inhibitor	Hot flushes, nausea, rashes, joint stiffness, vaginal dryness, raised cholesterol, osteoporosis
Anastrozole		
Letrozole		
Medroxyprogesterone	Progestogen	Nausea, fluid retention, weight gain
Megestrol		

An overview of hormone therapy in breast cancer is presented in Table 6.8.

PROSTATE CANCER

The basis of hormone therapy in prostate cancer is the dependence on androgen for its growth. The drugs used to treat prostate cancer therefore are anti-androgens working either directly by antagonism at the androgen receptor or by impairing intracellular androgen synthesis and utilization, or androgen deprivation agents working on the hypothalamic–pituitary axis regulation of androgen release. Similar effects are also achieved by surgical orchidectomy removing the main site of androgen production. An overview of androgen blockade is shown in Figure 6.4. The relative clinical merits of the available anti-androgen therapies are illustrated in Table 10.1.

None of the individual anti-androgen treatments offer complete blockade of both testicular and adrenal androgens. This may be achieved by combining a centrally acting gonadotrophin-releasing hormone agonist/antagonist, e.g. goserelin, with a peripherally acting drug such as cyproterone or bicalutamide, and this is known as 'maximal androgen blockade – MAB'. This may be slightly more effective than single drug therapy in advanced disease, particularly in younger patients, but it is associated with more severe toxicity from androgen withdrawal, including lethargy, hot flushes, gynaecomastia and loss of sexual interest and function.

An important distinction between the hormone response of prostate cancer and that of breast cancer is seen on relapse to first-line anti-androgen therapy; second responses with prostate cancer are seen only occasionally.

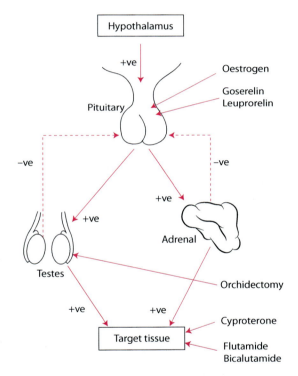

Figure 6.4 Mechanisms of androgen release and blockade.

ENDOMETRIAL CANCER

Endometrial cancer is recognized as a tumour related to high levels of circulating oestrogen. Both oestrogen and progesterone receptors can be demonstrated in the cells of endometrial cancer and treatment with progestogens or gonadotrophin-releasing hormone agonist/antagonists such as goserelin or leuprorelin can be effective in metastatic disease. Response is predicted by the presence of oestrogen or progestogen receptors with around 65% of patients having positive receptors responding to treatment. A reduction in oestrogen receptor concentration has been seen after progestogen treatment, suggesting that the efficacy of hormone treatment in endometrial cancer reflects the inhibition of oestrogenic stimulus at the tumour cell.

BIOLOGICAL THERAPY

A number of the chemicals produced by the body in response to injury or infection have been explored as potential new treatments to eradicate cancer cells. Unfortunately, only limited success has so far been achieved. Invariably such preparations are immunogenic and are therefore associated with side effects such as malaise and low-grade fever. These are often debilitating but major toxicities are rare with commercially available compounds.

MONOCLONAL ANTIBODY TREATMENTS

Monoclonal antibodies (MABs) are the equivalent of the magic bullet, their principle being to carry a toxic agent to a cell defined by specific surface antigens against which the antibody is targeted. In recent years, this approach has resulted in a number of new clinical agents becoming available.

Rituximab is targeted against the CD20 antigen on B-cell lymphomas; when added to standard chemotherapy it improves survival. Ibritumomab is an anti-CD20 antibody tagged with a radioisotope yttrium-90, which is highly effective in follicular lymphoma.

Herceptin is targeted against the HER2 antibody on breast cancer cells, and it is now a valuable additional treatment option for patients with breast cancer which is HER2 positive; this can be demonstrated immunohistochemically and the extent of staining can be graded to predict the likelihood of response, as shown in Figure 6.5.

Alemtuzumab is an anti-CD52 antibody, which is highly active in chronic lymphocytic leukaemia.

Bevacizumab, discussed earlier, is a monoclonal antibody targeting tumour vasculature through VEGF.

Erlotinib and gefitinib target EGFR receptor in lung cancer.

IMMUNOTHERAPY

In recent years, a number of drugs targeting the immune response provoked by tumour antigens have

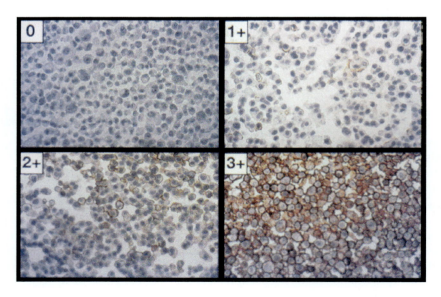

Figure 6.5 Histological section showing breast cancer cells with a range of positive staining for the HER-2 receptor, which may be seen to predict varying degrees of response to the monoclonal antibody transtuzumab (Herceptin®).

been developed. Tumour antigens binding to the cytotoxic T-lymphocyte-associated protein 4 (CTLA-4) and programmed death (PD)-1 binding sites on a CD8 T cell will result in the downregulation of the immune response to the tumour antigen enabling tumour growth. Immunomodulating drugs target PD-1 receptor and its ligands PD-L1 and PD-L2 or the CTLA-4 receptor by blocking this action of tumour antigens and enhancing the immune response.

Current agents include PD-1 antagonists:

- Pembrolizumab
- Nivolumab
- Atezolizumab

and CTLA-4 monoclonal antibody:

- Ipilimumab

Improvements in the outcome of treatment for advanced disease have been observed in melanoma, renal cancer, and lung and bladder cancers.

The use of these agents can result in a range of toxicities specific to their immune effects including pneumonitis, colitis, hepatitis, nephritis and endocrinopathies, in particular, hypophysitis resulting in hypopituitarism. Specific management of these events requires withholding the causative drug and high-dose steroids alongside supportive measures.

Specific contraindications include patients with CNS metastases and potentially latent infections such as HIV and hepatitis B or C.

GROWTH FACTORS

One of the major dose-limiting toxicities encountered in the use of chemotherapy is bone marrow toxicity. In recent years, the availability of colony-stimulating factors (CSF), in particular, granulocyte colony-stimulating factor (G-CSF), has enabled chemotherapy dose to be intensified within the limits of tolerance of bone marrow. G-CSF is an analogue of naturally occurring growth factors given by subcutaneous injection following exposure to chemotherapy. It stimulates the granulocyte production lines in the bone marrow, reducing the period of neutropenia after intensive chemotherapy. The growth factors currently available have no significant effect on platelet and red cell lines. Their use has also facilitated the process of peripheral blood progenitor cell (PBPC) harvesting, thereby simplifying the use of ultra-high-dose chemotherapy which is being increasingly applied to the treatment of solid as well as haemopoietic tumours.

EXPERIMENTAL CHEMOTHERAPY

The chemotherapy drugs and combination regimens widely used in routine oncological practice today have arisen out of carefully designed and regulated drug development programmes. From the discovery of a promising new drug in the laboratory to successful drug marketing and routine clinical use there is a lengthy and expensive period of evaluation starting with animal pharmacology and toxicology studies and leading into clinical trials. The phases of clinical studies within which new drugs are evaluated are outlined as follows and discussed in greater detail in Chapter 3.

- *Phase 1 studies*: These are studies in which a new agent is first tried in patients. Such agents are offered only to patients for whom there is no other recognized effective treatment and who may wish to try other drugs in the slim hope of benefit. In phase 1, the study of activity against the tumour is not an endpoint but these studies are designed to assess the maximum tolerated doses and define the toxicity profile in humans.
- *Phase 2 studies*: These are the earliest studies in which antitumour activity is sought, giving the drug in doses and schedules defined from phase 1 studies to patients who have failed previous conventional therapy or for whom there may be no effective recognized treatment.
- *Phase 3 studies*: With activity in phase 2 established, the new agent is compared with the standard best treatment (or, if there is none, with placebo) in a large prospective randomized trial. A large number of patients are entered into such trials in order to achieve statistically robust results, and most of these studies are therefore multicentre studies.

Only following satisfactory passage through the aforementioned steps is a drug incorporated into the routine treatment of cancer; this may be many years after the first identification of the compound and will be followed by further evaluation of the drug to establish its full potential and application in adjuvant and primary treatment and its role in palliation both alone and in combination. Its toxicity in wider use must also be continuously monitored and notified (*post-marketing surveillance*).

FURTHER READING

Butterfield LH, Kaufman HL, Marincola FM. *Cancer Immunotherapy: Principles and Practice*. Springer, New York, 2017.

ESMO Handbook on Clinical Pharmacology of Anti-Cancer Agents. https://oncologypro.esmo.org/Education-Library/Handbooks/Clinical-Pharmacology-of-Anti-Cancer-Agents 2012

Skeel RT, Khleif S. *Handbook of Cancer Chemotherapy*. Lippincott Williams and Wilkins, Philadelphia, 2011.

Young A, Rowett L, Kerr D (eds.). *Cancer Biotherapy: An Introductory Guide*. Oxford University Press, Oxford, 2006.

SELF-ASSESSMENT QUESTIONS

1. Which three of the following drugs are antimetabolite chemotherapy agents?
   a. Gemcitabine
   b. Topotecan
   c. Cisplatin
   d. Fludarabine
   e. Adriamycin
   f. Cyclophosphamide
   g. Cytosine arabinoside

2. Which of the following applies to intercalating agent in chemotherapy drugs?
   a. They act by alkylation of DNA
   b. They inhibit RNA synthesis
   c. They prevent separation of the DNA strands
   d. They are topoisomerase inhibitors
   e. They include irinotecan

3. Which of the following statements is true regarding chemotherapy agents acting on mitosis?
   a. They interfere with the synthesis of DNA
   b. They affect spindle formation
   c. They are independent of topoisomerase
   d. They include cisplatin
   e. They are independent of the cell cycle

4. Which of the following is true of signal transduction inhibitors?
   a. They act through tyrosine synthase
   b. They can inhibit angiogenesis
   c. They include bortezomib
   d. They are cell cycle dependent
   e. They act on cell division

5. Which three of the following are true of drugs targeting the tumour vasculature?
   a. They reduce blood flow to normal tissues
   b. They can act through VEGF
   c. They include thalidomide
   d. They cause extensive thrombosis
   e. Their effect is reversed by heparin
   f. They can alter blood vessel structure

6. Which three of the following are highly sensitive to chemotherapy?
   a. Breast cancer
   b. Non-Hodgkin lymphoma
   c. Small cell lung cancer
   d. Neuroblastoma
   e. Renal cell carcinoma
   f. Phaeochromocytoma
   g. Glioblastoma

7. For which three of the following drugs is neurological toxicity a major concern?
   a. Cyclophosphamide
   b. Carboplatin
   c. Paclitaxel
   d. Irinotecan
   e. Cisplatin
   f. Ifosphamide

8. For which of the following drugs must the renal function be measured before administration?
   a. Vincristine
   b. Adriamycin
   c. Carboplatin
   d. Etoposide
   e. Epirubicin

Self-assessment questions

9. Which of the following drugs are used for anti-androgen activity?
   a. Fluoxetine
   b. Tamoxifen
   c. Exemestane
   d. Bicalutamide
   e. Cyclophosphamide

10. Which three of the following are the monoclonal antibodies used in cancer treatment?
    a. Rituximab
    b. Bortezomib
    c. Herceptin
    d. Lapatinib
    e. Erythropoietin
    f. Combretastatin
    g. Bevacizumab

11. Immunotherapy targets which of the following?
    a. EGFR
    b. PD-2L
    c. VEGF
    d. P53
    e. PD-L1
    f. IL6

12. Which of the following are recognized toxicities of immunotherapy?
    a. Bone marrow depression
    b. Colitis
    c. Encephalopathy
    d. Neuropathy
    e. Hypopituitarism

Lung cancer and mesothelioma

LUNG CANCER

EPIDEMIOLOGY

Each year in the UK there are 46,000 cases of lung cancer, 24,800 cases in men and 21,600 cases in women, making it the third commonest form of cancer, accounting for 13% of all cancer cases. The incidence in males has fallen by 10% whilst in females it has increased by 18% in the past decade due to changes in smoking habits in recent decades. Most cases present at a late stage, leading to a very low 5-year survival rate (~5%) and nearly 36,000 deaths per annum. It is the commonest cause of cancer death in men accounting for 19,600 cancer deaths and in women 16,300. In line with the incidence, the mortality is declining in men, but increasing in women. Approximately 50% of cases occur in the over 75 age group.

AETIOLOGY

The majority of cases of lung cancer can be attributed to the exposure of the bronchial epithelium to inhaled carcinogens. There is a strong causal relationship between smoking and lung cancer, with 90% of cases attributable to the use of tobacco in males and 80% in females. The bronchial tree and alveoli are directly exposed to the inhaled smoke and it is the hydrocarbon carcinogens such as benzopyrene liberated by the combustion of tar that are responsible, rather than nicotine. These lead to metaplasia of the bronchial epithelium from a columnar pattern to a squamous one, eventually leading to dysplasia and carcinoma. The risk of developing lung cancer is related to the duration and intensity of smoking, increasing with the rise in the number of cigarettes or weight of tobacco smoked per day, increasing tar content, shorter cigarette stubs and use of non-filter brands. The tumours tend to be found adjacent to the larger airways of the lung comprising mainly squamous cell carcinoma and small-cell lung cancer (SCLC). Evidence suggests that passive smoking leads to an increased risk of lung cancer. The lung cancer risk declines towards that of non-smokers after 10–20 years of abstinence, although there is a persistent risk in those who have smoked more than 20 cigarettes per day. Smoking intake can be described in pack years, this is calculated by multiplying the number of packs of cigarettes smoked per day by the number of years the person has smoked (one pack = 20 cigarettes).

Particulate air pollution in cities is now associated with lung cancer, the WHO and others have flagged the problem of emission from diesel engines and many countries are now trying to act to reduce the exposure to such pollutants.

It is important to elicit a history of occupational asbestos exposure in patients with lung cancer as they may be eligible for industrial injuries compensation. The carcinogenic potential of asbestos is synergistic with that of tobacco smoking and, of the many types of asbestos, the blue variant is the most powerful carcinogen. Asbestos-induced cancers are more common in the lower lobes, usually squamous carcinomas, and may be multicentric.

During the nineteenth century, cobalt miners in Eastern Europe were noted to have a very high mortality from lung cancer owing to high levels of radon gas released from the granite-bearing rocks by the radioactive decay of naturally occurring uranium, which in turn had led to high doses of radiation exposure to the bronchial tree and eventual malignant transformation. There is evidence that the level of radon in dwellings may account for a small proportion of deaths from lung cancer each year, particularly in non-smokers. Previous therapeutic radiation exposure, e.g. spinal irradiation for ankylosing spondylitis (no longer practiced) or radiation received for lymphoma has also been shown to increase the risk of developing lung cancer later in life.

Nickel, arsenic and chromates have all been implicated as causes of lung cancer. Tuberculous scars, subpleural blebs/bullae or the site of a previous pulmonary embolus may occasionally account for peripheral carcinomas, particularly adenocarcinoma. Cytogenetic studies have shown loss of a tumour-suppressor gene on part of the short arm of chromosome 3 in some cases of SCLC.

A healthy diet high in fruit and vegetables may reduce the risk of developing lung cancer.

PATHOLOGY

Macroscopically, lung cancers arise within the bronchial epithelium and therefore usually have an endobronchial component. They may be multifocal and may arise anywhere in the bronchial tree, although squamous and small-cell carcinomas often arise centrally in the larger airways, while adenocarcinomas usually arise peripherally, particularly at the apices. Central necrosis leads to cavitation in the larger tumours. Microscopically, lung cancers may be divided into two groups:

- SCLC – 15%
- Non-small-cell lung cancer (NSCLC) – 85%:
  - Squamous cell carcinoma – 35%
  - Adenocarcinoma – 40%
  - Large-cell anaplastic carcinoma – 10%

Squamous cell carcinoma may be preceded by stepwise progression from squamous metaplasia to dysplasia followed by carcinoma *in situ* and frankly invasive cancer. The tumour cells have the morphology of squamous epithelial cells, stain for keratin, and intercellular bridges are visible under the electron microscope, these features being more evident in well-differentiated tumours.

Small-cell carcinoma arises from the Kulchitsky cells of the basal layer of the bronchial epithelium and is characterized histologically by small, uniform cells containing neurosecretory granules, and staining for neuron-specific enolase (NSE), reflecting their origin from cells derived from the neural crest of the foetus. The ectopic production of peptides and hormones will be reflected in their immunocytochemical staining.

Adenocarcinoma cells stain for mucin, reflecting their glandular origin, and may be arranged in an acinar pattern. Large-cell anaplastic carcinoma is poorly differentiated and cannot be recognized under the light microscope as belonging to any of the other subgroups. Clear cell and giant cell tumours are included in this group.

Molecular phenotyping has developed significantly over the last few years and now makes an impact on treatment decision. Tumours are routinely tested for EGFR (~15% of cancers) and EML4-ALK or ROS1 (5% of cancers), and for PDL1 expression. Testing for several more molecular pathways are being researched and may also be useful in guiding potential therapy options.

NATURAL HISTORY

The pattern of growth of a lung cancer is related to the histological subtype. The anaplastic carcinomas are the most rapidly growing tumours, while adenocarcinomas grow more slowly and may have been present over several years prior to diagnosis. SCLC has a propensity to early and widespread metastatic dissemination with 80%–90% having spread beyond the thorax by the time of diagnosis.

Lung cancer spreads circumferentially and longitudinally along the bronchus of origin, eventually leading to bronchial occlusion, which causes lobar or segmental pulmonary collapse owing to the resorption of air distal to the tumour. Stasis of pulmonary secretions in turn leads to secondary infection manifesting as pneumonia and occasionally lung abscess and empyema. Proximally the tumour may extend to the carina and trachea while distally it may reach the visceral pleura from where it may invade the chest wall, interlobar fissures or pleural space, resulting in

Lung cancer

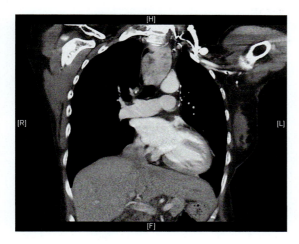

Figure 7.1 Mediastinal lymphadenopathy. Coronal CT image of the thorax. There is a large central mass of lymph nodes.

a blood-stained exudative pleural effusion. A pneumothorax may result from a tumour that breaches the visceral pleura and allows a direct connection between the pleural space and the bronchial tree, i.e. a bronchopleural fistula. Mediastinal structures such as the oesophagus, pericardium, heart and great vessels, and occasionally the vertebral bodies and diaphragm, may be invaded. The tumour frequently involves the regional lymphatics, spreading to ipsilateral peribronchial and hilar nodes, followed by subcarinal, contralateral hilar, paratracheal and supraclavicular nodes (Figure 7.1). Lung cancer has a propensity to disseminate widely via the bloodstream and can virtually involve any site. There is an unusual and unexplained involvement of the adrenal glands in a high proportion of cases. Other common sites include the liver, skeleton, brain (especially SCLC), skin and contralateral lung.

SYMPTOMS

A small proportion of patients will present with no symptoms, having been diagnosed on a chest x-ray either as part of a routine screening or as part of the investigation of another disease. Most, however, present owing to intrathoracic symptoms:

- Cough
- Haemoptysis
- Dyspnoea
- Chest pain
- Recurrent chest infections

Cough occurs due to bronchial irritation by the tumour and is often unproductive unless associated with secondary infection. The cough will have a 'bovine' character if there is also a vocal cord palsy.

Haemoptysis varies in severity from slight streaking of the sputum with blood to frank haemorrhage where there is a large intrabronchial component in the tumour with mucosal ulceration. It is a common presenting symptom. Massive intrapulmonary haemorrhage may occasionally lead to the death of the patient.

Dyspnoea reflects a deficiency in pulmonary ventilation owing to a restrictive defect (e.g. pleural effusion, diffuse parenchymal infiltration), obstructive defect (e.g. bronchial obstruction by tumour or secondary infection) or a combination of the two. It will be first noticed on mild exertion, progressing to dyspnoea at rest. It usually indicates locally advanced disease.

Chest pain may be pleuritic or aching in nature and localized to the involved hemithorax, reflecting pleural involvement by tumour, secondary infection of the pleura or direct invasion of the chest wall.

Recurrent chest infections are a common presenting feature and carcinoma of the lung should be considered in anyone of the appropriate age who has had recurrent chest infections for no apparent cause or an infection that has failed to resolve following one or more courses of the appropriate antibiotic.

Dysphagia may result from extrinsic compression from the primary tumour, particularly if the tumour is arising from the left main bronchus as the oesophagus has a close anatomical relationship with it posteriorly. A large mass of *involved lymph nodes* (usually subcarinal) should also be considered as a cause. A *hoarse voice* suggests invasion of the recurrent laryngeal nerve, giving rise to a vocal cord paralysis, which in turn results in a hoarse voice and 'bovine' cough owing to failure to adduct the vocal cords. Indirect laryngoscopy in the clinic or visualization of the cords at bronchoscopy will be diagnostic.

Tumours arising at the lung apex may cause nerve root pain as they lead to direct invasion of the T1 nerve root, leading to pain radiating down the ipsilateral arm to the medial aspect of the forearm, and

Lung cancer and mesothelioma

may lead to infiltration of the spinal cord itself. Non-specific extrathoracic symptoms include anorexia, weight loss, malaise and lethargy.

SIGNS

No physical signs at all may be elicited, particularly in those presenting without symptoms after a routine chest x-ray. Pulmonary collapse and/or consolidation is the most frequent finding. Examination of the hands may reveal clubbing, characterized by an increase in nail convexity in the transverse and longitudinal planes, loss of the nail fold angle and sponginess of the nail bed on compression of the nail. There may be nicotine staining of the fingers. The supraclavicular lymph nodes should be checked as these are the only palpable nodes that are in continuity with the regional lymphatics. The syndrome of superior vena cava obstruction deserves special mention (see Chapter 21). The involvement of the cervical sympathetic nerves at the level of T1 leads to Horner's syndrome characterized by partial ptosis, miosis (pupillary constriction), enophthalmos (indrawing of the globe of the eye relative to the orbit) and anhydrosis (loss of sweating on the ipsilateral side of the face). The ipsilateral hand may be warmer owing to vasodilation, and there will be wasting of the small muscles of the hand as these are partly innervated by the T1 nerve root.

A small proportion will present with one or more of a variety of clinical syndromes which are unassociated with metastases. These are the so-called non-metastatic manifestations of malignancy (Table 7.1). Other signs will depend on the tumour burden and sites of spread.

DIFFERENTIAL DIAGNOSIS

This includes:

- *Benign tumours*: Papilloma, hamartoma, carcinoid, fibroma, leiomyoma
- *Other malignant primary tumours*: Mesothelioma, bronchial gland carcinomas, soft-tissue sarcomas
- Metastases
- Non-neoplastic diseases, e.g. aspergilloma, chronic lung abscess, Wegener's granulomatosis
- Radiographic artefact, e.g. nipple shadow

Table 7.1 Non-metastatic manifestations of lung cancer

Type	Manifestations
Cutaneous	Dermatomyositis, acanthosis nigricans, erythema gyratum repens, hypertrichosis lanuginosa, clubbing
	Hypertrophic pulmonary osteoarthropathy (HPOA), scleroderma
	Herpes zoster
	Urticaria
Neuromuscular	Myositis
	Proximal myopathy, peripheral neuropathy, mononeuritis multiplex, cortical degeneration Progressive multifocal leucoencephalopathy, transverse myelitis, cerebellar degeneration
	Eaton–Lambert myasthenic syndrome
Ectopic hormone production	Hyponatraemia and water retention (ADH), hyperpigmentation and hypokalaemic alkalosis (ACTH), hypercalcaemia (PTH), carcinoid (5-HT), hypoglycaemia (insulin-like peptides)
	Hyperglycaemia (glucagon, growth hormone), gynaecomastia and testicular atrophy (gonadotrophins, HCG), hypertension (renin)
Haematological	Anaemia (may be sideroblastic), disseminated intravascular coagulation
	Eosinophilia
	Thrombocytosis, thrombocytopenia, leucocytosis/leukaemoid picture, red cell aplasia, Bone marrow plasmacytosis
Miscellaneous	Murantic endocarditis (may lead to systemic emboli), membranous glomerulonephritis, hypouricaemia, hyperamylasaemia
	Migratory thrombophlebitis (Trousseau's syndrome)

INVESTIGATIONS

Patients with suspected lung cancer should have investigations performed as early as possible after presentation with symptoms. Much work has been done to educate patients to report to their general practitioner (GP) if they have symptoms that could indicate a risk of lung cancer. The aim is to reduce the time from the development of symptoms to a diagnosis of lung cancer being made leading to more patients being diagnosed at an earlier stage, and so achieving better outcomes.

CHEST X-RAY

This provides a rapid, non-invasive, widely available means of ascertaining the position, size and number of tumours (Figure 7.2). For optimal assessment, a posteroanterior and lateral view should always be requested. Common features of lung cancer include a discrete opacity, which may be cavitating, hilar lymphadenopathy, pulmonary collapse, consolidation and pleural effusion. Associated intrathoracic complications owing to local invasion can be assessed, special care being taken to look for rib erosion in peripherally placed tumours. The hemidiaphragms should be inspected, looking for excessive elevation – the right is usually slightly higher than the left owing to the underlying liver. An elevated hemidiaphragm suggests palsy of the ipsilateral phrenic nerve, which in turn suggests mediastinal infiltration and therefore an inoperable tumour.

SPUTUM CYTOLOGY/CORE BIOPSY

These are rapid means of obtaining a tissue diagnosis with minimal patient inconvenience and distress. The sensitivity of the cytology testing increases with the number of sputum specimens collected and so at least three specimens are desirable. Samples should represent bronchial secretions rather than saliva and the best time for collection is early in the morning. Prior to collection, 5 mL of nebulized saline and physiotherapy might help a patient who has a non-productive cough. Central tumours are most likely to be detected in this way, particularly those associated with a large endobronchial component, e.g. squamous carcinoma. If possible the cytology sample may be cytospun to create a pellet so that additional molecular tests can be performed. It should be noted that sputum containing squamous carcinoma cells could be related to an underlying primary cancer of the upper respiratory tract, e.g. larynx. Core biopsy has become more important with the need to obtain cores of tissue so that both a histological and molecular diagnosis can be achieved. Transthoracic CT (computed tomography) guided biopsy is now a standard procedure and in many cases is an outpatient procedure.

BRONCHOSCOPY

This should be performed whenever active treatment is indicated. A fibreoptic bronchoscope is passed down the respiratory tract via the nose under topical anaesthesia, although rigid bronchoscopy under general anaesthesia is sometimes performed by the thoracic surgeon. Detailed anatomical information is gained regarding the precise location of the tumour within the bronchial tree, which is of value when

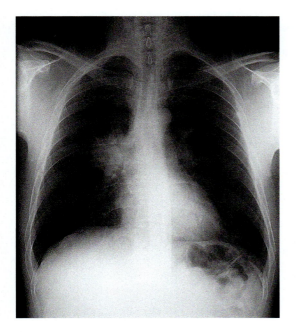

Figure 7.2 Chest radiograph showing a squamous carcinoma arising adjacent to the right hilum. In this example, there is no associated pulmonary collapse, suggesting patency of the bronchi.

Lung cancer and mesothelioma

surgery or radiotherapy is contemplated; vocal cord palsy also may be confirmed on entry into the lower respiratory tract with the scope. Once visualized, the tumour can be biopsied or, if the tumour is located too peripherally for the bronchoscope to reach it, saline can be injected and aspirated, and the 'washings' sent for cytology; a small brush can be used to obtain 'brushings' from the epithelial lining of the bronchi. Bronchoscopy also allows emergency procedures to be performed such as diathermy or laser of a bleeding tumour.

Endobronchial ultrasound-guided node biopsy (EBUS) enables biopsy of nodes in the mediastinum to help confirm the diagnosis and complete the staging of the patient.

COMPUTED TOMOGRAPHY

CT is indicated in all cases. The thorax is scanned to supplement the findings on plain x-rays and bronchoscopy, as the superior soft-tissue contrast of CT more precisely defines the local extent of the tumour (Figure 7.3) and distinguishes tumour from collapsed/consolidated lung tissue. It is the investigation of choice for detecting chest wall invasion, particularly in the case of apical tumours, which may not be well visualized with plain radiographs (Figure 7.4), and for detecting mediastinal lymphadenopathy, both of which individually are contraindications to surgical resection. The brain, liver and adrenals (Figure 7.5) are included to exclude distant metastases as they are frequent sites of soft-tissue spread. CT is also important to facilitate percutaneous needle biopsy, this technique has evolved so it is now frequently possible to perform these biopsies as an outpatient procedure.

MAGNETIC RESONANCE IMAGING

Magnetic resonance imaging (MRI) can be used in staging prior to surgery, providing images that are complementary to those obtained by CT. It is of particular value in providing high-resolution images of soft tissues, which may clarify the extent of local tumour invasion, e.g. when CT has suggested equivocal large blood vessel infiltration. MRI of the brain is important part of staging of lung cancer patients especially if radical treatment is proposed.

ISOTOPE BONE SCAN

This is performed to exclude bone metastases in those who are being considered for curative therapy.

POSITRON EMISSION TOMOGRAPHY

This is now routinely performed to complete the staging of the patient, especially when radical treatment is planned as shown in Figure 7.6. It has the advantage of disclosing the presence of metastatic disease at occult sites in the body (e.g. adrenal glands) and can show foci of active cancer in mediastinal lymph nodes or indeterminate pulmonary nodules, areas where CT can be equivocal or negative.

BIOPSY OF PALPABLE METASTASES

Biopsy of palpable metastatic deposits, such as a supraclavicular lymph node or a cutaneous nodule, is a relatively atraumatic means of obtaining a tissue diagnosis.

MEDIASTINOTOMY AND/OR MEDIASTINOSCOPY

These are invasive surgical investigations to determine whether the tumour is operable by allowing the surgeon to visualize and sample the mediastinal lymph nodes. Such procedures have largely been superseded by the CT scan and PET scan.

THORACOTOMY

This is the most invasive means of obtaining tumour tissue for histopathology, and is reserved for the very small proportion of patients who are not diagnosed after routine investigations. Unless the tumour has been shown to be inoperable during preoperative assessment, the surgeon will aim to proceed to radical resection after frozen section has been performed, particularly for non-small cell lung cancer.

LUNG FUNCTION TESTS

These are performed to assess the patient's ventilatory capacity with regard to the compliance of the lungs

Differential diagnosis

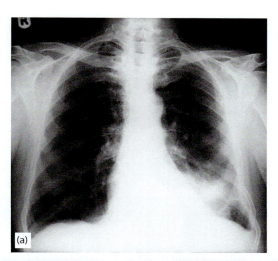
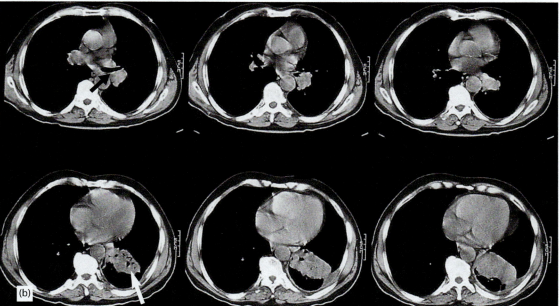

Figure 7.3 Locally advanced lung cancer. (a) Chest radiograph in a patient with a carcinoma causing obstruction of the left lower lobe bronchus leading to collapse and consolidation distally. (b) CT images of the thorax from the same patient demonstrating the primary tumour near the left hilum (top left arrow). The collapse and consolidation can be seen distal to this (bottom left arrow). There is also a left basal pleural effusion. These images demonstrate the greater detail seen with CT compared with plain radiographs.

and degree of airway obstruction, and are required only prior to definitive lung resection as a guide to how disabled the patient would be post-operatively. A simpler guide is the patient's exercise tolerance – inability to climb a flight of stairs without stopping would be considered a contraindication to surgery.

INDIRECT LARYNGOSCOPY

This is indicated if the patient has an unexplained vocal abnormality and entails visualization of the position and mobility of the two vocal cords using a laryngeal mirror in the ENT clinic. Partial or

Lung cancer and mesothelioma

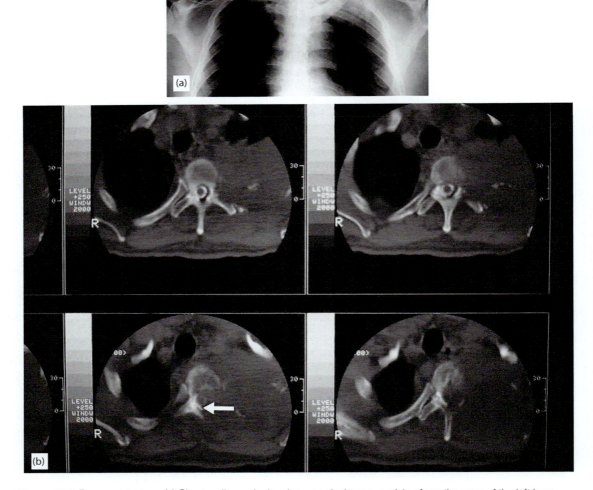

Figure 7.4 Pancoast tumour. (a) Chest radiograph showing an apical tumour arising from the apex of the left lung. Note the soft-tissue swelling in the supraclavicular fossa. There is pulmonary collapse leading to the narrowing of the intercostal spaces and destruction of the underlying posterior ribs. (b) CT images of the corresponding region. Note the enormous soft tissue mass destroying the rib and vertebral body. Such patients are at high risk of spinal cord compression (arrowed).

complete palsy suggests pressure on the recurrent laryngeal nerve.

STAGING

The TNM staging is the most frequently used and can be used as a guide to management and prognosis, this staging system is updated regularly to reflect the views of clinicians so that the staging reflects therapy choices and outcome:

- T: Extent of primary tumour
- Tis: Carcinoma *in situ*
- Tx: Positive cytology

Differential diagnosis

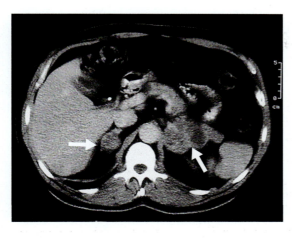

- T1a: The tumour is contained within the lung and is smaller than 2 cm
- T1b: The tumour is contained within the lung and is between 2 and 3 cm
- T2a: 3–5 cm (or tumour with any other T2 descriptors: main bronchus, >2 cm from carina, invades visceral pleura, partial atelectasis – but less than 5 cm)
- T2b: 5–7 cm
- T3: >7 cm or into chest wall, diaphragm, pericardium, mediastinal pleura, main bronchus and, 2 cm from carina, total atelectasis, phrenic nerve, more than 1 nodule in the same lobe

Figure 7.5 Bilateral adrenal metastases. CT image of the upper abdomen.

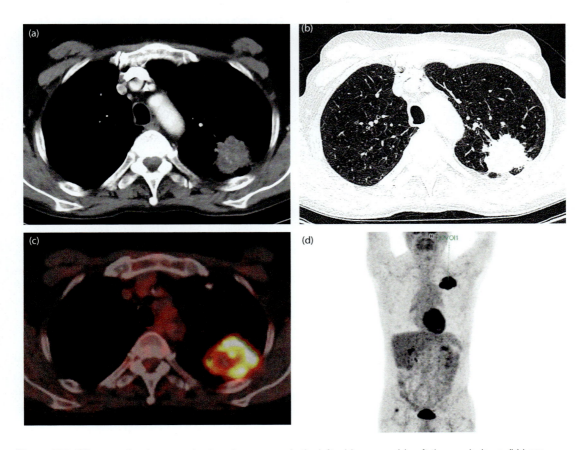

Figure 7.6 CT scans showing an early stage lung cancer in the left mid-zone on (a) soft tissue windows, (b) lung windows and (c) FDG PET. The whole body image of the FDG PET scan is shown in (d) demonstrating the absence of metastases elsewhere.

- T4: Into mediastinum, heart, great vessels, trachea, oesophagus, vertebral body, carina; or tumour nodules in more than one lobe
- N: Regional lymph nodes
- N0: No regional lymph node metastasis
- N1: Ipsilateral peribronchial, ipsilateral hilar lymph nodes
- N2: Ipsilateral mediastinal and/or subcarinal lymph node(s)
- N3: Contralateral mediastinal, contralateral hilar, ipsilateral or scalene, or supraclavicular lymph node(s)
- M: metastases
- MX: Distant metastasis cannot be assessed
- M0: No distant metastasis
- M1: Distant metastasis present

Stage groupings:

- *Occult*: TX, N0, M0
- *Stage 0*: Tis, N0, M0
- *Stage IA*: T1a and b, N0, M0
- *Stage IB*: T2a, N0, M0
- *Stage IIA*: T1a or b – T2a, N1, M0 or T2bN0M0
- *Stage IIB*: T2b, N1, M0 – T3, N0, M0
- *Stage IIIA*: T1 or 2, N2, M0 – T3, N1 or 2, M0 – T4, N0 or1, M0
- *Stage IIIB*: Any T, N3, M0 – T4, N2, M0
- *Stage IV*: Any T – Any N – M1a or b

With SCLC, the TNM classification is used and frequently a two-category staging system is also used, which correlates well with prognosis and serves as a guide to determining the most appropriate therapy in clinical trials:

- *Limited (30%)*: Extent of tumour as defined by physical examination and radiological investigations is confined to the ipsilateral hemithorax and ipsilateral supraclavicular nodes; most 2-year survivors will be in this group
- *Extensive (70%)*: Defined as disease other than limited stage.

MANAGEMENT

The management of lung cancer is based on the stage at diagnosis. A 5-year overall survival rate reduces dramatically as the stage of disease increases.

NSCLC stage	% of patients at diagnosis	5 year OS	Treatment options
1	15%–20%	50%	Surgery/radical radiotherapy including stereotactic/percutaneous thermal ablation
2	5%–10%	25%	Surgery/radical radiotherapy
3	30%–45%	10%–20%	Chemoradiotherapy/primary chemo followed by surgery or RT
4	30%–40%	2%	Palliative therapy, chemotherapy or biological agents Palliative radiotherapy for symptom control

RADICAL TREATMENT OF NSCLC
Surgery

Complete surgical excision is desirable and offers the best chance of cure, although only about 25% of patients will be suitable candidates. Surgery will involve either lobectomy or pneumonectomy depending on the site of the tumour, its size and the patient's respiratory reserve. Both procedures have a significant risk of mortality, but with correct patient selection this is now less than 5%. A more conservative segmental resection could be considered for those with very small tumours or limited respiratory reserve, although the rate of local recurrence is higher than that following lobectomy, especially for larger cancers. Complete mediastinal lymph node dissection seems superior to node sampling when combined with definitive lung resection. Only 25% of those selected for radical resection will be cured because of either occult persistence of local disease or distant metastases at the time of surgery. The survival rate following surgery varies greatly from series to series but is in the range 20%–50% at 5 years, and reflects the selection criteria used by the surgeon to determine which patients undergo surgery and the skill of the surgeon concerned. Table 7.2 outlines the contraindications to surgery.

Radiotherapy

Comparisons of radiotherapy versus surgery have often been confounded by the majority of poor

Table 7.2 Contraindications to radical surgery for lung cancer

Patient parameter	Preoperative investigation
Poor lung function	Routine lung function test
Phrenic nerve palsy	Diaphragmatic screening
Recurrent laryngeal nerve palsy	Indirect laryngoscopy
Invasion of trachea, aorta, heart, superior vena cava, oesophagus	CT/MRI scan of thorax
Distant metastases	Relevant imaging studies and/or biopsies

performance status patients being treated with radiotherapy. This is partly because radiotherapy has the advantage of treating tumours adjacent to or directly involving vital thoracic structures, which cannot be sacrificed at operation.

Radical radiotherapy for lung cancer remains a very important treatment for patients with early stage disease. Changes in radiation technique and fractionation have also made important improvements in outcome.

CHART (continuous, hyperfractionated, accelerated radiotherapy): This regimen was developed to exploit the radiobiological advantages conferred by rapid completion of treatment and avoidance of breaks in radiotherapy at weekends (a good example of translational research, where work in the laboratory in radiobiology led to trials and a change in clinical practice). This entails treatment three times daily, 7 days a week for 2.5 weeks (54 Gy in 36 fractions). In the pivotal randomized trial of CHART, which enrolled over 500 patients with NSCLC, the 2-year survival was 29% for CHART versus 20% for conventional (2 Gy/day) radiotherapy. The acute side effects were similar apart from a rapid onset of severe dysphagia in the CHART group.

Stereotactic ablative radiotherapy (SABR): This is the delivery of very high doses of radiotherapy (ablative) in very few fractions to a small volume. SABR techniques have been developed and are now the radiotherapy treatment of choice for stage 1–2 disease in patients not suitable for surgery. For peripheral tumours radiotherapy is typically given in three fractions, with more central tumours requiring the fractionation to be extended up to eight fractions. SABR results suggest that outcomes are directly comparable to that of surgery.

Standard fractionation radical radiotherapy – This remains important for stage 3 disease and benefit has been shown with the delivery of concurrent chemotherapy (see the section 'Chemotherapy').

Pre-operative and post-operative radiotherapy has not produced any significant prolongation of survival and is not routinely practiced. Indeed, meta-analysis of the randomized trials of post-operative radiotherapy suggest a 7% 2-year survival disadvantage for this approach. Post-operative radiotherapy should be used where the benefit is felt to outweigh the risk, e.g. positive post-operative resection margin.

CASE HISTORY

LUNG CANCER 1

A 65-year-old female smoker with no prior history of pulmonary disease presents to her GP during the winter months with a chest infection manifest as cough productive of purulent sputum and mild shortness of breath on exertion. She received a course of amoxycillin to good effect but remained slightly short of breath, which she attributed to her age. Four weeks later, the cough and sputum return. This return of symptoms in a patient with a smoking history is an indication to refer the patient for further investigation. A chest x-ray is arranged and this reveals collapse and consolidation of the right middle lobe. The referral to the chest physician triggers the appropriate further tests of CT scans and bronchoscopy. Bronchoscopy indicates a polypoid tumour almost completely obstructing the right middle lobe bronchus with some ulceration and bleeding. Biopsies are taken and laser resection used to restore patency to the bronchus and achieve haemostasis. Histology confirms small-cell carcinoma.

Lung cancer and mesothelioma

Staging CT scan of the brain, thorax and abdomen shows bulky right hilar lymphadenopathy and small volume metastases to the liver. Following the scan, she complains of headache and lethargy. Serum biochemistry profile indicates a sodium level of 118 mmol/L. Serum osmolarity is low at 230 mmol/L (normal range 275–295 mmol/L) and urine osmolarity inappropriately low at 300 mmol/L (normal range 400–1000 mmol/L). A diagnosis of inappropriate antidiuretic hormone secretion is made and she is commenced on fluid restriction and demeclocycline to good effect.

She commences systemic chemotherapy with cisplatin and etoposide. After three cycles, CT scan of the thorax shows re-expansion of the right middle lobe and a dramatic reduction in the size of the hilar lymphadenopathy and complete resolution of the liver metastases. After a further three cycles, there is no further measurable disease. The demeclocycline is withdrawn and the fluid restriction successfully relaxed. Her excellent response to induction chemotherapy is therefore consolidated by a course of radiotherapy to the site of the original bronchial tumour and adjacent hilum, given concurrently with a course of prophylactic cranial irradiation (PCI).

She remains well until 8 months later when she experiences further cough and dyspnoea. This is now associated with malaise and lethargy, and her performance status is rapidly deteriorating. CT scans confirm recurrent bronchial obstruction and new liver and adrenal metastases. She declines further chemotherapy. She requires two bronchoscopic laser treatments within a 2-week period. In order to reduce the need for continual bronchoscopies, she is treated with endobronchial brachytherapy as a day-case procedure. This successfully palliates the local symptoms of her disease. She is referred to the community multidisciplinary team affiliated to her local hospice and dies 6 weeks later.

Chemotherapy

Platinum agents are still considered the cornerstone of chemotherapy for NSCLC. Meta-analysis indicates that cisplatin-based chemotherapy leads to small but consistent improvements in overall survival in all patient groups. In early NSCLC, chemotherapy in combination with surgery yields a 13% reduction in the odds of death and 5% absolute survival advantage at 5 years compared with surgery alone. Comparable benefits are seen for the comparison of radiotherapy and chemotherapy versus radiotherapy alone. Adjuvant chemotherapy after surgery may be indicated in patients who are node positive and/or have large tumours.

As with other solid tumours, synchronous chemoradiotherapy (CRT) protocols are in widespread use to maximize locoregional control and to treat occult metastatic disease at distant sites. Meta-analyses of trials of CRT versus radiotherapy alone for locally advanced disease indicate an improvement in local and distant progression-free survival translating into a 7% reduction in the odds of death at 2 years at the expense of short-term increases in oesophagitis and anaemia. Concurrent chemotherapy is considered to be superior to sequential chemoradiotherapy with a meta-analysis showing an absolute overall survival benefit of 4.5% at 5 years.

RADICAL TREATMENT OF SCLC

Surgery

Surgery is not the usual treatment for SCLC, but may have a role as part of multimodality treatment in certain situations.

Radiotherapy

Thoracic radiotherapy is of value in the combined modality treatment of those with limited stage disease (b.d. radiotherapy over 3 weeks). It has also gained wider acceptance in decreasing the risk of intrathoracic recurrence in those who have had induction chemotherapy, and is associated with a 5% absolute 3-year survival advantage.

Of those with controlled local, regional or visceral disease, 60% will sustain an intracerebral relapse within 2 years. This is often the sole site of disease relapse and frequently proves to be a fatal manifestation of their disease. Prophylactic cranial irradiation (PCI) decreases the incidence of cerebral metastases by approximately 50%. Meta-analysis data suggest a 5% absolute 3-year survival advantage for PCI. There is evidence suggesting some neuropsychiatric sequelae from PCI, and the dose and fractionation of PCI is such as to make this risk as low as possible.

Chemotherapy

The propensity for SCLC to disseminate early and its inherent chemosensitivity means that systemic treatment with chemotherapy is the most appropriate initial management for both limited and extensive stages of disease. Median survival for untreated limited SCLC is only 14 weeks, falling to 7 weeks for those with extensive disease. Combination therapy is more efficacious than single-agent chemotherapy. Objective responses in the order of 70%–80% have been reported for a variety of schedules, the active drugs being cisplatin/ carboplatin, cyclophosphamide, ifosfamide, etoposide, vincristine, doxorubicin and irinotecan. Complete responses of 30%–40% can be expected in limited stage disease, and 20%–30% for extensive stage disease. There is no benefit in prolonging chemotherapy beyond 6 months in duration. Chemotherapy improves the median survival significantly to 6–12 months in extensive stage disease and 16–24 months in limited stage disease. In recent years, published data have emerged suggesting a benefit for chemotherapy (e.g. etoposide and cisplatin) given concurrently with thoracic radiotherapy for limited stage disease. Chemotherapy drugs do not cross the blood–brain barrier to a substantial degree, hence the need for PCI in complete responders.

PALLIATIVE TREATMENT

The priority of treatment is to relieve symptoms for the patient's remaining lifespan with as little inconvenience and discomfort as possible. There is published evidence confirming that immediate chemotherapy confers a survival advantage for patients with metastatic disease versus best supportive care.

Radiotherapy

Radiotherapy is employed for local symptoms from both NSCLC and SCLC when chemotherapy is deemed inappropriate, and is very effective at relieving cough, chest pain and haemoptysis with palliation lasting for much of the patient's remaining lifespan. Dyspnoea can be helped if it is due to bronchial obstruction. Treatment can be delivered using external beam radiotherapy or high-dose rate brachytherapy using an endobronchial catheter placed adjacent to the tumour under bronchoscopic guidance. Large single doses of thoracic radiation are as effective as a more prolonged course, e.g. 10 fractions in 2 weeks, in terms of onset, quality and duration of response, at least for patients in poor general condition. Median survival in such cases is only 6 months, with a 1-year survival of 20% falling to 5% at 2 years. Palliative thoracic irradiation can be repeated if symptoms recur, provided care is taken not to exceed the radiation tolerance dose of the spinal cord. Radiotherapy to the brain has a role in patients with limited spread to the brain but may have little benefit in patients with extensive spread and poor performance score. Molecular phenotype is also likely to be important in deciding if radiotherapy to the brain is beneficial.

Chemotherapy

A rather pessimistic aura has pervaded the management of advanced NSCLC for too long. The emergence of new drugs and the resulting combination therapy has led to increased response rates, disease-free survival and overall survival prolongations. Cisplatin/carboplatin remains the standard treatment for NSCLC. In advanced NSCLC, cisplatin-based chemotherapy reduces the risk of death at 1 year by 27% (10% absolute survival advantage, increase in median survival of 6 weeks) compared with best supportive care. Combination chemotherapy yields an approximate doubling in response rates compared with single agents, but is significantly more toxic. In recent years, a number of other agents used alone or in combination with cisplatin have demonstrated activity in NSCLC:

- Vinorelbine
- Gemcitabine
- Paclitaxel/docetaxel
- Pemetrexed

For non-squamous histology (with no EGFR or ALK mutations) cisplatin and pemetrexed is the more active combination, with maintenance pemetrexed in patients who have responded to treatment. Objective responses are often lower than the rate of symptom relief in lung cancer patients.

For SCLC, the drug regimens are similar to those used for primary treatment. It is sound practice to use drug combinations with constituent drugs to which the patient has not previously been exposed.

Lung cancer and mesothelioma

Biological therapies

Tyrosine kinase inhibitors (TKIs) such as gefitinib and erlotinib are orally delivered treatments that inhibit intracellular pathways. Patients with EGFR sensitizing mutations (15% of non-squamous lung cancer) have improved response rates, PRS and QOL (quality of life) when treated with these agents compared to initial chemotherapy. An increasing number of these agents are becoming available, often termed second- or third-generation TKIs. These agents have different activity and side-effect profiles such that when a patient's cancer has stopped responding to one agent it may respond to another – indeed it is recognized that further mutations can arise and should be tested for with new biopsies when possible (e.g. T790M), as if present different TKIs may still be active. There is also significant interest as some agents have been shown to have activity in patients with metastases to the brain, this is exciting as traditionally the brain has been a sanctuary site and many systemic therapies do not penetrate the brain. Crizotinib is active in ALK mutated tumours and further agents in this class of drug are being developed allowing further therapy options.

Immunotherapy is another exciting line of therapy in certain lung cancers. Trials have shown that patients who have significant expression of PDL1 respond to the agent pembrolizumab and do so with better response and survival than to conventional chemotherapy. Research continues to try to understand which patients should be treated with which agent (chemo, TKI, immunotherapy) and in what order – the therapy options in lung cancer are changing very quickly – and for some patients this is altering their survival significantly.

OTHER TREATMENT MODALITIES

Endobronchial laser therapy

This is particularly useful for proximal endobronchial tumours in relieving haemoptysis by permitting direct coagulation of the bleeding tumour and in relieving bronchial obstruction by acting as a cutting diathermy. It is frequently used in patients who have already received a maximal dose of radiation to the thorax.

Endobronchial stent insertion

This can provide instantaneous symptomatic relief when a tumour is occluding one of the main bronchi. By the opening up of an obstructed bronchus, the collapsed lung distally can re-expand.

Vocal cord apposition

Teflon injection into the posterior two-thirds of the vocal cord leads to the approximation of vocal cords. It is indicated for recurrent laryngeal nerve palsy when there is persistent aspiration of food and pharyngeal secretions into the bronchial tree, leading to recurrent chest infections or respiratory distress.

Pleuropericardial aspiration

Drainage of pleural and pericardial effusions will rapidly relieve dyspnoea and sometimes any associated chest pain or dry cough. Talc or bleomycin may be instilled into the pleural cavity to obliterate the pleural space (pleurodesis), thereby preventing further fluid accumulation.

Other medical measures include:

- Antibiotics for chest infections
- Codeine or methadone linctus as a cough suppressant
- Analgesics for chest pain
- Treatment of biochemical abnormalities resulting from non-metastatic manifestations

TUMOUR-RELATED COMPLICATIONS

Complications can be divided into thoracic and extrathoracic. Thoracic complications include:

- Pneumonia
- Pleural effusion
- Lung abscess
- Empyema
- Pneumothorax
- Massive pulmonary or pleural haemorrhage
- Atrial fibrillation
- Pericardial effusion
- Dysphagia
- Broncho-oesophageal fistula
- Sudden death from rupture of one of the great vessels
- Horner's syndrome

Differential diagnosis

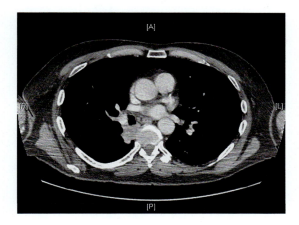

Figure 7.7 Vertebral body erosion from lung cancer. CT image of the thorax. A tumour arising from the right main bronchus has invaded posteriorly causing incipient spinal cord compression.

- Spinal cord compression (Figure 7.4 and 7.7)
- Superior vena cava obstruction

Extrathoracic complications can be inferred from Table 7.1. Ectopic hormone production is most common with SCLC although squamous carcinomas may produce a parathyroid hormone-like peptide leading to hypercalcaemia or a syndrome of inappropriate antidiuretic hormone secretion (SIADH).

TREATMENT-RELATED COMPLICATIONS

RADIOTHERAPY

Radiation oesophagitis is characterized by a feeling of retrosternal discomfort on swallowing food or fluids, particularly if hot or spicy, and beginning 2 weeks after commencing radiotherapy. Sucralfate and local anaesthetic lozenges may be of symptomatic benefit. Symptoms are rarely severe enough to interfere significantly with the patient's nutrition and usually subside within 2 weeks of finishing radiotherapy. Radiation pneumonitis has an acute phase beginning 6 weeks to 3 months after radiotherapy and is characterized by dry cough, fever, dyspnoea and chest pain. Radiologically there is a diffuse opacification of the lung corresponding to the applied radiation fields, which is often more severe than the symptoms would suggest. Mild cases resolve spontaneously but more severe cases will require treatment with a broad spectrum antibiotic together with prednisolone 20–40 mg daily. Some will progress to a chronic phase characterized by increasing pulmonary fibrosis leading to a restrictive defect and some degree of permanent respiratory compromise. The probability of pneumonitis can be minimized by using a small radiation dose per fraction and treating as small a lung volume as possible. As a consequence of the large doses per fraction used for palliative radiotherapy, some patients surviving long enough can be at risk of developing radiation myelitis.

SURGERY

Potential complications include:

- Empyema owing to infection within the pleural space
- Decrease in respiratory reserve owing to resection of lung tissue
- Persistent bronchopleural fistula
- Seeding of the tumour into the thoracotomy scar and subcutaneous tissues; and
- Discomfort related to the scar, which may lead to an unremitting neuralgia

CHEMOTHERAPY

Many drugs used for SCLC cause alopecia. Radiotherapy can increase the toxicity of drugs such as cyclophosphamide leading to pulmonary fibrosis and Adriamycin leading to heart failure.

PROGNOSIS

The prognosis from lung cancer remains poor and, despite advances in surgery, radiotherapy and chemotherapy, it has not changed for several decades. The three main poor prognostic factors include:

- Advanced stage, e.g. large tumour size, extrathoracic disease
- Small-cell histology
- Poor performance status

Patients with disease not amenable to radical therapy have a median survival of 6 months or less. Only about 5% of SCLC patients survive 5 years. The pretreatment prognostic factors that consistently predict for prolonged survival include good performance status, female gender and limited stage disease. Patients with the involvement of the central nervous system or liver at the time of diagnosis have a significantly worse outcome. Median survival with current treatment of limited stage SCLC is 18–24 months, compared with 6–12 months for those with extensive disease.

Overall, 10%–20% of patients with NSCLC survive 5 years. Stage at presentation is the most important prognostic factor in this disease, and molecular phenotype is now providing prognostic information.

Among surviving smokers, there is a significant risk of second primary cancers of 3%–4% per annum, about half of which will be second lung primary cancers.

SCREENING

It is clear that if the screening detects lung cancer at an earlier stage then patients should be suitable for radical treatment options that should lead to better survival. Several studies have suggested that screening individuals at high risk of developing lung cancer can alter their outcome. Trials in the United Kingdom, and Europe (Netherlands and Belgium) have been performed using low-dose CT scans – these suggest a reduction in lung cancer mortality compared with CXR screening of higher risk patients. Further data are awaited from these trials and it may be that combining lung cancer screening with assessment for cardiovascular disease (similar risk factors) will prove to be cost effective.

PREVENTION

Lung cancer is predominantly caused by smoking tobacco, implicated in 90% of cases. Better health education, legislation to reduce cigarette advertising and punitive taxes on tobacco may decrease consumption and in turn reduce the incidence significantly. Avoidance of passive smoking in the social and work environment is of benefit, with legislation altering the behaviours of society (no smoking in public buildings, or cars with children in). Public health medicine stopping smoking programmes are making an impact on patient's ability to stop smoking. The use of e-cigarettes as an alternative to actual cigarettes remains controversial and further research into their safety is ongoing.

Ventilation of dwellings in regions where radon gas levels are high and avoidance of industrial carcinogens can also contribute to a reduction in lung cancer incidence, particularly for non-smokers. Reducing particulate air pollution in our cities could also have a small impact. There is currently no evidence to support recommending vitamins such as α-tocopherol, β-carotene or retinol, alone or in combination, to prevent lung cancer.

RARE TUMOURS

CARCINOID

Bronchial carcinoids are the most common benign tumours arising in the major bronchi. They are more common in the right lung and usually metabolically inactive but can produce carcinoid syndrome without liver metastases. They occasionally are the site of ectopic ACTH production.

THYMOMA

This arises from the adult remnants of the thymus rather than the lung parenchyma; 90% are found in the anterior mediastinum. They are often detected incidentally when the thorax is surveyed by imaging, such as CT, for another purpose. There is a mixture of lymphocytic and epithelial components. Atypical cells or frank malignant change in the latter alters the diagnosis to thymic carcinoma. Thymomas are often slow-growing tumours with invasion and expansion at the site of origin. Thymomas are associated with paraneoplastic autoimmune syndromes such as myasthenia gravis (50%), polymyositis, lupus erythematosus, rheumatoid arthritis, thyroiditis, Sjögren syndrome and autoimmune pure red cell aplasia. Thymic carcinoma is potentially more aggressive with a tendency to metastasize. Both are best treated by surgical thymectomy. Post-thymectomy radiotherapy is reserved for individuals with more advanced stages of thymic carcinoma. There is an increased risk of second malignancies.

Mesothelioma

CASE HISTORY

LUNG CANCER 2

A 44-year-old male smoker presents with two episodes of haemoptysis. A chest x-ray shows a 2 cm rounded density adjacent to the right hilum. Bronchoscopy indicates a localized mucosal roughening 4 cm distal to the origin of the right main bronchus, which is biopsied and found to be squamous cell carcinoma. CT scan of the brain, thorax and abdomen shows no evidence of distant metastases and a bone scan is clear. A PET scan is also normal apart from a focus of hyper-metabolism corresponding to the primary lung tumour. Lung function tests show normal levels of FVC and FEV1. He is referred to a thoracic surgeon. A lobectomy is performed. Pathology indicates a 2.5 cm squamous cell carcinoma. The margins of excision are clear.

Two years later, he presents with a 2-week history of nausea, increasing confusion and polyuria. The corrected serum calcium is measured at 3.85 mmol/L. After a dose of zoledronic acid to correct the calcium, his condition improves. A CT scan confirms metastatic disease in the left adrenal gland and liver. There are no bone metastases on an isotope bone scan suggesting a retrospective diagnosis of inappropriate parathyroid hormone secretion. Rather than electing to be treated with best supportive care, the patient elects to be treated actively. After an EDTA clearance scan to determine the glomerular filtration rate, he receives six cycles of gemcitabine in combination with carboplatin. Prospective imaging confirms disease stabilization. After stopping chemotherapy, he remains on 4-weekly infusions of zoledronic acid; 3 months after stopping chemotherapy, a surveillance CT scan confirms significant hepatic disease progression and bilateral adrenal metastases. He feels very weak to a degree out of context with his disease activity and this precludes further active treatment. A random cortisol analysis suggests a very low value. A diagnosis of adrenal insufficiency is made. He is started on hydrocortisone replacement therapy and regains his strength with a corresponding improvement in performance status. He is then started on second-line chemotherapy with single agent vinorelbine. He responds to this by RECIST criteria but develops cerebral metastatic disease. He derives some benefit from whole brain radiotherapy but profound somnolence precludes further active treatment. He is referred to the community palliative care team and dies of progressive disease 3 years after diagnosis.

MESOTHELIOMA

EPIDEMIOLOGY

Each year in the United Kingdom, there are 2700 cases of mesothelioma accounting for 0.8% of all cancer cases and leading to a total of 2500 deaths per annum. They can arise at any age but are most common in the 50–70-year age group. There is a male predominance (5:1) reflecting occupational exposure to asbestos, e.g. in miners, builders, naval dockyard workers. Only three-quarters of patients actually give a history of asbestos exposure. Case clustering has been described around asbestos mines (e.g. central Turkey, Cyprus, Greece) and in those who used to live near asbestos processing factories in the United Kingdom.

AETIOLOGY

Mesothelioma is not caused by smoking. It is now recognized that asbestos exposure is the main risk factor for both pleural and peritoneal mesothelioma. Blue asbestos (crocidolite) is more carcinogenic than white and brown types, and this is due to the size and shape of the asbestos fibres. Not only asbestos workers, but their spouses are also at risk as the fibres are carried home on their clothing. There is a long latent period (often 30–40 years) between asbestos exposure and development of mesothelioma, and cancer risk depends on duration and intensity of fibre exposure. Most patients have no evidence of asbestosis. About half will give a history of occupational exposure to asbestos. Patients with a possible occupational history of asbestos exposure should be identified as they may be eligible for industrial injuries compensation. Such patients should have a post-mortem examination.

PATHOLOGY

Mesothelioma arises from mesothelial cells of the pleura, much less commonly from the peritoneum, and rarely from the pericardium or tunica vaginalis around the testicle. Pleural tumours are slightly more common on the right side, probably owing to the greater surface area of pleura at risk. Evidence of pulmonary asbestosis is more common in those with peritoneal mesothelioma, who often have a history of heavy asbestos exposure. Macroscopically, there are multiple, small, pale tumour nodules diffusely involving visceral and parietal layers of the pleura, particularly at the cardiophrenic angle medially. These nodules coalesce to form plaques, which encase the underlying lung and infiltrate into the fissures and intralobular septae. Eventually, the pleural space is obliterated. There may be an associated pleural effusion, usually rich in protein and blood-stained.

Microscopically, the tumours contain varying proportions of epithelial and spindle cell elements (resembling adenocarcinoma and sarcoma, respectively). Three subtypes are described: epithelioid (60%), sarcomatoid (15%) and mixed biphasic epithelial/sarcomatous (25%). Asbestos bodies might be found in the underlying lung, and asbestos fibres identified in the tumour by electron microscopy. The commonest mesothelial markers are calretinin, cytokeratin 5/6, WT1 and podoplanin.

NATURAL HISTORY

Mesothelioma relentlessly invades adjacent thoracic structures such as the underlying lung, overlying chest wall, pericardium and contralateral hemithorax. The tumour eventually invades through the diaphragm to involve the peritoneum and abdominal viscera. It also has a propensity to invade the chest wall and skin at the site of a previous thoracocentesis owing to direct implantation of tumour cells. Sarcomatous tumours have a more rapidly progressive natural history compared with epithelial types. Lymphatic spread is uncommon. Symptomatic distant metastases are also uncommon, even during the terminal phase of the disease, but are of a greater problem for those with sarcomatous histology and very few, highly selected patients treated by radical surgery.

SYMPTOMS

Ninety percent of patients with pleural mesothelioma present with increasing dyspnoea on exertion and/or chest discomfort on the affected side: 70% will have symptoms of less than 6 months in duration at presentation. Dry cough and systemic symptoms, such as anorexia, weight loss and fever, may occur. Haemoptysis is very uncommon, in contrast to lung cancer.

SIGNS

Finger clubbing and signs of chronic respiratory compromise can occur if there has been prior asbestosis. There is usually reduced expansion, dullness to percussion and reduced breath sounds over the affected region of the chest. This can be difficult to distinguish from a pleural effusion.

DIFFERENTIAL DIAGNOSIS

Asbestos can also cause a primary lung cancer, which may present with similar symptoms and signs. Other cancers, particularly adenocarcinomas, occasionally demonstrate a pleural pattern of spread and are difficult to distinguish on pleural fluid cytology alone or on analysis of small fragments of pleura.

INVESTIGATIONS

CHEST X-RAY

This usually shows a lobulated pleural mass with loss of volume of the affected hemithorax and there can be an associated pleural effusion (Figure 7.8). The changes are more common in the lower zones and may be bilateral. An underlying asbestosis may be seen. The chest x-ray is best taken after the drainage of an effusion, which may obscure the subtle signs of pleural thickening.

PLEURAL FLUID CYTOLOGY

This can be performed in the outpatient clinic by inserting a hypodermic needle into an intercostal space under local anaesthetic. The fluid is often heavily blood-stained and high in protein. A high (>50 ng/L) level of hyaluronic acid is common. Cytological examination may reveal malignant mesothelial cells, although the sensitivity is not high (approximately 40%).

Mesothelioma

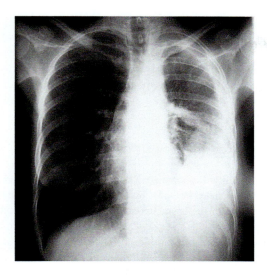

Figure 7.8 Mesothelioma. Chest radiograph showing encasement of the left lung. There is an associated pleural effusion.

PLEURAL BIOPSY

This is more invasive than obtaining fluid for cytology. It does, however, give a more reliable tissue diagnosis. A needle technique can usually be performed under local anaesthetic. Ultrasound or CT can be used to obtain better localization of pleural plaque for sampling. In difficult cases, an open biopsy at thoracoscopy or thoracotomy is necessary. Surgical biopsy has the advantage of yielding a larger specimen for histological analysis, drainage of pleural fluid and even simultaneous talc pleurodesis.

ULTRASOUND OF THORAX

This is a useful investigation for localizing the best place to perform a percutaneous pleural biopsy or aspiration of a loculated pleural effusion.

CT SCAN OF THORAX AND ABDOMEN

This is much better than plain radiographs for demonstrating pleural plaques (Figure 7.7) and assessing the degree of local invasion. It can be useful for localizing a suitable site for needle biopsy. It is also useful in excluding gross involvement of the peritoneum.

STAGING

There is no formal staging system in widespread clinical use. The modified Butchart staging classification shown here is an example:

- *Stage I*:
  - 1a: Tumour limited to ipsilateral parietal pleura
  - 1b: As 1a but with focal visceral pleural involvement
- *Stage II*: As stage 1a or 1b plus confluent involvement of diaphragm, visceral pleura or lung
- *Stage III*: Locally advanced tumour with nodal involvement
- *Stage IV*: Locally advanced unresectable or contralateral nodes or distant metastatic disease (Figure 7.8)

TREATMENT

Comparative studies show a survival advantage for active treatment versus observation only. Very few patients are suitable for radical surgical resection. Pleuropneumonectomy (excision of lung, pleura, hemidiaphragm and ipsilateral half of pericardium) followed by high-dose hemithoracic radiotherapy in selected patients has shown promising results but is yet to be tested in a randomized trial. Mortality (20%–30%) and morbidity is high. The less radical procedure of pleurectomy (mortality 2%) may palliate selected patients with severe, recurrent pleural effusions. Patients can derive much symptomatic relief

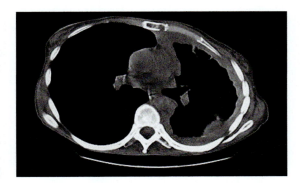

Figure 7.9 Mesothelioma. CT image of the patient in Figure 7.8 after the drainage of the pleural effusion. Note the confluent plaque of tumour surrounding the lung.

from simple drainage of a pleural effusion (Figure 7.9). Radiotherapy is of value in palliating chest pain. Treatment is usually given to the involved hemithorax. Two-thirds of patients will respond symptomatically, although it is difficult to demonstrate any objective tumour response to the moderate doses used. Cisplatin is an active drug in this disease and is usually combined with pemetrexed. Research continues with other agents including immunotherapy agents.

TUMOUR-RELATED COMPLICATIONS

Many patients succumb to respiratory failure from uncontrolled local disease. Pericardial constriction can occur owing to extrinsic tumour pressure, and malignant pericarditis can cause atrial fibrillation. Direct invasion of the myocardium can also compromise cardiac function. Mediastinal compression can lead to dysphagia and superior vena cava obstruction. Seeding of tumour cells along the path of an intercostal needle is common and can lead to subcutaneous and skin nodules. Peritoneal involvement can lead to intestinal obstruction and ascites. Non-metastatic manifestations include hypercoagulability of the blood, autoimmune haemolytic anaemia, phlebitis, hypoglycaemia and the syndrome of inappropriate ADH secretion leading to hyponatraemia.

TREATMENT-RELATED COMPLICATIONS

Pleuropneumonectomy has a mortality of approximately 20%. Treatment of the whole hemithorax with radiotherapy can lead to oesophagitis, nausea owing to irradiation of the stomach and/or liver and pneumonitis owing to the irradiation of large volume of lung.

PROGNOSIS

The disease runs a variable natural history, and therefore prognosis is unpredictable. In retrospective series of pleural mesothelioma patients, important prognostic factors have been found and are age, performance status and histology. Epithelial variants have a better prognosis than sarcomatoid ones. For patients treated with aggressive surgical approaches, factors associated with improved long-term survival include: epithelial histology, negative lymph nodes and negative surgical margins. Prognosis is usually very poor with a mean survival of 9 months, only 30% surviving to 1 year, falling to <5% at 2 years.

SCREENING/PREVENTION

The dangers of asbestos exposure are now appreciated. Asbestos is used much more sparingly in industry. Care must still be taken when older buildings are renovated, with careful isolation of the working area and use of respirators. High-risk individuals should be offered regular chest radiographs.

FURTHER READING

Bibby AC, Tsim S, Kanellakis N, Ball H, Talbot DC, Blyth KG, Maskell NA, Psallidas I. Malignant pleural mesothelioma: An update on investigation, diagnosis and treatment. *Eur Respir Rev*. 2016; 25: 472–486.

Kim J, Bhagwandin S, Labow DM. Malignant peritoneal mesothelioma: A review. *Ann Transl Med*. 2017 Jun; 5(11): 236.

Maconachie R. Lung cancer: Diagnosis and management: Summary of updated NICE guidance. *BMJ*. 2019; 364: l1049

Roth JA, Hong WK, Komaki RU. *Lung Cancer*. 4th edn. Wiley, New Jersey, 2014.

SELF-ASSESSMENT QUESTIONS

1. Which three of the following statements are true about the epidemiology of lung cancer?
   a. It is one of the commonest cancers in the UK
   b. It is far less common in women
   c. Might be caused by asbestos exposure
   d. Might be caused by alcohol consumption
   e. Not proven to be caused by smoking tobacco
   f. Associated with a high fat diet
   g. Might be caused by environmental radiation exposure

Self-assessment questions

2. Which one of the following statements is true about the pathology of lung cancer?
   a. Most are small-cell cancers
   b. Adenocarcinomas tend to be fast growing
   c. Small-cell carcinoma rarely spreads outside the lung
   d. Many patients present with symptoms caused by brain metastases
   e. Adrenal metastases are characteristic

3. Which three of the following statements are true about the presentation of lung cancer?
   a. Usually diagnosed on a routine chest x-ray in asymptomatic individuals
   b. Usually presents with symptoms of metastatic disease
   c. Palpable lymph nodes are usually present at diagnosis
   d. Cough is a common symptom
   e. Might present with recurrent chest infections
   f. Haemoptysis is rare
   g. Dyspnoea implies locally advanced disease

4. Which one of the following statements is true about the staging of lung cancer?
   a. Staging is only undertaken in those being considered for surgery
   b. Pulmonary angiography should be performed in all cases
   c. Bone marrow trephines are routinely performed
   d. PET imaging is of value in those being considered for curative surgery
   e. CT imaging is performed in selected cases

5. Which three of the following statements are true about the treatment of lung cancer?
   a. Adriamycin is the most active chemotherapy agent
   b. An attempt at curative surgery will be undertaken in the minority
   c. Small-cell lung cancer is best treated with chemotherapy
   d. Radiotherapy is more effective for small-cell carcinoma than non-small-cell carcinoma
   e. Women have a higher response rate to chemotherapy than men
   f. Trastuzumab is an active agent
   g. Cranial radiotherapy is useful for early stages of small-cell lung cancer

6. Which one of the following statements is true about the prognosis of lung cancer?
   a. 10%–20% will be cured
   b. Non-small cell lung cancer cannot be cured by radiotherapy
   c. Small-cell histology is a poor prognostic factor
   d. The median survival of untreated small-cell lung cancer is 12 months
   e. Adenocarcinomas with an EGFR mutation have a particularly poor prognosis

7. Which three of the following statements are true about mesothelioma?
   a. There is an association with asbestos exposure
   b. Most cases are not caused by smoking
   c. Presents with haemoptysis
   d. Most patients will be considered for surgery
   e. Chemotherapy is most important first-line treatment at diagnosis
   f. Distant metastases are uncommon
   g. Prophylactic cranial radiotherapy may be considered

Breast cancer

EPIDEMIOLOGY

Each year in the United Kingdom there are 55,000 new cases of breast cancer (16% of all cancer cases), and 12,000 deaths per annum. It is the most common malignancy in females, on an average approximately one in seven middle-aged women have a risk of developing the disease at some point during their lifetime. Left-sided cancers are slightly more common compared to right-sided ones (relative risk 1.05). The age of incidence increases throughout life and the risk prevails into the 80s. Only 0.5%–1% of cases occur in men. It is a disease most commonly occurring in the Western world and being much less prevalent in the Far East, particularly Japan. There is an increased rate of incidence in higher socioeconomic groups.

AETIOLOGY

The majority of cases are sporadic, and only 5% cases are due to a known genetic mutation. Hormonal influences are well recognized; breast cancer is more common in women with an early menarche or a late menopause. The use of combined oral contraceptive pill for around 10 years is associated with an relative risk of around 1.25 after its cessation. Hormone replacement therapy (HRT) is also associated with an increased risk of breast cancer (14 in 1000 women aged 50–64 not taking HRT develop breast cancer over 5 years, compared to 15.5 in 1000 taking oestrogen-only HRT for 5 years and 20 in 1000 for those taking combined [oestrogen/progestogen] HRT for 5 years).

An artificial menopause (surgical oophorectomy or radiation ovarian ablation) before the age of 35 years, increasing parity, young age (<30 years) at first pregnancy and breastfeeding are protective factors reducing the risk of developing breast cancer. Obesity is associated with an increased risk of breast cancer, with weight >82 kg associated with a relative risk of 3 compared with those weighing <59 kg. Regular strenuous exercise is protective by itself. The relative risk for women consuming four alcoholic drinks per day compared with non-drinkers is 1.3; it increases according to the amount of alcohol consumed.

Japanese women have a low risk of developing breast cancer. Japanese migrants in the United States eventually acquire the risk faced by the indigenous population, suggesting that there is an unknown environmental cofactor involved.

Exposure to radiation increases the risk. The increased incidence is being observed in the survivors of atomic bombs, in women treated with radiotherapy for postpartum mastitis, or ankylosing spondylitis, and in women who underwent regular chest fluoroscopies to monitor the progress of iatrogenic pneumothorax as treatment for tuberculosis. The carcinogenic effect of radiation on the breast varies inversely with age at the time of exposure and is dependent on the radiation dose. The increased risk of breast cancer in patients receiving radiotherapy to the chest for Hodgkin disease has led to specific screening in this population and to the reduced use of radiotherapy in favour of chemotherapy in the treatment of Hodgkin disease.

Common benign lumps such as fibroadenomata do not progress to carcinoma, but atypical ductal hyperplasia confers an increased risk of breast cancer and such patients should be kept under regular surveillance. Both ductal carcinoma *in situ* (DCIS) and lobular carcinoma *in situ* (LCIS) are precursors to invasive malignancy (see sections 'Ductal carcinoma *in situ*' and 'Lobular carcinoma *in situ*'), and therefore their presence in a breast biopsy is a significant risk factor.

Only 5% of cases are due to inheritable genetic abnormalities (e.g. *BRCA* gene mutations). The relative risk (RR) of breast cancer has significantly increased when first-degree relatives have previously been affected:

- One first-degree relative (RR 2)
- First-degree relative diagnosed at <40 years (RR 3)
- Two first-degree relatives (RR 4)
- Bilateral breast cancer (RR 4)

The inheritance of mutated *BRCA* genes confers an 80%–90% lifetime risk of breast cancer. The chance of a woman without a history of breast/ovarian cancer carrying such a mutation is 1 in 500 (0.2%); it rises to 1 in 50 (2%) if she has a history of breast cancer and 1 in 11 (9%) if this was diagnosed at <40 years of age.

The *BRCA1* gene mutation is located on chromosome 17 (17q12–21). *BRCA1* carriers are more likely to develop the uncommon 'medullary' histological subtype of breast cancer and exhibit less *in situ* disease. Many *BRCA1* tumours are derived from the basal epithelial layer of cells of the normal mammary gland, which characteristically exhibit high-grade features, areas of necrosis, are typically oestrogen receptor-negative, HER2-negative and stain positive for cytokeratins 5/6, 14 or 17, which are the markers of basal epithelium. *BRCA1* mutation carriers also have an increased risk of developing early onset carcinoma of the ovary and fallopian tube.

The *BRCA2* gene mutation is located on chromosome 13. *BRCA2* gene mutations also lead to an increased risk of pancreatic cancer, testicular cancer and early-onset prostate cancer.

Two specific *BRCA1* mutations (185delAG and 5382insC) and a *BRCA2* mutation (6174delT) have been reported to be common in the families of Ashkenazi Jewish descent – and can be tested for in this patient group. Other genetic abnormalities associated with familial breast cancer are as follows:

- *TP53* mutations in Li–Fraumeni families (associated with leukaemia, gliomas, adrenocortical carcinomas and soft-tissue sarcomas)
- *PTEN* mutation in Cowden disease (macrocephaly, mucocutaneous hamartomas, thyroid disease)
- *STK11* in Peutz–Jeghers' syndrome
- Heterozygotes for the ataxia–telangiectasia gene

PATHOLOGY

Macroscopically, most carcinomas arise in the upper outer quadrant of the breast and are usually solitary, although multifocal tumours can occur in the same or opposite breast. The tumour can be well circumscribed or diffusely infiltrating. The cut surface and texture vary depending on the tumour type. For example, a scirrhous tumour has a gritty texture and grey/white cut surface, while a colloid carcinoma has a more gelatinous texture. Conversely, a diffusely infiltrating lobular cancer tumour might be invisible to the naked eye.

Microscopically, breast cancers are classified as 'lobular', arising in the lobules at the termination of the duct system of the breast, or 'ductal' arising from the extralobular ducts themselves. *In situ* carcinoma is diagnosed when all the malignant cells are confined to the lumen of the duct or lobule and do not breach the basement membrane. This contrasts with invasive carcinoma where malignant cells breach the basement membrane. The vast majority are ductal carcinomas but there are a number of variants such as papillary, scirrhous, colloid, medullary and comedo carcinomas. Oestrogen and progesterone receptors are detectable, usually reaching high levels in well-differentiated tumours.

The molecular make up and understanding of breast cancer is advancing. Currently four intrinsic subtypes of invasive disease are described:

Luminal A and luminal B tumours: These are ER-positive tumours and tend to have the better prognosis.

HER2 enriched: Covering tumours that can be ER positive or negative but express the HER2 receptor. These tumours grow and spread faster than luminal tumours. HER2-targeted agents are active and used in the treatment of these cancers.

Basal-like: These are usually ductal carcinomas that are 'triple negative', i.e. oestrogen and progesterone receptor negative and HER2-negative. In younger women, they may suggest an increased probability of an underlying genetic predisposition.

DUCTAL CARCINOMA *IN SITU* (DCIS)

This is more common than lobular carcinoma *in situ*. About 90% cases are asymptomatic and detected by breast screening, and only a small percent present with a lump or nipple discharge or Paget disease of the breast (see the section 'Paget disease of the breast'). Indeed the introduction of breast screening led to an increase in the diagnosis rate. Central necrosis leads to calcium deposition and this calcification can be detected by mammography. Two percent of surgically staged patients have spread to the axilla owing to the areas of unrecognized invasive carcinoma. About 40% will progress to invasive carcinoma after biopsy alone and treatment is aimed at preventing progression to invasive disease.

LOBULAR CARCINOMA *IN SITU* (LCIS)

This could be an incidental finding in a biopsy performed for benign breast disease or associated with an invasive cancer; 70% of cases arise in premenopausal women and it is frequently bilateral. It is usually undetectable clinically and might not be seen on a mammogram owing to the lack of necrosis (and therefore calcification) in the lesion. It is a marker of a higher probability of subsequent invasive cancer. About one-third will develop invasive cancer in the same or contralateral breast within 20 years of diagnosis. The rate of progression to carcinoma after biopsy alone is approximately 1% per annum.

INFLAMMATORY CARCINOMA

This comprises only 2% of all cases of breast cancers. Clinically, there is ill-defined erythema, tenderness, induration and oedema (Figure 8.1). It may be misdiagnosed as a breast abscess. Microscopically, there is invasion of dermal lymphatics by tumour cells. It behaves aggressively with a high rate of local recurrence and distant metastases.

PAGET DISEASE OF THE BREAST

This is a premalignant condition affecting the nipple and areola and arises in older women. Clinically there is erythema, dryness and fissuring of the nipple, sometimes with exudation of fluid, resembling eczema (Figure 8.2). Unlike eczema, it is very rarely bilateral; it is confined to the nipple/areola, less itchy and not associated with vesicle formation. It is microscopically characterized by large, pale Paget cells within the epidermis, which do not invade the dermis. All patients have an associated ductal carcinoma. Half have an associated lump, more than 90% of which are invasive carcinomas. If no lump is palpable, 30% will have an underlying invasive carcinoma and 70% ductal carcinoma *in situ*.

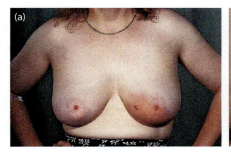 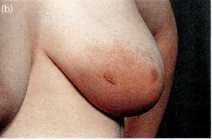

Figure 8.1 (a) Inflammatory breast cancer. (b) Note the small skin biopsy scar. The tissue removed confirmed dermal lymphatic invasion by carcinoma cells. This type of breast cancer can be confused with an infective process, particularly in lactating women.

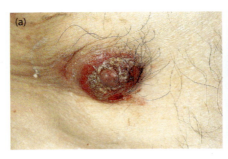
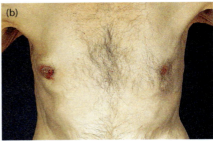

Figure 8.2 (a) Paget's disease of the nipple (male patient). Note the resemblance to eczema. (b) Note the large breast mass in the same patient suggestive of the underlying carcinoma.

BILATERAL BREAST CANCER

This is more common in those with a strong family history of breast cancer and those diagnosed at an early age. Synchronous primaries (i.e. two tumours occurring simultaneously) are rare, occurring in <1% of cases, while a metachronous primary (i.e. diagnosed 6 months or more after the original tumour) has an incidence of 1%–2% per year on follow-up. A second primary tumour is suggested by its being of a different histological type and differentiation to the original tumour with surrounding *in situ* changes.

MALE BREAST CANCER

This cancer is rare. There is an association with inherited *BRCA2* gene mutations. The tumours are morphologically the same as those seen in women and have a similar natural history. There is a high incidence of oestrogen receptor positivity. The management is largely comparable to that in female breast cancer.

NATURAL HISTORY

Public health medicine and patient awareness campaigns and breast screening has led to more patients with breast cancer being diagnosed at an earlier stage, and better outcome. As a primary tumour enlarges it invades adjacent breast tissue, eventually leading to fixation to the pectoral fascia, serratus anterior muscle and ribs. The parietal pleura might be breached in neglected cases leading to transcoelomic spread within the pleural cavity. The dermal lymphatics can be invaded leading to 'peau d'orange' or satellite lesions. The dermis and epidermis can become infiltrated directly leading to nodules (Figure 8.3), plaques, ulceration or inflammatory changes (Figure 8.4). In the neglected cases, the whole

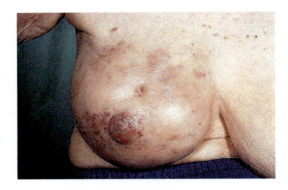

Figure 8.3 Locally advanced breast cancer. The breast is diffusely infiltrated by tumour. Multiple nodules are erupting over the surface of the breast.

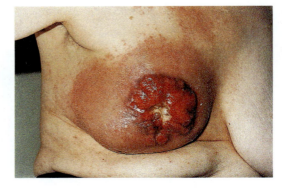

Figure 8.4 Locally advanced breast cancer. There is ulceration of the overlying skin. There are inflammatory changes in the surrounding skin suggesting invasion of the dermal lymphatics.

Symptoms

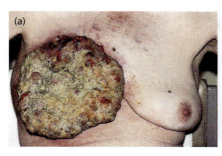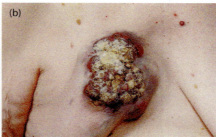

Figure 8.5 Examples of fungating breast cancer. (a) An enormous fungating tumour. This patient suffered from schizophrenia, which contributed to the late presentation. (b) Vascular tumour mass.

breast can be replaced by tumour with tumour growing externally as an exophytic mass (Figure 8.5). In exceptional cases, the breast can be completely replaced by the cancer (Figure 8.6).

The likelihood of lymphatic involvement increases with increasing tumour size, decreasing tumour differentiation and lymphatic channel invasion within the primary tumour. Approximately one-third will have macroscopic or microscopic spread to the axillary nodes at the time of diagnosis; less commonly infra- and supraclavicular nodes will also be involved. Medial tumours can involve the internal mammary nodes in the parasternal region (Figure 8.7), particularly if large and if the axillary lymph nodes are involved.

The most common site for distant metastases is the skeleton. Other sites include liver, lung, brain and skin. Bone metastases may be predominantly lytic (Figure 8.8), sclerotic (Figure 8.9) or a mixture of the

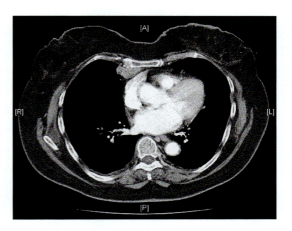

Figure 8.7 Internal mammary lymph node recurrence. CT image of the thorax. There is an expansile mass in the right parasternal region.

two types. The disease can remain confined to the skeleton for much of its natural history and the burden of skeletal disease considerably (Figure 8.10). Some patients present years after their original breast cancer diagnosis with respiratory symptoms from pleural disease (Figure 8.11). Breast cancer occasionally spreads to both ovaries, giving rise to 'Krukenberg tumours', a phenomenon also seen in stomach cancer when both ovaries are involved in metastases due to transcoelomic spread across the peritoneal cavity. Lobular cancers have a particular propensity for gastrointestinal and genitourinary involvement.

SYMPTOMS

For those patients not diagnosed by screening, the majority present with a painless breast lump

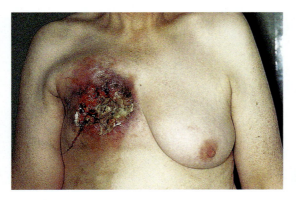

Figure 8.6 Neglected breast cancer. The woman had not undergone mastectomy – the breast has been consumed by the malignant process over years.

93

Breast cancer

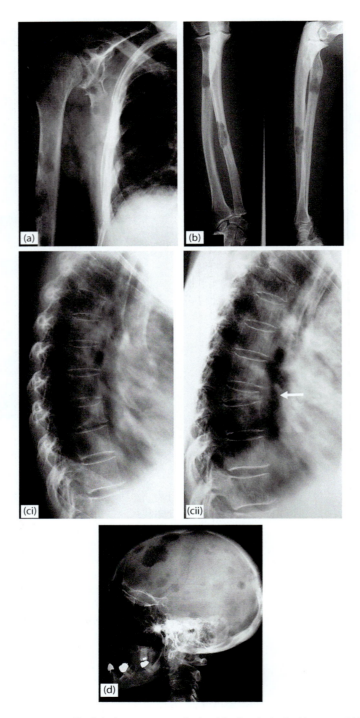

Figure 8.8 Lytic bone metastases. Such lesions are at particular risk of pathological fracture. (a) Humerus, scapula and clavicle. (b) AP and lateral views of forearm. (c) i and ii: Vertebrae. Sequential lateral radiographs of the thoracic spine taken nearly 2 months apart showing development of a wedge collapse. (d) Skull.

Signs

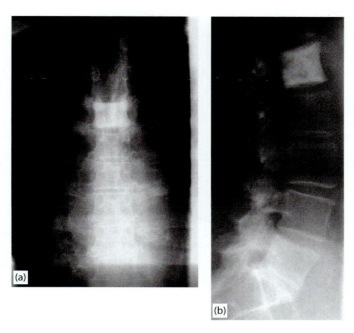

Figure 8.9 (a) Plain radiograph of the thoracic spine showing a sclerotic metastasis from breast cancer. (b) Lateral view of lumbar spine.

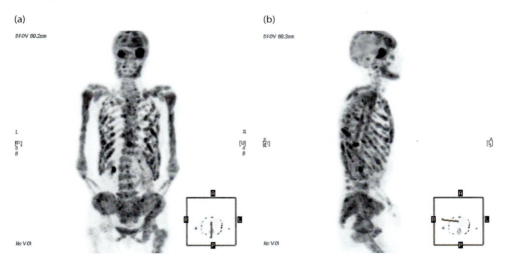

Figure 8.10 Widespread bone metastases. Whole body PET survey. (a) Coronal view. (b) Lateral view.

or distortion of the breast, which might be associated with a blood-stained nipple discharge. Patients detected by screening are likely to be asymptomatic. Less frequently, the presentation is with diffuse enlargement or reddening of the breast, and occasionally lymphadenopathy or symptoms from distant metastases.

SIGNS

The lump is usually non-tender, well-defined and most likely located in the upper outer quadrant, which contains the majority of the breast tissue. Breast discomfort is occasionally a presenting

Breast cancer

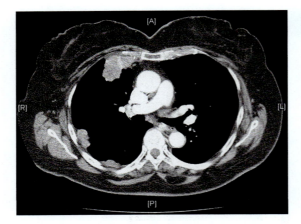

Figure 8.11 Pleural spread. CT image of the thorax. There is nodular involvement of the pleura on the right side.

symptom. In advanced cases, the overlying skin can be dimpled or frankly invaded by tumour leading to reddening, induration and nodular irregularity. Fixation to the skin or chest wall with limited mobility of the lump should be sought by the clinician during physical examination. A very large lump will lead to obvious asymmetry of the breasts. There may be enlargement of the ipsilateral axillary lymph nodes, the mobility of which should be assessed as part of the clinical staging, and less frequently enlargement of the supraclavicular lymph nodes. Hepatomegaly could suggest metastatic infiltration while intrathoracic signs of collapse, consolidation or pleural effusion could suggest pulmonary or pleural metastases. Bone metastases are most frequent in the thoracic and lumbar spine and can lead to tenderness when pressure is applied to the affected vertebrae.

DIFFERENTIAL DIAGNOSIS

A number of benign breast lumps are clinically indistinguishable from carcinoma such as fibroadenoma, duct papilloma, breast abscess, fat necrosis, haematoma and galactocoele. Many such cases will be diagnosed as non-malignant during preoperative investigations. Rarer malignant tumours of the breast may occasionally cause confusion ('rare tumours').

INVESTIGATIONS

'Triple assessment' comprises physical examination, radiological assessment, mammography and ultrasonography, and pathology obtained by fine needle aspiration or core biopsy.

MAMMOGRAPHY

This comprises radiographic examination of the breasts using low-energy x-rays to allow definition of the soft-tissue detail and breast architecture. Two views are taken of each breast, usually in craniocaudal and oblique projections. These may substantiate the clinical diagnosis of carcinoma, detect ductal carcinoma *in situ* in both the affected and contralateral breasts and localize the tumour, to assist the planning of a biopsy or definitive surgical procedure. Carcinoma is suggested by an irregular mass lesion containing areas of microcalcification, sometimes with distortion of the surrounding breast architecture (Figure 8.12).

BREAST ULTRASOUND

This enables the radiologist to determine whether a lump is solid or cystic, the former being more likely to be malignant, and facilitates fine-needle aspiration or preferably needle biopsy of small lumps under direct vision, reducing the risk of a geographical miss and thereby increasing the sensitivity of the procedure. It provides images that are complementary to those obtained by mammography (Figure 8.13). The axilla can also be assessed and abnormal nodes biopsied.

MAGNETIC RESONANCE IMAGING

This is reserved for the investigation of younger women with more dense breast tissue or more difficult cases such as a suspicious lump arising in a breast augmented with a tissue expander or silicon implant, where mammography can be impractical. It is also useful in excluding multifocal disease in mammographically dense breasts and in helping to define the extent of the cancer and checking for occult contralateral breast cancer in those with invasive lobular carcinoma.

Investigations

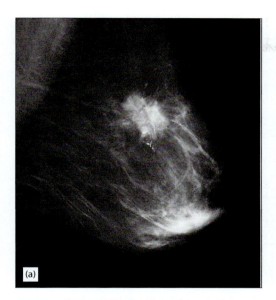

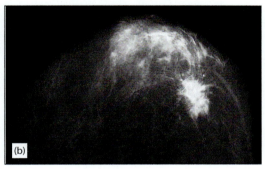

Figure 8.12 Two-view mammogram. There is a spiculate density with flecks of microcalcification typical of carcinoma. (a) Oblique view. (b) Craniocaudal view.

FINE-NEEDLE ASPIRATION (FNA) CYTOLOGY AND NEEDLE CORE BIOPSY

These are rapid, safe, relatively non-traumatic procedures which can be performed at an outpatient consultation and can provide a tissue diagnosis within hours. Core biopsy is favoured as cores allow histological analysis, distinguishing between invasive cancer and DCIS, and enables grading, and determination of receptor status (ER = oestrogen receptor, PR = progesterone receptor and Her2 status). Biopsy should be performed whenever a palpable lump or

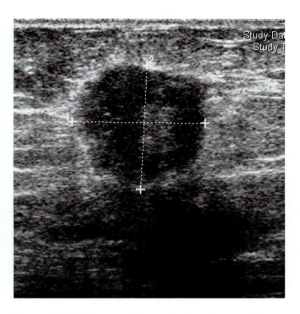

Figure 8.13 Ultrasound image of a breast cancer. The lesion is a sonographically rounded mass with complex echoes within it and a transmission void beyond the main mass.

suspicious area of induration is found, and is applicable to the primary tumour, regional lymph nodes or suspicious skin lesions. Small, impalpable lesions might have to be localized by stereotactic mammogram or ultrasound.

NIPPLE DISCHARGE CYTOLOGY

This is useful in women presenting with a bloody nipple discharge in the absence of a palpable lump.

EXCISION BIOPSY

An excision biopsy is mandatory when it is not possible to obtain a tissue diagnosis by FNA or core biopsy. This is now an uncommon procedure as a diagnosis is usually made by core biopsy. Excision biopsy is usually performed under general anaesthetic and the specimen can be sent for instant frozen section so that if a more radical operation is deemed necessary, it can be performed immediately. Small, impalpable lesions are first localized with a 'guidewire' under radiological control, which

Breast cancer

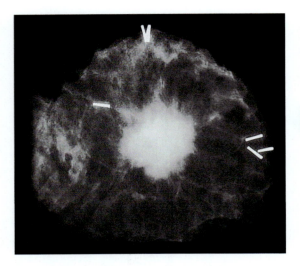

Figure 8.14 Specimen radiograph showing the tumour excised with a good margin of clearance all round. The radio-opaque markers allow the pathologist to orientate the specimen.

can be used to determine which piece of tissue should be excised. A specimen radiograph (Figure 8.14) is useful to confirm preoperatively that the area under suspicion has been fully excised. This guidewire localization is important in the surgical removal of impalpable lesions.

EXCLUSION OF METASTATIC DISEASE

In many patients presenting with early breast cancer there is no need to perform staging investigations. In patients presenting with features that put them at increased risk of having distant disease, it is important to complete staging tests to exclude such disease and act as valuable baseline assessments. Such risk features include T3/T4 cancers, or those patients with lymph node involvement at diagnosis. Patients with concerning systemic symptoms should also be investigated. The most usual investigations are:

- CT scan of the brain, thorax, abdomen and pelvis and in some circumstances a PET/CT scan
- Isotope bone scan or whole-body MRI scan

Tumour markers (CEA and CA15-3) should not be routinely performed, but can be useful in assessing the effect of treatment in patients with known metastatic disease, especially in patients with metastases to the bone only

STAGING

The TNM staging is the most frequently used and can be used as a guide to management and prognosis:

- T0: No evidence of primary tumour
- TX: Primary tumour cannot be assessed
- Tis: Carcinoma *in situ*
- T1: 2 cm or less in greatest dimension
  - 1a: 0.5 cm or less in greatest dimension
  - 1b: >0.5 cm but not >1 cm in greatest dimension
  - 1c: >1 cm but not >2 cm in greatest dimension
- T2: >2 cm but not >5 cm in greatest dimension
- T3: >5 cm in greatest dimension
- T4: Tumour of any size with extension to chest wall and/or skin
  - 4a: Invasion of chest wall (ribs, serratus anterior, intercostal muscles)
  - 4b: Oedema/'peau d'orange', ulceration, satellite nodules confined to the same breast
  - 4c: Both 4a and 4b
  - 4d: Inflammatory carcinoma
- N0: No lymphadenopathy
- N1: Ipsilateral mobile axillary nodes
- N2: Ipsilateral axillary nodes fixed to one another or to adjacent structures or ipsilateral internal mammary node metastases
- N3: Involvement of ipsilateral infra- or supraclavicular nodes
- M1: Distant metastases

TREATMENT

The aims of treatment are:

- Locoregional control with optimal cosmesis
- Reduction of risk of developing distant metastatic disease
- Minimization of short- and long-term treatment-related morbidity

Treatment

The treatment of breast cancer for an individual depends on the clinical stage of the disease, menopausal state and performance status of the patient. Ideally, the patient should be assessed in a multidisciplinary breast clinic by both the surgeon and the oncologist prior to any definitive treatment so that the optimum treatment can be instituted at the outset. Patients with no evidence of spread are treated with curative intent, whereas those with distant metastases are not curable but depending on the type and extent of the disease may live for a long time with treatment.

TREATMENT OF LOCAL DISEASE

DUCTAL CARCINOMA *IN SITU* (DCIS)

DCIS is curable in the vast majority of patients. However, local treatment must ensure that it is eradicated as there is a high risk of local recurrence; this recurrence may be invasive in breast cancer (approximately half of recurrences after treatment for DCIS are invasive cancer and half DCIS). Traditionally, simple mastectomy was the treatment of choice, and this is still the case for multifocal disease or when clear surgical margins cannot be attained. However, in recent years, the experience of breast conservation for invasive cancers has been extrapolated to DCIS. Whilst small foci of low/intermediate-grade DCIS can be treated with excision alone, if adequate margins of clearance are attained, local excision and adjuvant radiotherapy to the breast alone is now the standard treatment in many centres for unifocal DCIS that has been completely excised. There remains a debate about the role of tamoxifen after definite surgery and radiotherapy for DCIS. It may further reduce the risk of local recurrence within the breast after breast-conserving treatment if, as is usually the case, the DCIS is oestrogen receptor-positive. Pure DCIS should not spread to regional lymph nodes and therefore no axillary surgery is necessary. Similarly, DCIS has no potential for systemic spread, and therefore there is no role for chemotherapy in the management of DCIS.

CASE HISTORY

BREAST CANCER 1

A 43-year-old premenopausal woman presents with a 6 cm diameter lump arising within her left breast with no clinically palpable axillary lymph node enlargement. Mammography and ultrasound are suspicious for carcinoma in the breast and ultrasound shows an abnormal axillary node. Core biopsy of breast indicates a grade 3 invasive ductal carcinoma, which is hormone receptor negative and Her2 negative and core biopsy of the axillary node is positive for cancer. Staging investigations indicate no evidence of metastatic disease. The tumour is therefore staged as T3N1M0. The only surgical option is mastectomy. The patient requires chemotherapy after mastectomy, so opts to receive it as neoadjuvant (i.e. preoperative) treatment. A radio-opaque marker is inserted under ultrasound guidance to mark the site of the tumour radiologically. After three cycles of chemotherapy using epirubicin and cyclophosphamide (100 and 600 mg/m^2 repeated every 21 days with GCSF support), the lump clinically measures 2 cm in diameter. Three cycles of docetaxel chemotherapy (100 mg/m^2 with GCSF support) are then administered and the mass becomes almost impalpable clinically but still visible on mammography. A breast-conserving operation is now feasible and she undergoes a wire localized excision of the residual disease and axillary lymph node dissection. Histopathological examination confirms a 1 cm diameter area of residual grade 2 ductal carcinoma and DCIS, representing tumour that has been downgraded by chemotherapy. Two of 12 axillary lymph nodes removed are involved. The tumour is confirmed as negative for oestrogen receptors, progesterone receptors and HER2. Postoperative radiotherapy is delivered to the breast and supraclavicular fossa. No further adjuvant therapy is appropriate as hormone manipulation will confer no advantage.

The woman remains well for 18 months after completing her treatment but then presents with a persistent aching pain in the right upper quadrant of the abdomen. Examination reveals tenderness and fullness in the right subcostal region. Liver function tests indicate γ-glutamyltransferase (GGT) of 470 U/L (normal <42) and alkaline phosphatase (ALP) of 350 U/L (normal range 38–126). The CA15-3 breast cancer marker is also elevated at 400 U/mL (normal <50). Preliminary liver ultrasound confirms multiple hypoechoic lesions suggestive of metastases. The CT scan of the thorax/abdomen and isotope bone scan are undertaken as staging investigations. These confirm multiple metastases throughout both lobes of the liver but no disease elsewhere. This metastatic disease is incurable but palliation of symptoms and potential prolongation of life is achieved by further chemotherapy – weekly paclitaxel chemotherapy is offered, and the patient proceeds with treatment. Three cycles are given with resolution of the woman's presenting symptoms. Repeat examination is normal and CT of the liver shows a partial response. The CA15-3 is 75 U/mL and there has been more than 50% decrease in GGT and ALP. A further three cycles of chemotherapy are given with further clinical, biochemical and radiological responses. CA15-3 falls to 40 U/mL by the end of chemotherapy and a baseline scan 6 weeks after the last cycle shows a further response compared with the previous one.

Six months later, she presents with increasing dyspnoea on exertion. Clinically, there are no signs of note. Chest x-ray shows bilateral perihilar opacification suggestive of lymphangitis. CT scan confirms miliary-type metastases throughout both lung fields and a further increase in the number and size of liver metastases. Further chemotherapy is delivered using vinorelbine on days 1 and 8 of a 21-day cycle. G-CSF growth factor support is necessary because of significant myelotoxicity. An interval scan after three cycles shows no response and her performance score has reduced to 3. It is decided that further active oncological treatment is inappropriate and that symptom control should be the priority. The woman dies approximately 3 years after presentation.

INVASIVE CANCER

Surgery

Surgery facilitates total clearance of the primary tumour and pathological examination of the primary tumour and regional lymph nodes. The operation used depends on the size of the lump, its location within the breast, the size of the breast, the presence of multifocal disease or extensive carcinoma *in situ* in the surrounding breast tissue.

Breast-conserving surgery (wide local excision, lumpectomy, therapeutic mammoplasty) is offered whenever possible but mastectomy with immediate or delayed reconstruction will be required in some patients.

Breast-conserving surgery excises the tumour with a small margin of uninvolved surrounding breast tissue. This gives an excellent cosmetic result as it preserves the bulk of the breast and nipple/areola complex, even in women with small breasts. It is unsuitable for very large tumours (>5 cm in maximum dimension), particularly if located centrally, although with successful preoperative chemotherapy (or in some cases preoperative endocrine therapy) such surgery may become possible. Inflammatory carcinomas are never treated with breast-conserving surgery. Even if the excision margins are clear after microscopic examination of the specimen, there is up to 25% risk of local recurrence without further local treatment – this risk varies with tumour size, grade, node status and age, reducing significantly with small, low grade node-negative tumours in patients over the age of 65.

Simple mastectomy involves complete removal of the disease-involved breast. The pectoral muscles are preserved. The procedure is often combined with a breast reconstruction using either a tissue expander (Becker implant) or an autologous flap, e.g. latissimus dorsi (LD) muscle or TRAM flap. If reconstruction is not undertaken, the physical appearance of the chest wall will be far superior to that after a more radical mastectomy.

Radical (Halstead) mastectomy involves en bloc removal of the breast, pectoralis major and minor muscles and the axillary contents. It is not indicated in the current era unless the tumour is directly invading the underlying pectoral muscle to a significant degree.

Treatment

Mature trial data have shown that breast-conserving surgery and postoperative radiotherapy have the same local control and survival rates compared to mastectomy, making breast-conservative surgery the treatment of choice in many patients. Mastectomy is still the treatment of choice in certain situations:

- When the patient wishes to have the breast removed for psychological reasons or in women who are known BRCA mutation carriers where there is a higher ongoing risk of further breast cancer
- Extensive ductal carcinoma *in situ*
- Paget disease of the nipple with an occult primary
- Multifocal primaries
- Inflammatory carcinoma
- Treatment of malignant phylloides tumour or sarcoma
- A very large tumour in a small breast, particularly if centrally located
- Salvage treatment after failure of conservative therapy
- As a toilet procedure for a fungating tumour

The psychosexual trauma and disturbance of body image that breast surgery can inflict should be considered. Patients for whom a mastectomy is planned should have the opportunity to see a trained breast care nurse counsellor prior to their surgery so that the implications of the operation can be sympathetically and skilfully discussed. Patients may wish to be fitted with a prosthesis to maintain their chest contour or undergo immediate/subsequent surgical reconstruction of the breast using either a tissue expander or autologous muscle flap transposition (Figure 8.15). Patients undergoing conservative treatment should also be offered counselling, as studies suggest these patients experience psychological trauma similar to that of mastectomy patients.

The axilla is frequently a site for lymph node metastases, which in many cases cannot be detected clinically. The risk increases with increasing tumour size and grade, and the presence of lymphovascular invasion. The presence of lymph node metastases is a valuable prognostic factor, and correlates with the risk of the patient subsequently developing distant metastases. The management of the axilla with a conventional axillary dissection does cause

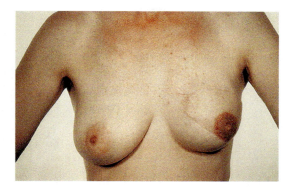

Figure 8.15 Reconstruction of the left breast using a latissimus dorsi (LD) flap. Note the nipple reconstruction.

morbidity (longer recovery, shoulder stiffness and a small risk of lymphoedema), and trial data have shown that for a clinically and radiologically negative axilla, the lesser procedure of sentinel lymph node biopsy has a similar outcome. An axillary dissection is still usually indicated in patients with positive nodes at initial assessment.

Sentinel lymph node biopsy entails preoperative injection of a vital dye and/or radio-labelled technetium colloid around the tumour. These visual and radioactive markers are then taken up by the regional lymphatic vessels and concentrated initially within the sentinel lymph node(s) (Figure 8.16). The rationale is that, if this node(s) is removed alone and found histologically not to contain malignant cells, it is highly (>95%) likely that no other regional lymph nodes are involved and therefore no further surgery is necessary.

Axillary sampling entails the removal of the lower lymph node group up to the level of the lower border of the pectoralis minor muscle. It has largely been superseded by sentinel lymph node biopsy. At least four nodes should be obtained for histological examination. If these nodes are not involved by cancer, it is unlikely that nodes higher in the axilla will be either. Conversely, if a node is positive, a full axillary lymph node dissection may be necessary.

Axillary dissection is a more extensive surgical procedure comprising the removal of the axillary contents at least up to the level of the upper border of the pectoralis minor muscle (level 2) or even axillary vein (level 3). Twenty to thirty nodes may be retrieved by the pathologist, giving more detailed

Breast cancer

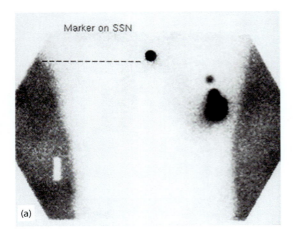
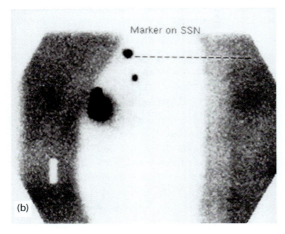

Figure 8.16 Sentinel lymph node scintigram. Radioactive technetium has been infiltrated around the breast cancer. The sentinel lymph node is shown (the midline spot is a sternal notch reference marker). (a) Front view. (b) Lateral view.

prognostic information. It also has the advantage of being a one-stop therapeutic manoeuvre in its own right, lessening the risk of axillary recurrence. It has the disadvantage of increasing the surgical morbidity, resulting in local sensory loss, stiffness of the shoulder and a risk of lymphoedema of the ipsilateral arm.

Radiotherapy

Breast conservation

Radiotherapy is indicated in nearly all patients treated by breast-conserving surgery. Such an approach produces long-term survival equivalent to that of mastectomy. External beam radiotherapy to the breast alone typically comprises a 3-week course of treatment to the whole breast to reduce the risk of recurrence at the site of the original primary tumour and also the possibility of recurrence elsewhere within the breast arising from occult foci of DCIS and LCIS. An extra 'boost' can be delivered specifically to the tumour bed when the margins of excision are narrow or focally involved, and is recommended in all women under 50 years of age. Despite data from studies initiated prior to 1975 indicating an excess risk of cardiovascular death for women treated with radiotherapy, this has not been shown to be the case for more recent studies, presumably reflecting more careful planning to exclude the myocardium. CT planning for breast cancer patients is now standard and enables avoidance of the myocardium and lung; modern radiotherapy techniques now allow reduce radiotherapy dose to the heart by treating in deep inspiration, a technique known as deep inspiratory breath hold.

CT imaging is also helpful for very large-breasted women where it allows more sophisticated treatment methods such as modulation of the beams to deliver a more homogeneous dose distribution.

Radiotherapy to the whole breast remains the standard of care for most patients. Research evidence is being produced to evaluate the role of:

- Partial breast irradiation (either by external beam, intraoperative or brachytherapy approaches)
- Shorter (hypofractionated) radiotherapy schedules
- IMRT techniques that define different doses to different parts of the breast defined by the disease characteristics
- The avoidance of radiotherapy in patients older than 65 years with low risk cancers

Postmastectomy

Simple mastectomy alone is associated with a local recurrence rate of 5%. Radiotherapy reduces the risk of chest wall recurrence (Figure 8.17) but is used more selectively for those at particularly high risk of chest wall relapse.

The risk factors recognized for local recurrence after mastectomy are follows:

- T3 and T4 tumours
- Poorly differentiated tumours

Treatment

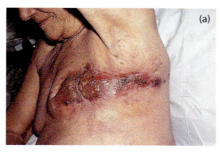 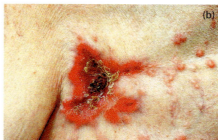

Figure 8.17 Chest wall recurrence after mastectomy. Showing tumour nodules change with satellite lymphatic spread.

- Lymphovascular invasion
- Involved axillary lymph nodes
- Incomplete microscopic excision, usually at the deep margin

Lymph node regions

The axilla is not routinely irradiated after axillary dissection. The risk of lymphoedema of the arm, and of arm and shoulder stiffness increases significantly if both axillary surgery and radiotherapy are given.

Radiotherapy may be given to the axilla in those patients who have not undergone axillary surgery and in whom the risk of lymph node involvement justifies further therapy to the axilla.

The supraclavicular fossa can be irradiated after a significantly positive (four or more involved nodes) axillary node dissection, and is frequently treated in patients who have had primary chemotherapy and were node positive prior to chemotherapy.

Chemotherapy/hormone manipulation as initial treatment for locally advanced disease

Inoperable tumours and in cases where breast-conserving surgery may become possible with tumour shrinkage are initially treated with systemic therapy. Chemotherapy (termed 'neoadjuvant' or 'primary') is the treatment of choice for most women. Those unfit or unsuitable for chemotherapy will be considered for hormone therapy alone providing the tumour has been confirmed as oestrogen receptor positive. Once maximal response to systemic therapy has been attained, the breast can be treated by surgically and followed by radiotherapy as appropriate. Preoperative systemic therapy has been established as a means of decreasing the mastectomy rate, although it has no significant survival advantage over postoperative chemotherapy.

ADJUVANT SYSTEMIC THERAPY

Adjuvant systemic therapy complements the role of radiotherapy or surgery to the breast. The former acts on cancer cells that have already metastasized outside the breast and its regional lymphatics, while the latter reduces the local relapse rate. It is now widely accepted that adjuvant systemic therapy has proven benefit in reducing the risk of distant relapse from metastatic spread, and that this translates into a significant benefit in disease-free and overall survival. Breast cancer is statistically an important cancer accounting for much morbidity and mortality among women, and therefore only a little increase in these parameters will be worthwhile. There are two main types of adjuvant systemic therapy.

HORMONE THERAPIES

Adjuvant hormone therapy can reduce the risk of distant metastatic relapse. Adjuvant hormonal therapy agents include tamoxifen and the aromatase inhibitors. Tamoxifen, an antioestrogen, which acts by blocking the action of oestradiol on its receptors has been used for many years and trial data now suggest that greater benefit is seen with longer duration of use, i.e. from 5 years up to 10 years. The dose is 20 mg once daily. There is no evidence that a higher dose is any more effective.

In women with oestrogen receptor-positive tumours, 5 years use of tamoxifen reduces:

- The odds of recurrence by approximately 40%, an absolute reduction of approximately 13% by 15 years of follow-up

Breast cancer

- The odds of dying from breast cancer by approximately 30%, an absolute reduction of approximately 9% by 15 years of follow-up

In the same group of patients, the addition of chemotherapy to tamoxifen produces a further benefit in terms of recurrences and deaths from breast cancer versus tamoxifen alone. These benefits are also independent of age and lymph node status. Tamoxifen also halves the risk of developing a contralateral primary breast cancer over 5 years it is taken and for up to 5 years afterwards.

The aromatase inhibitors anastrozole, letrozole and exemestane have been investigated in trials looking at a comparison of efficacy with tamoxifen and in trials looking at combinations and duration of therapy. The aromatase inhibitors have some side effects in common with tamoxifen but importantly also have some differences in the side effects, e.g. less risk of thromboembolism. However, they do not have the bone protective action of tamoxifen and bone mineral health should be assessed and actively managed during their use. The aromatase inhibitors are appropriate only in postmenopausal patients, where they have slightly higher efficacy than tamoxifen and may be the treatment of choice upfront or used after tamoxifen (e.g. switch after 2–5 years of tamoxifen). Trial data have also shown that aromatase inhibitors used in combination with ovarian suppression are more effective than tamoxifen in premenopausal patients who are at a high risk of recurrence, but this combination is also associated with greater side effects. An explanation of benefits versus side effects of these various options must be discussed with each individual patient.

Adjuvant bisphosphonate therapy is recommended for postmenopausal patients who have cancers with a higher risk of recurrence, and may be required in patients who have poor bone mineral density measurements.

CHEMOTHERAPY

The criteria used to determine whether a patient should receive adjuvant chemotherapy are based on the risk of recurrence — a low risk of recurrence does not warrant the use of chemotherapy whereas a moderate to high risk does. Defining this risk of recurrence and understanding the concerns and wishes of each patient makes the decision to use chemotherapy an individual one. A typical set of criteria are presented, any one of which would be sufficient to recommend chemotherapy as standard treatment:

- Premenopausal women:
  - Age <35 years
  - Tumour 20 mm or greater in maximum microscopic diameter
  - Poorly differentiated (grade 3) tumour of any size
  - Axillary lymph node involvement
  - Oestrogen receptor negativity
- Postmenopausal women 50–69 years:
  - Axillary lymph node involvement
  - Poorly differentiated tumours >20 mm
  - Oestrogen receptor negativity
- For women <50 years of age, adjuvant chemotherapy has been proven to reduce:
  - The odds of recurrence by approximately 35%–40%, an absolute reduction of approximately 11% by 15 years of follow-up
  - The odds of dying (due to breast cancer and other causes) by approximately 25%–30%, an absolute reduction of approximately 5% for node-negative cases and 11% for node-positive cases by 15 years of follow-up
- For women 50–69 years of age, adjuvant chemotherapy has been proven to reduce:
  - The odds of recurrence by approximately 20%, an absolute reduction of approximately 5% by 15 years of follow-up
  - The odds of dying from breast cancer by approximately 10%, an absolute reduction of approximately 2%–4% by 15 years of follow-up

Adjuvant chemotherapy therefore confers greater benefit to younger patients. Its effect is independent of hormone receptor status. There are comparatively few data available for the use of adjuvant chemotherapy in the >70-year age group. Women of this age group should be considered for chemotherapy if their cancer is hormonally insensitive and very adverse risk factors are present.

Trials continue to look at the optimum chemotherapy combination and duration in the adjuvant treatment of breast cancer.

TARGETED THERAPY / IMMUNOTHERAPY

Approximately 15% of women with early breast cancer will have tumours that test positive for human epidermal growth factor receptor 2 (HER2) oncogene overexpression. The monoclonal antibody trastuzumab (Herceptin®) has revolutionized the treatment of breast cancer. Trastuzumab is a humanized murine antibody that specifically targets the HER2-positive cells. Randomized trials in women with early breast cancer have confirmed that, when it is used in combination with chemotherapy, trastuzumab given for 1 year halves recurrence and reduces breast cancer mortality by one-third compared to the same chemotherapy used alone. The only significant toxicity is a small risk of reducing left ventricular ejection fraction of the heart leading to a risk of congestive cardiac failure in susceptible individuals. Regular cardiac assessment (ECHO or MUGA) detects cardiac changes early and at a reversible stage. The development of subcutaneous trastuzumab (initially only available in intravenous form) has also made therapy easier for patients. Trials with further HER2-targeting agents alone or in combination with trastuzumab in the adjuvant setting have been performed and results are awaited.

TREATMENT OF METASTATIC DISEASE

The disease is incurable at this stage, and treatment is aimed at palliating symptoms and maintaining the patient as active as possible with minimal side effects and the least inconvenience. As for other solid tumours, active treatment will have a superior outcome to best supportive care. The serum tumour markers (e.g. CA15-3) are surrogates for the whole body breast cancer activity for a given individual, and can be useful in assessing response to treatment, providing information complementary to that available from imaging.

SURGERY

There is rarely a role for breast surgery in the patient with metastatic disease provided a tissue diagnosis has already been obtained and satisfactory local control of the breast tumour can be achieved by other treatment modalities. Toilet mastectomy is occasionally performed for symptomatic locally uncontrollable disease. Thoracoscopic talc pleurodesis is sometimes of value in the treatment of recurrent malignant pleural effusions, and internal fixation is indicated if fracture of a weight-bearing bone has occurred or is imminent. In selected patients who are fit, with a long disease interval and a solitary cerebral metastasis as sole site of disease, neurosurgical removal may be indicated.

RADIOTHERAPY

The natural history of breast cancer dictates that many patients with metastatic breast cancer will have symptomatic bone metastases, and some will also be troubled by brain, cutaneous or rarely choroidal metastases. Radiotherapy is the treatment of choice for metastases causing local symptoms.

Radiotherapy for metastatic breast cancer may be as simple as a single fraction to a painful bone metastasis or as complicated as stereotactic radiotherapy for a patient with a limited number of brain metastasis. A significant percentage of patients will require some form of palliative radiotherapy while living with their disease.

Recurrent local disease in the breast or on the chest wall may also be treated with radiotherapy to avoid fungation and bleeding; this may mean retreatment if previous postoperative treatment has been given and careful consideration of cumulative radiation damage to the skin and ribs must be part of discussion with the patient when deciding upon such measures. In some cases brachytherapy will provide the best way of delivering local radiation limited to the tumour.

HORMONE THERAPY

The aromatase inhibitors (non-steroidal; letrozole and anastrozole and steroidal; exemestane) and tamoxifen are important agents in the treatment of ER+ metastatic breast cancer (Figure 8.18). Other hormonal agents include fulvestrant, progestogens (megestrol acetate 80 mg bd or medroxyprogesterone acetate 400 mg bd). Responses to second-line or third-line hormone therapy are more likely in those who have responded convincingly to initial hormone therapy.

Breast cancer

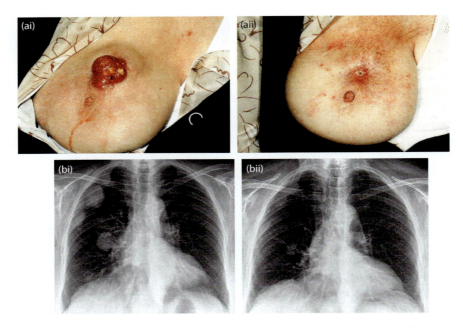

Figure 8.18 Examples of dramatic responses to endocrine therapy alone. (ai): Locally advanced disease at presentation. (aii): After 6 months' endocrine therapy. (bi): Chest radiograph. Lung metastases at presentation. (bii): After 4 months' endocrine therapy.

CHEMOTHERAPY

Chemotherapy is effective against soft-tissue metastases but is less effective compared to radiotherapy for palliating bone metastases. The choice of first-line metastatic regimen depends on that used for adjuvant therapy (if any). At least six cycles are administered unless chemoresistance is demonstrated by progression during treatment. After six cycles, the treatment can be continued for as long as some objective response is obtained, unless toxicity is so severe as to compromise the patient's quality of life and warrant termination of treatment.

- Anthracycline regimes:
  - Doxorubicin 60 mg/m^2 repeated every 21 days
  - Epirubicin 60–90 mg/m^2 repeated every 21 days
- For anthracycline refractory patients, a taxane should be considered:
  - Paclitaxel 80 mg/m^2 repeated weekly
  - Docetaxel 75 mg/m^2 repeated every 21 days
- Other options include:
  - Vinorelbine 25 mg/m^2 at days 1 and 8 of a 21-day cycle, an oral preparation is also available
  - Capecitabine 2500 mg/m^2 divided into two oral doses per day for days 1–14 of a 21-day cycle
  - Eribulin 1.23 mg/m^2 at days 1 and 8 of a 21 day cycle
  - Carboplatin (AUC 6) repeated every 21 days
  - Methotrexate 35 mg/m^2 and mitoxantrone 11 mg/m^2 (MM) repeated every 21 days

BIOLOGICAL THERAPIES

Approximately 20% of those individuals developing metastatic disease will have tumours that overexpress HER2. In combination with certain cytotoxic agents such as paclitaxel, docetaxel, capecitabine, vinorelbine and carboplatin, trastuzumab increases overall response rates and leads to a significant improvement in median survivals without any

Treatment

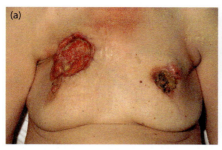
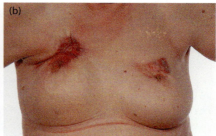

Figure 8.19 Response to single agent trastuzumab (Herceptin®). (a) Locally advanced bilateral breast cancer at presentation. (b) After 6 months' treatment. Both tumours were HER-2 positive.

significant increase in toxicity. In those who respond to treatment, trastuzumab is continued after chemotherapy until proven disease progression. In certain circumstances, chemotherapy may be deemed inappropriate for a woman with HER2-positive metastatic breast cancer and if so, trastuzumab can be used alone for good effect (Figure 8.19). Women on long-term trastuzumab are at significantly increased risk of developing brain metastases.

Other 'anti-Her2' agents have been developed and are active when the disease has progressed on trastuzumab and some have shown additional response rates when combined with trastuzumab; for example, pertuzumab is an anti-Her2 monoclonal antibody that has shown little useful activity on its own but when given with trastuzumab leads to a significant improvement in response.

Trastuzumab emtansine is an antibody drug conjugate (trastuzumab linked to the cytotoxic agent emtansine) and has also shown efficacy when patients have progressed on trastuzumab alone. This is an exciting concept as the trastuzumab targets cancer cells leading to targeted delivery of the cytotoxic agent.

Lapatinib is a dual (HER1 and HER2) kinase inhibitor that can be used in combination with capecitabine. Both of these are orally delivered. Being a relatively small molecule, lapatinib has the advantage over trastuzumab of crossing the blood–brain barrier. Diarrhoea is the most common toxicity with this combination.

Other newer agents

Everolimus (an mTOR inhibitor) has shown activity when combined with the aromatase inhibitor exemestane.

Palbociclib, ribociclib and abemaciclib (are small molecule inhibitors of cyclin-dependent kinases 4 and 6) they act by preventing DNA synthesis, blocking progression of the cell cycle from G1 to the S phase. They have shown exciting activity, and are now routinely used in combination with hormonal treatment in patients with metastatic ER+ disease.

Bevacizumab (a monoclonal antibody with activity against the vascular endothelial growth factor [VEGF] receptor) has been shown to have effect with weekly paclitaxel chemotherapy in ER-Her2-breast cancer.

PARP inhibitors are being researched, and may have a role especially in BRCA mutation patients.

CASE HISTORIES

BREAST CANCER 2

A 49-year-old premenopausal woman presents with a painless lump in the left breast. Clinical examination, mammography and ultrasonography suggest a malignant tumour approximately 2.1 cm in diameter. She proceeds to core biopsy, which indicates a grade 2 invasive ductal carcinoma that is oestrogen receptor strongly positive and HER2 positive (3+) on immunohistochemistry. She undergoes wide local excision and sentinel lymph node biopsy. Definitive histology confirms a 2.5 cm maximum diameter grade 3 invasive ductal carcinoma, the sentinel lymph node is clear.

She receives three cycles of EC chemotherapy (epirubicin 100 mg/m^2, cyclophosphamide 500 mg/m^2 repeated every 21 days) followed by three cycles of docetaxel (100 mg/m^2 repeated every 21 days) with trastuzumab (cardiac function has been assessed as good with an ECHO). This is immediately followed by a 3-week course of radiotherapy to the breast and a boost to the tumour bed using CT planning and deep inspiratory breath hold radiotherapy to avoid the myocardium. Adjuvant tamoxifen is also started. She continues to receive the adjuvant trastuzumab thrice weekly (s/c) for a total of 18 doses over a period of 12 months to complete her adjuvant therapy.

She remains well over the next 2 years, but then presents with increasing shortness of breath. Staging CT and bone scan confirm lung metastases have developed. She started on further palliative systemic treatment with docetaxel 75 mg/m^2 and the anti-HER2 agents trastuzumab and pertuzumab (after confirming adequate cardiac functioning with an ECHO and that blood tests are satisfactory). After just two cycles of treatment she is feeling much better. Chemotherapy is continued to a total of six cycles and the trastuzumab and pertuzumab are continued thrice weekly — these drugs will be continued until the breast can progress again. Cardiac function is monitored regularly with ECHO.

After 15 months she complains of a headache and sight weakness in her left arm. An MRI of the brain shows a solitary metastases and CT scan of body shows that no other new disease has developed. The case is reviewed at the breast and neurosurgery multidisciplinary meetings and it is felt that the solitary brain lesion is best managed by stereotactic radiotherapy rather than surgery as the metastasis is in an eloquent part of the brain. The patient is informed that she must not drive with this diagnosis.

She responds well to this stereotactic radiotherapy with no side effects and the follow-up MRI shows almost complete resolution of the solitary brain metastasis. As there has been no change in the systemic disease she continues on trastuzumab and pertuzumab.

The patient is fully aware that she needs to stay on follow-up with monitoring of her disease and that her breast cancer will get worse at some stage. Patients that have a good response to such initial treatment will have further palliative treatment options with other HER2 agents when their disease does get worse.

BREAST CANCER 3

A 59-year-old postmenopausal healthy woman presents with a painless lump in the right breast. Clinical examination, mammography and ultrasonography suggest a malignant tumour approximately 2.5 cm in diameter. She proceeds to core biopsy, which indicates a grade 3 invasive ductal carcinoma that is oestrogen receptor positive and HER2 negative. She undergoes wide local excision and sentinel lymph node biopsy. Definitive histology confirms a maximum diameter of 2.1 cm grade 3 invasive ductal carcinoma, the sentinel lymph node is clear. Using a risk assessment programme it is estimated that she has a borderline benefit to chemotherapy (3% increase in OS at 5 years). She would prefer to avoid chemotherapy and accepts testing by an Oncotype DX test. The recurrence score is 14 and supports the avoidance of chemotherapy. She proceeds to a 3-week course of radiotherapy to the right breast and a boost to the tumour bed using CT planning. A baseline DEXA scan shows both spine and hip are in the osteopenic range. She starts endocrine therapy with letrozole, starts calcium and vitamin D supplement and is encouraged to continue weight-bearing exercise. DEXA scan will be repeated at 2 years and annual mammograms are planned for the next 5 years.

She remains well over the next 4 years, but then presents with increasing pain arising from the mid-thoracic spine. A plain radiograph confirms collapse of the seventh thoracic vertebra. An isotope bone scan confirms isolated uptake in T7. In order to confirm the diagnosis a magnetic resonance scan is performed, which in fact confirms bone metastases at T7 and at other levels in the spine. A vertebroplasty is performed and leads to immediate pain relief. With bone only metastatic disease she is started on second-line endocrine treatment with exemestane and zoledronic acid, a bisphosphonate (consent includes discussion on the risk of osteonecrosis of jaw). Palliative radiotherapy to the T7 metastasis (8 Gy 1#) is also given. Although not curable it is likely that this patient will live a good quality of life with her disease controlled for many months.

OTHER DRUGS

Bisphosphonates such as zoledronic acid and ibandronic acid have a role in those with skeletal metastatic disease. Denosumab (a humanized monoclonal antibody to RANKL) is also an active agent. Regular administration of such therapies may reduce:

- Risk of bone pain
- Risk of hypercalcaemia
- Risk of pathological fracture
- Need for palliative radiotherapy
- Tumour-related complications

Patients must be consented for risks of use in particular osteonecrosis of the jaw which is rare (1%–2%) but can be very troublesome (Figure 8.19).

Fungating tumours can become infected causing an offensive discharge or lead to chronic blood loss. Uncontrolled disease in the axilla can lead to brachial plexopathy and lymphoedema of the arm. Hypercalcaemia, spinal cord compression and pathological fracture are seen in patients with widespread skeletal metastases (see Chapter 21). Pulmonary spread can lead to pleural effusion and lymphangitis (Figure 8.20). Mediastinal lymph node spread can lead to local complications such as superior vena cava obstruction, oesophageal compression or recurrent laryngeal nerve palsy (Figure 8.21). Occasionally, pericardial invasion will lead to a pericardial effusion, which may in turn lead to cardiac tamponade (Figure 8.22). Disseminated intravascular

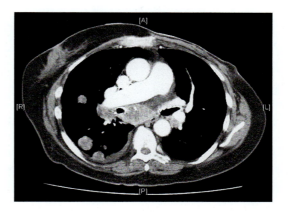

Figure 8.21 Mediastinal lymphadenopathy. CT image of the thorax. There is a mass of bulky lymph nodes compressing the oesophagus posteriorly. Note also the lung metastases and right pleural effusion.

coagulation is a rare complication of advanced disease when the tumour burden is high and usually heralds the terminal phase of the disease. It arises due to mucin production by the tumour which can activate the clotting cascade causing uncontrolled coagulation coupled with a physiological thrombolysis leading to occlusion of both small and large blood vessels. Consumption of clotting factors deranges thrombin time and activated partial thromboplastin time resulting in a bleeding tendency, while platelet consumption leads to thrombocytopenia manifested as epistaxis, petechiae and bruising. Fibrin degradation products are elevated.

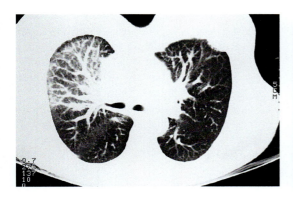

Figure 8.20 Pulmonary lymphangitis. CT image of the thorax. Note the widened lymphatic channels emanating from the hila bilaterally.

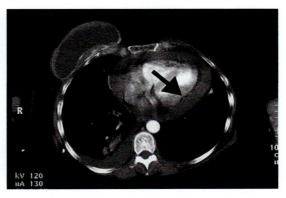

Figure 8.22 Pericardial effusion. CT image of the thorax showing a thick layer of fluid around the myocardium.

TREATMENT-RELATED COMPLICATIONS

RADIOTHERAPY

Breast radiotherapy leads to breast erythema, swelling, skin irritation and tenderness, which settle within 4–8 weeks of completing treatment. The skin may temporarily break down in areas subject to friction such as the inframammary fold. Late complications of radiotherapy are uncommon and include chronic breast or chest wall discomfort, breast shrinkage, breast swelling, breast firmness, telangiectasia of the skin, rib fractures, radiation costochondritis and pulmonary fibrosis. Data from randomized trials initiated prior to 1975 have suggested an increased risk of death from cardiovascular disease, confined to those women with left-sided breast cancers, possibly relating to irradiation of the coronary arteries rather than the myocardium itself — this should be avoided with modern radiotherapy techniques. Axillary irradiation (and surgery) is associated with late morbidity such as lymphoedema of the arm, stiffness of the shoulder and exceptional radiation injury to the brachial plexus and radionecrosis of the irradiated skeleton. With current techniques the incidence is very low.

CHEMOTHERAPY

Infertility, as evidenced by amenorrhoea, is a frequent complication of chemotherapy. This will be permanent and associated with menopausal symptoms in many. The age at receiving chemotherapy is the most important factor for predicting the chance of spontaneous recovery of the menstrual cycle. Many studies with long-term follow-up have suggested an increased risk of leukaemia and myelodysplasia in long-term survivors who have received chemotherapy. Anthracyclines such as epirubicin and doxorubicin can cause a reduction in left ventricular function. This is more likely to become manifest in those with severe hypertension or co-existing cardiac conditions, and leads to an increased risk of congestive cardiac failure later in life.

HORMONE THERAPY

Menopausal symptoms, particularly vasomotor symptoms such as hot flushes, are the main problems with endocrine therapies. Vasomotor symptoms are particularly difficult to treat. Many oncologists remain reluctant to prescribe hormone replacement therapy, although there is no direct evidence of it being detrimental. Megestrol acetate at low doses of 40 mg daily is a useful treatment. Some SSRI antidepressants have also shown activity. Acupuncture is also worthwhile for some patients.

Tamoxifen is associated with a three- to four-fold increase in the risk of thromboembolic phenomena (deep vein thrombosis, pulmonary embolism) and endometrial cancer in postmenopausal women. The aromatase inhibitor drugs (anastrozole, letrozole and exemestane) are associated with a risk of osteoporosis and an assessment of bone mineral density is advisable in those on these as an adjuvant treatment. They are also associated with troublesome musculoskeletal symptoms such as joint stiffness and sexual dysfunction (vaginal dryness, loss of libido).

IMMUNOTHERAPY

Trastuzumab can cause allergic reactions at the time of infusion and potentially reversible declines in baseline cardiac contractility. Lapatinib can cause diarrhoea, rashes and pneumonitis. Bevacizumab can cause hypertension, proteinuria and abnormalities in blood clotting.

PROGNOSIS

The prognosis from breast cancer has improved significantly in a stepwise manner decade on decade.

Breast cancer is a good example of how cancer outcomes can be substantially improved by combining together a number of small advantages from a variety of treatment improvements over the years. Approximately one in three women diagnosed with breast cancer would die if no adjuvant therapy was administered. The combination of radiotherapy and systemic therapies will lead to a significant improvement in survival by independently contributing additional odds reductions in recurrence and in turn mortality. The following adverse prognostic factors should be considered:

- Young age (<35 years) at diagnosis
- Increasing TNM stage

- Poorly differentiated tumours
- Lymphatic vessel and/or vascular channel invasion
- Oestrogen and progesterone receptor negativity
- Positivity for the *HER2* oncogene

Prognostic models that incorporate these prognostic factors are available, e.g. predict breast cancer (https://breast.predict.nhs.uk/). These are widely used across the world to provide a consistent guide to 10-year disease outcomes. Figure 8.23 illustrates its usefulness in providing an objective and evidence-based insight into 10-year outcomes. There is now

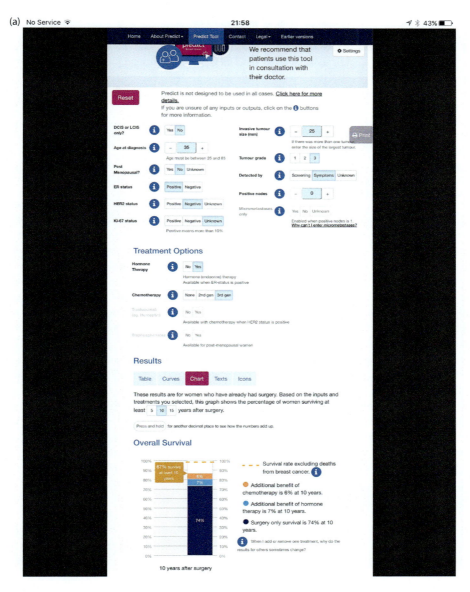

Figure 8.23 Examples of prognosis estimation using the Adjuvant software. (a) Example of a 35-year-old woman with a 2–3 cm Grade 3 node-negative oestrogen receptor-positive HER 2 negative cancer, showing the relative and absolute advantages of hormone therapy alone, chemotherapy alone and combined treatment versus no treatment. *(Continued)*

Breast cancer

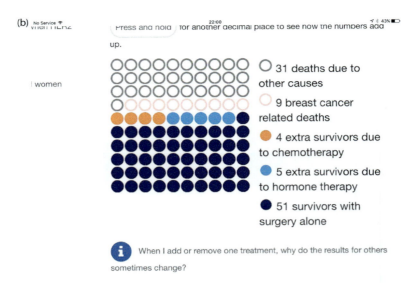

Figure 8.23 (Continued) Examples of prognosis estimation using the Adjuvant software. (b) Same scenario but for a 75-year-old woman. Note the much higher risk of dying of other causes over the next 10 years. Note also the smaller absolute survival advantage for each treatment option.

increasing use of gene 'signature' profiling to aid in prognostication. Examples include Oncotype DX®, Mammaprint®, Prosigna (PAM50), Mammatype, NexCourse Breast (IHC4-AQUA) and IHC4. The test involves probing a sample of the primary cancer for a panel of genes, looking for a pattern of amplification or suppression that has been validated against known breast cancer outcomes. These tools are now used to aid decision-making in certain circumstances, e.g. whether to use chemotherapy or not in a patient with early breast cancer that is ER+ and node negative. Trials are ongoing to see if these tests can also be used to predict benefits of chemotherapy or patients that can avoid chemotherapy based on a low risk of recurrence determined by their gene profile in node-positive patients.

SCREENING

Screening should permit the diagnosis of a higher proportion of early stages of the disease. As early stage at diagnosis is an important favourable prognostic factor, and breast cancer has a defined non-invasive phase that is readily detectable by imaging; this should translate into a reduction in mortality from invasive breast cancer.

Breast self-examination (BSE) should be routinely practised by women at the same time each month to take account of the variation in breast size and consistency with the menstrual cycle. However, to date BSE has not conclusively been shown to have decreased breast cancer mortality and there has been concern about the stress of such a practice, together with the inevitably high false-positive rate and false-negative rate.

Mammography is a sensitive means of detecting carcinomas, often before the lump is palpable by the patient or clinician, thereby facilitating the detection of early breast cancers with a particularly good prognosis. In the United Kingdom, the National Breast Screening Programme screens all women aged 50–70 years with 3-yearly mammograms. This age range is being extended to 47–73 over the next few years. Women older than this can be screened on request. Such a programme should result in a mortality reduction of 20%–30%. There is at present no consensus as to what age premenopausal women should be included in a screening programme, as they tend to have dense breasts, which can obscure the radiological signs of early breast cancers; studies to date have indicated a much smaller impact on survival than in the >50 year age group. However, young women with a family history of breast cancer should be offered regular clinical assessments and mammographic screening at an earlier age. Digital mammography seems to lead to fewer false-positive results than traditional film-based mammography and is superior for young women with dense breasts. Ultrasonography is a poor substitute for mammography. In younger women with dense breasts, particularly those with *BRCA* gene mutations, magnetic resonance mammography is the optimum screening modality.

PREVENTION

Patients with a strong family history of breast cancer should be referred to a specialist genetics clinic for risk assessment, counselling and identification of other susceptible family members. Those shown (by gene testing or by statistical modelling) to be *BRCA* gene mutation carriers are at sufficient lifetime risk of developing breast cancer to be considered for bilateral mastectomy, which very substantially reduces the risk, although it does not eliminate it completely.

Breast cancer is sufficiently common to make prevention a worthwhile exercise. Any method of prevention must be easy to comply with, free of short- and long-term adverse effects and be cost effective. The difference in dietary fat intake between the Western world and Africa and Asia contributes to the geographical variation in incidence. A reduction in the proportion of daily calories obtained from dietary fat could make a significant impact on the incidence of breast cancer. Dietary manipulation has the advantage of being inherently cost effective, and can reduce morbidity and mortality from cardiovascular and cerebrovascular diseases and colorectal cancer. Uncertainty exists as to when such a dietary adjustment should be instituted and for how long, although its other advantages make it a desirable lifelong commitment. Reducing body mass index and alcohol consumption, and regular strenuous exercise may all help prevent breast cancer, although this is yet to be proven in prospective trials.

Breast cancer is one of the few malignant diseases for which a large randomized trial has shown that chemoprevention is not only feasible but also effective. Tamoxifen 20 mg daily as adjuvant therapy has been conclusively shown to decrease the risk of contralateral breast cancer. This observation has been extrapolated to the prevention setting where a large (15,000 women) placebo-controlled, double-blind, randomized trial has shown this regimen to significantly reduce the risk of developing DCIS and invasive breast cancer. There is an increased risk of thromboembolic disease and endometrial cancer in women receiving tamoxifen. Tamoxifen incidentally reduces cholesterol levels and helps maintain bone mineral density in postmenopausal women, and could therefore have additional health benefits. The osteoporosis-prevention drug raloxifene has also been shown to reduce substantially the risk of developing breast cancer, and has the advantage of not causing hyperstimulation of the endometrium. The aromatase inhibitor anastrozole also reduces the risk of contralateral breast cancer in women receiving the drug as treatment for metastatic breast cancer. Anastrozole could therefore be a promising prevention strategy for postmenopausal women.

FURTHER READING

NCCN Clinical Practice Guidelines in Oncology (NCCN Guidelines®) Breast Cancer Version 4. 2018 https://www.nccn.org/patients/guidelines/content/PDF/stage_0_breast.pdf.

NICE guideline [NG101] 2018: Early and locally advanced breast cancer: Diagnosis and management. https://www.nice.org.uk/guidance/ng101.

Primary breast cancer: ESMO clinical practice guidelines for diagnosis, treatment and follow up. *Ann Oncol*, 2011, 22 (suppl 6) vi22–vi24.

3rd ESO-ESMO international consensus guidelines for advanced breast cancer (ABC3). *Ann Oncol*, 2017, 28 (1), 16–33.

SELF-ASSESSMENT QUESTIONS

1. Which three of the following statements are true about the epidemiology of breast cancer?
   a. It is the third commonest cancer in the United Kingdom
   b. 1 in 1000 cases will arise in men
   c. Environmental factors are important causes
   d. Genetic predisposition is an uncommon causative factor

Breast cancer

e. There is no association with smoking tobacco
f. Hormonal influences are important causes
g. Radiation exposure does not cause breast cancer

2. Which one of the following statements is true about the pathology of breast cancer?
   a. Lobular carcinomas are more common than ductal
   b. Paget disease of the nipple is almost always associated with an underlying cancer
   c. Most are squamous carcinomas
   d. LCIS is frequently detected by a mammogram
   e. Inflammatory cancers account for 10% of cases

3. Which three of the following factors are associated with an increased probability of lymph node spread?
   a. Increasing tumour size
   b. Tumours arising in men
   c. Lymphovascular invasion in and around the primary tumour
   d. Medial quadrant breast cancers
   e. Screen-detected cancers
   f. High-grade cancers
   g. Cancers arising close to the nipple

4. Which one of the following statements are true about the spread of breast cancer?
   a. Distant relapses can occur more than 10 years after presentation
   b. The brain is the commonest site for metastatic spread
   c. Bone metastases may be lytic or sclerotic
   d. Lobular cancer is more likely to spread to the lymph nodes
   e. PTS with bone metastases only have a better prognosis that PTS with lung metastases only

5. Which three of the following statements are true about the presentation of breast cancer?
   a. There will always be a palpable lump
   b. A breast lump in a woman will usually be malignant
   c. Most cases will present with palpable lymph nodes
   d. The cancer is usually painful
   e. The supraclavicular lymph nodes could be enlarged
   f. Can cause a blood-stained nipple discharge
   g. There might be distant metastases at diagnosis

6. Which one of the following is true about the use of trastuzumab in breast cancer?
   a. Most patients benefit from it
   b. Heart toxicity is common
   c. It is only used in advanced forms of the disease
   d. Brain metastases are a particular problem
   e. Cannot be used concurrently with chemotherapy

7. Which three of the following statements are true about hormone treatments for breast cancer?
   a. Progesterone is contraindicated in women with a history of breast cancer
   b. Letrozole and exemestane are both aromatase inhibitors
   c. Adjuvant hormone therapy reduces the risk of distant metastatic relapse
   d. Aromatase inhibitors cause endometrial cancer
   e. Tamoxifen is associated with an increased risk of ovarian cancer
   f. Hormone therapy is not usually necessary if the patient receives chemotherapy
   g. Tamoxifen reduces the risk of contralateral breast cancers

8. Which one of the following is not an important prognostic factor?
   a. Tumour size
   b. Histological grade
   c. Centrally located tumour
   d. TNM stage
   e. Age at diagnosis

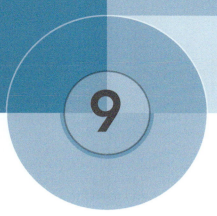

Gastrointestinal cancer

CARCINOMA OF THE OESOPHAGUS

EPIDEMIOLOGY

Each year in the United Kingdom there are around 9000 cases of oesophageal cancer, 6200 cases in men and 3000 cases in women, accounting for 3% of all cancer cases and leading to a total of 8000 deaths per annum. Tumours of the upper third of the oesophagus are much more common in females. The highest incidence is over the age of 85 years with a lifetime risk of 1 in 50 for males and 1 in 96 for females in the United Kingdom. Geographically, the highest incidence is found in Russia, Turkey, China, Iran and southern Africa.

AETIOLOGY

Around 60% of cases of oesophageal cancer are due to preventable causes:

- One-third is caused by *tobacco smoking*; smokers in Europe have a relative risk of 4.2 compared to never smokers for squamous oesophageal cancer. It is also higher in non-smoking tobacco users, e.g. betel nut, snuff and snus.
- Thirteen percent by *alcohol* drinking and there is synergy between smoking and alcohol consumption. Carcinogenic contaminants of alcoholic drinks have also been implicated in some cases, e.g. the home-made beer consumed by the Xhosa people in Transkei.
- *Obesity* is related to over a quarter of cases.
- In *achalasia* there is chronic stasis and pooling of food and secretions in a dilated oesophagus owing to a loss of oesophageal motility. The increased risk of cancer is due to the prolonged contact of the mucosa with carcinogens within the food or produced from food by the action of bacteria.
- *Patterson–Brown–Kelly syndrome* (Plummer–Vinson syndrome) is characterized by koilonychia, iron-deficiency anaemia, the presence of an 'oesophageal web' in the upper third of the oesophagus on barium swallow, and is usually seen in women. It leads to a carcinoma of the upper third of the oesophagus typically in the postcricoid region.
- *Tylosis* is a very rare, dominantly inherited condition characterized by palmar and plantar hyperkeratosis and a strong predisposition to oesophageal carcinoma.
- *Barrett's oesophagus* is characterized by glandular metaplasia of the squamous epithelium of the lower third of the oesophagus, usually in response to chronic gastro-oesophageal reflux from a hiatus hernia. Patients are at risk of developing an adenocarcinoma of the oesophagus.

PATHOLOGY

Approximately 40%–50% of tumours arise in the middle third of the oesophagus, 40%–50% in the lower third and less than 10% in the upper third; the tumour appears nodular, ulcerating or diffusely infiltrative. If there is oesophageal obstruction, the proximal oesophagus is frequently dilated and contains food debris. A fistula can exist between the oesophagus and trachea or bronchial tree, and there may be evidence of an aspiration pneumonia particularly in the lower lobes of the lungs. Cancers of the upper two-thirds of the oesophagus are invariably squamous cell carcinomas. Cancers in the lower third are most commonly squamous but one-third is adenocarcinomas, which may have arisen in an area of metaplasia such as Barrett's oesophagus. These must be distinguished from adenocarcinoma of the proximal stomach that has infiltrated the oesophagus. The histological spectrum of oesophageal cancer is changing with an increasing proportion being classified as adenocarcinomas.

NATURAL HISTORY

The tumour will spread within the oesophagus both longitudinally and circumferentially, eventually resulting in complete oesophageal obstruction. Invasion through the deeper layers of the oesophageal wall results in spread to the surrounding mediastinal structures such as the trachea, main bronchi (especially left), pleura, lung, vertebrae and great vessels. Insidious spread along the submucosa is common and can lead to skip lesions some distance from the main tumour. The pattern of lymphatic involvement reflects the complex blood supply to the oesophagus. Tumours of the upper third spread to the deep cervical and supraclavicular nodes, those of the middle third to the mediastinal, paratracheal and subcarinal nodes and those of the lower third to the nodes of the coeliac axis below the diaphragm. The venous drainage of parts of the oesophagus is into the portal circulation and so the liver is the most common site of distant metastases, although the lungs and skeleton may also be involved.

SYMPTOMS

Dysphagia is the most common presenting symptom. A middle-aged or elderly patient complaining of this symptom should be considered to have oesophageal cancer until proven otherwise and referral to a gastroenterologist is mandatory. The symptom begins insidiously as a sensation of food sticking, usually when solids such as meat have been eaten, progresses so that there is difficulty with softer foods/liquids, and can be associated with retrosternal discomfort owing to stretching of the oesophagus and increased peristalsis. Regurgitation usually accompanies severe dysphagia. Retrosternal discomfort is followed by effortless regurgitation of the oesophageal contents. These do not taste sour as they have not entered the stomach. This contrasts with gastro-oesophageal reflux where there will be a strong taste of acid.

Weight loss is due to both reduced caloric intake owing to dysphagia and/or regurgitation and the non-specific effects of malignancy.

Recurrent aspiration is a problem in patients with proximal tumours leading to overflow into the upper respiratory tract or with a fistula connecting the oesophagus to the lower respiratory tract. The patient experiences a severe bout of coughing within a short time of swallowing, and may expectorate solid material from the food bolus. Both predispose to recurrent chest infections that can be fatal.

In the United Kingdom around 20% of cases present as an emergency.

SIGNS

There is often evidence of malnutrition, the degree of which is dependent on the duration and severity of dysphagia and whether there has been a history of alcoholism. In cases of oesophageal obstruction the patient could even be dehydrated owing to poor fluid intake. Women with Plummer–Vinson syndrome can appear anaemic and have koilonychia, while alcoholics may have stigmata of chronic liver disease. There is usually no palpable evidence of disease although an epigastric mass is sometimes palpable in tumours of the lower third of the oesophagus and if there are large intra-abdominal lymph nodes. The cervical and supraclavicular lymph nodes should be palpated carefully. Hepatomegaly suggests metastatic disease but also fatty infiltration or cirrhosis in heavy drinkers.

DIFFERENTIAL DIAGNOSIS

Care has to be taken not to confuse a tumour arising from the oesophageal mucosa with a tumour arising from an adjacent structure and invading into the oesophagus, e.g. carcinoma of the left main bronchus (most often squamous or small cell carcinoma), carcinoma of the fundus of the stomach or gastro-oesophageal junction (adenocarcinoma). Other differential diagnoses include a benign oesophageal stricture owing to chronic gastro-oesophageal reflux, achalasia and hysteria, a diagnosis made only after excluding all other possible causes.

INVESTIGATIONS

BLOOD TESTS

Routine blood tests including full blood count, urine and liver function will be taken.

ENDOSCOPY

This is the investigation of choice. The oesophagus starts at the lower border of the cricoid cartilage at the level of the sixth cervical vertebra, approximately 15 cm from the incisor teeth. It is 25 cm in length, entering the stomach at the level of the tenth thoracic vertebra (i.e. approximately 40 cm from the incisors). Endoscopy allows a thorough assessment of the whole oesophagus. The tumour can be visualized directly, a biopsy taken for histology and brushings for cytology. It also allows a thorough evaluation of the stomach, which is particularly important in tumours of the lower third of the oesophagus, and is the most sensitive means of detecting small primary tumours and skip lesions. Endoscopic ultrasound is also a useful tool, allowing direct imaging of the tumour. It is particularly sensitive for determining the depth of invasion and involvement of first station lymph node groups.

Endoscopic mucosal resection should be undertaken to complete staging of small T1 oesophageal cancers and as definitive treatment of associated Barrett's oesophagus.

COMPUTED TOMOGRAPHY (CT) OF THE THORAX AND UPPER ABDOMEN

This provides information on the local extent of the disease with respect to invasion beyond the oesophagus and is of value in planning radiotherapy or surgery because it will also allow an assessment of the regional lymph nodes, liver, lungs and adrenals (Figure 9.1).

MRI OF THE THORAX AND UPPER ABDOMEN

This will be useful in the preoperative assessment of candidates for radical surgery. The improvement in soft-tissue contrast will aid in patient selection and surgical planning.

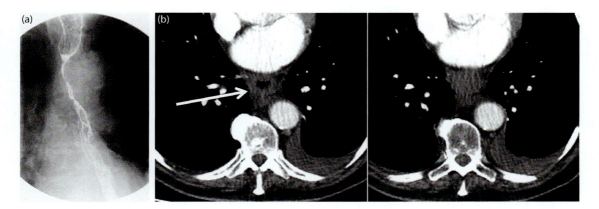

Figure 9.1 Carcinoma of the oesophagus. (a) Barium swallow showing an irregular, malignant stricture of the middle third of the oesophagus. Note the small pool of barium at the top of the stricture. (b) Sequential CT scans showing oesopahgeal cancer (arrowed) and on subsequent scan complete occlusion of the oesophageal lumen.

POSITRON EMISSION TOMOGRAPHY (PET)

This is routinely performed to complete whole-body staging prior to curative surgery. It has the advantage of disclosing the presence of metastatic disease at occult sites in the body (e.g. adrenal glands, perigastric, mediastinal and coeliac lymph nodes) and can show foci of active cancer in other areas where CT can be equivocal (e.g. liver).

BRONCHOSCOPY

This could be necessary to exclude direct invasion of the posterior tracheal wall and left main bronchus when the operability of a tumour of the upper or middle third is being considered.

STAGING

The TNM staging system is most frequently used:

- Tis: Carcinoma *in situ*
- T0: No evidence of primary
- TX: Primary cannot be assessed
- T1: Involving lamina propria/submucosa
- T2: Involving muscularis propria
- T3: Involving adventitia
- T4: Involving adjacent structures
- N0: No regional lymphadenopathy
- N1: Regional lymph node involvement
- M0: No distant metastases
- M1: Distant metastases

TREATMENT

Many patients will be poorly nourished, which lessens their tolerance of radical treatment and therefore referral to a dietician is advisable in all cases. A liquidizer may help the patient to continue eating food prepared at home. It may be necessary for the patient to be given liquid dietary supplements to maintain calorie intake, and enteral feeding via a nasogastric tube or a percutaneous gastrostomy catheter might be the only means of maintaining nutrition.

RADICAL TREATMENT

Surgery

Surgery should be offered to patients with stage IbN0 adenocarcinoma and may also be considered for stage Ib squamous carcinoma. Around 20% of patients diagnosed with oesophageal cancer will undergo primary resection. This is stage-related and almost 50% of stage I patients will have primary surgery.

Specific contraindications to surgery include:

- Poor performance status
- Severe malnutrition
- Vocal cord palsy, indicating infiltration/pressure on the recurrent laryngeal nerve from tumour spreading beyond the oesophagus
- Broncho-oesophageal fistula
- Invasion of great vessels (aorta, superior vena cava), pericardium
- Cervical/coeliac node involvement clinically or radiologically
- Distant metastases

Tumours of the middle third have historically been treated by an 'Ivor Lewis' two-stage oesophagectomy. The stomach is mobilized via upper abdominal incision, the oesophagus approached via the right fifth intercostal space, the tumour resected allowing a 5 cm margin of macroscopically normal oesophagus, and the oesophagus then re-anastomosed.

For tumours of the lower third, oesophago-gastrectomy is more usual with re-anastomosis of the transected oesophagus. In experienced hands and with appropriate patient selection, the operative mortality will be <5%. Minimally invasive techniques using thoracoscopic or a combined thoracoscopic–laparoscopic approach should be considered with which postoperative recovery and rehabilitation are faster.

Radiotherapy

Curative treatment uses chemoradiation, delivering concurrent chemotherapy with the course of radiation. This should be considered preoperatively for patients who should undergo surgical resection for adenocarcinomas greater than T1N0 and as a definitive treatment option instead of surgery in squamous carcinomas. It can also be used for tumours that are not amenable to surgery. Around 30% of patients with oesophageal cancer receive radiotherapy. Although distant metastases are a contraindication to radical radiotherapy, extra-oesophageal invasion can still be encompassed within the radiation high-dose zone. Treatment is given daily over 5–6 weeks.

Chemotherapy

Chemotherapy should be offered to patients before (neoadjuvant) or before and after having radical surgery. The common drugs used are a combination of epirubicin, cisplatin and continuous venous infusion of 5FU.

PALLIATIVE TREATMENT

Dysphagia and regurgitation are the symptoms most often requiring treatment. Both are extremely distressing and can erode the quality of life significantly.

Surgery

Endoscopic dilatation and insertion of a self-expanding stent give rapid relief of dysphagia. Laser therapy can be given to coagulate a bleeding tumour or to unblock an obstructed oesophagus. An endoprosthesis such as a rigid Atkinson tube can be inserted to maintain oesophageal patency and is particularly useful in relieving recurrent aspiration because of a fistula.

Radiotherapy

A short course of radiotherapy relieves dysphagia in most patients with acceptable short-term morbidity and can usually be repeated if necessary. This may be given as a course of external beam irradiation or intraluminal brachytherapy whereby a high-activity radiation source is inserted directly into the oesophagus through a plastic tube called an applicator. This may be positioned directly using an endoscope or with imaging via a nasogastric tube. Radiotherapy should also be considered after insertion of a stent for longer term disease control.

Chemotherapy

This should be offered to patients with advanced oesophageal cancer and good performance status. Capecitabine or 5FU with cisplatin or oxaliplatin and epirubicin (ECX or EOX) are used as first-line treatment in the palliative setting.

Patients with metastatic adenocarcinoma of the lower oesophagus should have their tumour tested for HER-2, and if positive trastuzumab be given with chemotherapy.

CASE HISTORY

OESOPHAGEAL CANCER

A 60-year-old man with a history of chronic bronchitis develops dysphagia. He experiences retrosternal discomfort when he swallows solid foodstuffs, e.g. meat and bread. He has a long history of gastro-oesophageal reflux and had a barium swallow some years earlier which confirmed a hiatus hernia. He initially self-medicates himself with a proton pump inhibitor in addition to a mucosal surface protectant. His discomfort temporarily improves but then worsens and is accompanied by regurgitation of food.

He is referred to a gastroenterologist. Endoscopy reveals a polypoid tumour at 32–36 cm obstructing the lumen of the oesophagus with no extension into the stomach. Biopsy confirms a poorly differentiated adenocarcinoma with some evidence of an underlying Barrett's oesophagus and chronic oesophagitis. CT scan shows no evidence of mediastinal or abdominal lymphadenopathy and no evidence of liver metastases.

He is initially treated with chemoradiation over a 5-week period during which time his symptoms improve significantly. A repeat endoscopy 6 weeks later reveals no obvious mucosal abnormality and random biopsies show chronic inflammatory cells alone. At this time, his shortness of breath is worse than usual and he has a dry cough. Chest x-ray confirms opacification corresponding to the radiation fields suggesting a degree of radiation pneumonitis. In view of an apparent pathological complete response, and his respiratory compromise, he is not deemed a suitable candidate for major surgery.

Gastrointestinal cancer

> Eighteen months later, he presents with recurrent dysphagia. He is referred to a dietician for dietary advice. Endoscopy confirms a recurrence at the same level as previously, which is dilated. Adenocarcinoma is confirmed histologically; 6 weeks later, his symptoms have recurred. An oesophageal stent is inserted that provides good symptom control for 3 months. He then develops right upper quadrant pain and anorexia. Liver ultrasound confirms hepatic metastases. He declines further chemotherapy. There is a symptomatic improvement with dexamethasone but he dies of his disease 4 weeks later.

TUMOUR-RELATED COMPLICATIONS

Malnutrition can be caused by chronic dysphagia. Invasion of tumour into the adjacent main bronchi sometimes leads to a broncho-oesophageal fistula (Figure 9.2). Aspiration of food into the respiratory tract leads to pneumonia, which may be further complicated by lung abscess and empyema. Haemorrhage is a rare but potentially fatal local tumour complication.

TREATMENT-RELATED COMPLICATIONS

SURGERY

Loss of oesophageal integrity after surgical resection can lead to a fistula or mediastinitis which is often fatal, while pneumothorax, pulmonary collapse and pneumonia can complicate a thoracotomy.

RADIOTHERAPY

During treatment, it is inevitable that the patient will experience some worsening of dysphagia owing to a radiation oesophagitis. This can be minimized by avoidance of very hot or cold food/fluids, and relieved by local anaesthetic mucilage. Anorexia, nausea and vomiting are likely if stomach or liver is included in the radiation fields, and will be helped by a regular anti-emetic. Radiation pneumonitis is uncommon and usually subclinical, although it can cause a dry cough, fever and dyspnoea. Oesophageal stricture can occur 6 months or more after radiotherapy giving rise to dysphagia, and needs to be distinguished from a recurrent tumour. This will be confirmed by endoscopy when dilatation can be performed simultaneously.

CHEMOTHERAPY

Apart from drug-specific toxicity, combined modality treatment with chemotherapy and radiotherapy leads to more severe acute oesophageal reaction, which can compromise nutrition and require supportive therapy.

PROGNOSIS

Survival rates in the United Kingdom have tripled over the past 40 years. Overall 5-year survival is 15% and 12% will survive for more than 10 years after diagnosis. Survival rates decline with age.

SCREENING/PREVENTION

Patients with Barrett's oesophagus and achalasia should be offered annual endoscopic examination, particularly those with high-grade dysplastic

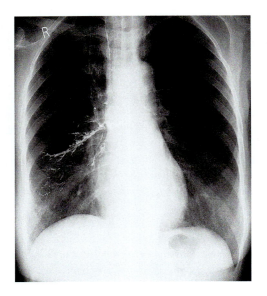

Figure 9.2 Broncho-oesophageal fistula. Chest radiograph taken after a gastrografin swallow. Contrast has leaked into the right side of the bronchial tree.

features because of their high risk of developing carcinoma. Routine endoscopic screening of a population is not a proven strategy, and should be balanced against the risks of the procedure such as perforation, aspiration, vasovagal events and bleeding.

Informing the public of the risks of tobacco and alcohol could reduce the incidence of oesophageal cancer. Other factors associated with reducing the risk of oesophageal cancer include a diet rich in green vegetables and long-term use of non-steroidal anti-inflammatory drugs.

RARE TUMOURS

ADENOID CYSTIC CARCINOMA

This is a tumour arising from the mucous glands of the mucosa and is of the same type as that arising in the parotid salivary glands and elsewhere.

SMALL CELL CARCINOMA

Although infiltration from an underlying lung primary should be considered, a primary tumour of this type has been described.

MELANOMA

This is a rare site for mucosal melanoma. Prognosis will be very poor owing to advanced stage at presentation.

CARCINOID

This is an uncommon site for this rare tumour. It should be treated as elsewhere by surgical resection.

LEIOMYOSARCOMA

This tumour arises from the smooth muscle fibres of the oesophageal wall. It is best treated by radical surgery combined with radiotherapy.

CARCINOMA OF THE STOMACH

EPIDEMIOLOGY

Each year in the United Kingdom there are 6700 cases of stomach cancer, 4400 cases in men and 2400 cases in women, accounting for 2% of all cancer cases and leading to a total of 4400 deaths per annum. Incidence rates are highest in those over 85 years. The incidence of stomach cancer in the United Kingdom has fallen by more than a quarter in the past 10 years and is forecast to fall by another 17% over the next 20 years. The O blood group confers some protection against developing stomach cancer while the A blood group is associated with a higher incidence of the diffuse form of stomach cancer. It is associated with a deprivation index in the United Kingdom and more common in black races compared to white with the lowest incidence in Asians. The incidence is however very high in Japan and Chile.

AETIOLOGY

Around one-half of all cases in the United Kingdom are preventable:

- Fifteen percent are due to *smoking*.
- Six percent are associated with *obesity*.
- Forty percent are related to chronic infection with *Helicobacter pylori* infection.
- Around 9% of stomach cancers are positive for *Epstein–Barr virus*; its role in cancer development in the stomach being unclear.
- *Nitrosamines* have been implicated in stomach cancer, as has a diet rich in *smoked and pickled foodstuffs*.
- Excessive *dietary salt* has been implicated.
- *Occupational exposure* to asbestos and chromium has been related to increased incidence of stomach cancer.
- Both *atrophic gastritis* and *achlorhydria* increase the risk of developing stomach cancer, in the case of pernicious anaemia five-fold. This could be related to bacterial overgrowth and increased production of endogenous carcinogens.
- *Partial gastrectomy* or *gastroenterostomy* is also associated with an increased cancer risk, probably owing to a chronic reflux of bile salts into the stomach.

An adenoma–carcinoma sequence has been seen but is much rarer than in the large bowel.

Gastrointestinal cancer

PATHOLOGY

Stomach cancers usually form discrete ulcerating lesions, but can be nodular or polypoid. They are occasionally diffusely infiltrating leading to obliteration of the stomach lumen. Fifty percent arise in the pyloric region while, of those arising in the body, most are found along the lesser curvature; 90% are adenocarcinomas, subclassified into intestinal (well differentiated) and diffuse (undifferentiated). Around 5% are squamous carcinoma or adenoacanthoma (adenocarcinoma with areas of squamous metaplasia). There is, sometimes, evidence of prior intestinal metaplasia and carcinoma *in situ* in the surrounding mucosa.

NATURAL HISTORY

Cancers spread longitudinally and circumferentially within the stomach and, as with carcinoma of the oesophagus, insidious submucosal spread is frequent. Occasionally, this leads to diffuse infiltration of the whole stomach with luminal narrowing and rigidity of the stomach wall, and is known as 'linitis plastica'. Progressive invasion into the muscle layer of the stomach wall eventually leads to invasion of the serosa and in turn invasion of adjacent viscera, such as the omentum, pancreas, spleen, left kidney and adrenal glands. Invasion superiorly by a tumour of the fundus can result in occlusion of the lower third of the oesophagus leading to dysphagia and regurgitation. There is a propensity for transcoelomic spread with diffuse peritoneal seeding leading to ascites (Figure 9.3) and ovarian deposits (Krukenberg tumours – Figure 9.4), particularly with the signet ring variant. Spread to the regional lymph nodes (gastric, gastroduodenal, splenic and coeliac groups) occurs early in the natural history, and Virchow's node in the left supraclavicular fossa can be involved (Troisier's sign). Distant spread occurs in the liver via the portal venous circulation, lungs, bone, brain and skin.

SYMPTOMS

About one-third of patients in the United Kingdom present as an emergency most commonly with haematemesis. Others may present with non-specific gastrointestinal symptoms such as epigastric discomfort, anorexia, nausea, vomiting and weight loss, which are frequently confused with a benign condition such as peptic ulceration or gastritis, and can even be relieved by the antacids, H2-antagonists or proton pump inhibitors prescribed for these conditions. There may be symptoms of iron-deficiency anaemia, and stomach cancer should always be considered in the assessment of such patients. A more acute presentation can occur with stomach perforation, haematemesis and melaena.

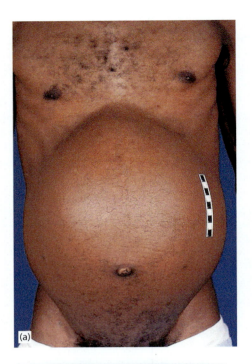
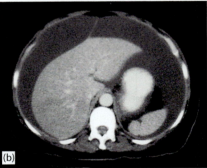

Figure 9.3 Massive ascites. (a) Frontal view of abdomen. (b) Transverse CT image of abdomen.

Carcinoma of the stomach

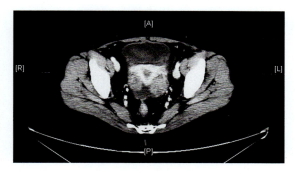

Figure 9.4 Krukenberg tumours. CT image of the pelvis. There are bilateral ovarian masses representing metastatic spread from gastric cancer.

SIGNS

Signs of weight loss and cachexia are a frequent finding. An epigastric mass might be palpable as can be lymph nodes in the left supraclavicular fossa. The liver is sometimes enlarged, tender and knobbly, suggesting metastatic infiltration, and there may be ascites. Non-metastatic manifestations such as dermatomyositis and acanthosis nigricans might also be seen.

DIFFERENTIAL DIAGNOSIS

This includes:

- Inflammatory conditions, e.g. peptic ulcer
- Other malignant gastric tumours, e.g. lymphoma and leiomyosarcoma
- Benign gastric tumours, e.g. leiomyoma and carcinoid

INVESTIGATIONS

ROUTINE BLOOD TESTS

These include evaluation of full blood count, renal and liver function.

FIBREOPTIC ENDOSCOPY

This allows direct visualization of the gastric mucosa with a more accurate assessment of the macroscopic appearances of an abnormality. It also allows biopsy and brushings for cytology to give a tissue diagnosis.

CT SCAN OF THE THORAX AND ABDOMEN

This provides information regarding invasion beyond the stomach and whether the regional lymph nodes are enlarged, and thereby helps determine whether the tumour is operable (also see the next section). It will also screen for distant metastases in liver, lungs and peritoneum.

LAPAROSCOPY

This facilitates direct visualization of the stomach, regional lymph nodes, liver and peritoneal surfaces. It is complementary to high-quality cross-sectional imaging and is important in a condition with a high rate of lymphatic involvement and transcoelomic spread. The revelation of an otherwise occult disease might in turn spare the patient unnecessary surgery.

STAGING

The TNM system is widely used:

- Tis: Carcinoma *in situ*
- T0: No evidence of primary
- TX: Primary cannot be assessed
- T1: Involving lamina propria/submucosa
- T2: Involving muscularis propria/muscularis mucosa
- T3: Penetrates serosa invading subserosa
- T4: (a) has just grown through stomach wall; (b) has invaded nearby structures involving adjacent structures
- N0: No regional lymphadenopathy
- N1: 1 to 2 regional lymph nodes involved
- N2: 3 to 6 regional lymph nodes involved
- N3: 7 or more regional lymph nodes involved
  - M3a: 7–15 regional lymph nodes involved
  - M3b: 16 or more regional lymph nodes involved
- M0: No distant metastases
- M1: Distant metastases

TREATMENT

RADICAL TREATMENT

Surgery

Curative surgery is undertaken in a little over 20% of patients in the United Kingdom. Surgery may be attempted in stage 1B–III tumours in the absence of metastatic disease. Early well-differentiated stage Ia tumours ≤2 cm may be treated by endoscopic resection. Otherwise partial or total gastrectomy is performed in operable cases depending on the size and site of the tumour to achieve a 5–8 cm clear margin. It is recommended that when undertaking curative surgery a D2 nodal resection is also considered which will remove perigastric lymph nodes plus those along the left gastric, common hepatic and splenic arteries and coeliac axis with a minimum of 15 nodes.

Laparoscopic surgery is an alternative to open gastrectomy. There are fewer cases of ileus and postoperative chest infections after laparoscopic surgery but it might result in fewer lymph nodes being removed. Long-term outcomes from ongoing trials are therefore awaited.

Radiotherapy

Radiotherapy has no curative role in treatment owing to the dose-limiting toxicity induced in the stomach and adjacent structures such as the small bowel and transverse colon when a high dose of radiation is administered. Adjuvant postoperative radiotherapy does not significantly improve survival but does reduce the risk of local recurrence approximately three-fold. One large, randomized trial indicated that postoperative chemoradiation (CRT) substantially improved overall survival in high-risk completely resected locally advanced adenocarcinoma of the stomach and gastroesophageal junction. In the United States, CRT regimen is now the standard of care, but less widespread elsewhere.

Chemotherapy

Preoperative chemotherapy is the standard of care. A common schedule is epirubicin, cisplatin and capecitabine (ECX). Adjuvant chemotherapy postoperatively may be an alternative but is more commonly combined with radiotherapy in the adjuvant setting.

PALLIATIVE TREATMENT

Surgery

Intestinal bypass surgery (e.g. gastrojejunostomy) is effective at relieving gastric outflow obstruction while gastrectomy may be justified in the presence of metastatic disease when massive bleeding cannot be controlled by less invasive methods.

Laser therapy is particularly useful for the photocoagulation of a persistently bleeding tumour or debulking of a large tumour that is narrowing the oesophageal lumen. An oesophageal endoprosthesis is occasionally of benefit for a tumour of the upper stomach occluding the oesophagus from below.

Radiotherapy

Radiotherapy is valuable in relieving the local symptoms of inoperable disease such as dysphagia, haemorrhage or pain owing to retroperitoneal infiltration.

Chemotherapy

As with other solid tumours, there is some evidence suggesting that immediate chemotherapy confers a survival advantage compared with best supportive care and is of value in relieving symptoms from metastatic disease, particularly for lung and liver metastases. Common schedules are epirubicin, cisplatin, 5FU (ECF), epirubicin, oxaliplatin, 5FU (ECX) or epirubicin, oxaliplatin and capecitabine (EOX), which appear broadly equivalent to each other. Second-line chemotherapy should be considered for progressive disease using taxane or irinotecan.

About 10%–15% of gastric cancers are HER-2 positive, and in these cases trastuzumab should be added to any chemotherapy regime.

TUMOUR-RELATED COMPLICATIONS

Haemorrhage can be life threatening if a major gastric vessel is eroded, while chronic blood loss will lead to iron-deficiency anaemia with a reduced serum ferritin. Invasion through the stomach wall into the peritoneal cavity sometimes leads to leakage of gastric contents and an acute peritonitis. Pyloric stenosis can lead to gastric outflow obstruction, eventually leading to episodes of projectile vomiting, visible peristalsis, a 'succussion splash' and obstruction. Mucin secretion by the tumour might rarely result in activation of the plasmin/plasminogen cascade, leading to a disseminated intravascular coagulation manifested by abnormal clotting, thrombocytopenia and raised fibrin degradation products (see Chapter 8).

TREATMENT-RELATED COMPLICATIONS

SURGERY

Loss of stomach volume will lead to a feeling of fullness after small portions of food, while loss of gastric acidity can predispose to iron deficiency. Impaired intrinsic factor production leads to vitamin B12 deficiency secondary to impaired absorption at the terminal ileum resulting in a macrocytic anaemia, while impaired digestion can result in malabsorption and a 'dumping syndrome' owing to hypoglycaemia. Sternal ulceration and ultimately a second malignancy might occur.

RADIOTHERAPY

During treatment the patient will experience some degree of anorexia, nausea and vomiting. High doses of radiation to the stomach can result in chronic gastritis. The left kidney might receive a dose sufficient to impair its function permanently, but this will only be relevant if the right kidney function is subnormal. Radiation enteritis is also a recognized complication.

CHEMOTHERAPY

Drug-specific toxicity.

PROGNOSIS

Overall, around 20% of patients will survive for 5 years and 15% will survive for 10 years or more after a diagnosis of stomach cancer. The survival rates have increased dramatically from around 5%–15% in the past 40 years. Early gastric cancer has a 5-year survival of over 70%. Adverse prognostic factors include increasing tumour stage at presentation, unresectable disease, diffuse morphology and poor tumour differentiation. It also decreases with age from 35% for <50 years to only 8% for over 80 years.

SCREENING/PREVENTION

A screening programme of double contrast barium examination of the stomach and gastroscopy has been successfully implemented in Japan. This has led to a greater proportion of early cancers being detected, resulting in a decline in mortality. The efficacy of screening in Western populations has yet to be proven.

RARE TUMOURS

GASTROINTESTINAL STROMAL TUMOUR (GIST)

GISTs are mesenchymal neoplasms occurring in later life: 70% arise in the stomach and 25% in the small intestine. They express a growth factor receptor with tyrosine kinase activity (c-kit) which can be detected with CD117 immunohistochemistry. Their uncontrolled cell proliferation makes them highly malignant tumours that are relatively resistant to conventional treatments. They typically take up glucose avidly and therefore PET imaging is a sensitive way of visualizing them (Figure 9.5). However,

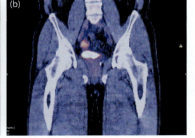

Figure 9.5 GIST tumour. PET scan showing high glucose metabolism within a GIST tumour arising just above the bladder superimposed on the CT anatomy for spatial reference. (a) Transverse view. (b) Coronal view.

significant responses and long-term survivors are achieved with the antibody imatinib (Glivec®) which targets c-kit. Consideration should therefore be given to identifying such tumours when usual sites or histological patterns of gastrointestinal malignancy are diagnosed, so that the few individuals with this disease can be identified and treated appropriately.

LEIOMYOMA

This is a benign tumour arising from smooth muscle of the stomach wall, often found incidentally during investigation of the upper gastrointestinal tract but it may ulcerate leading to haematemesis.

CARCINOID

The stomach is a very uncommon site for carcinoid tumours, which are best treated surgically (see Chapter 14).

LYMPHOMA

The stomach is a common site for extranodal lymphoma – usually a low-grade tumour mucosal associated lymphoid tissue (MALT-oma). This is associated with *H. pylori* infection and remissions can be obtained by helicobacter eradication treatment before considering standard lymphoma management (see Chapter 16).

CARCINOMA OF THE PANCREAS

EPIDEMIOLOGY

Each year in the United Kingdom there are almost 10,000 cases of pancreatic cancer, evenly distributed between men and women, accounting for 3% of all cancer cases and leading to over 9000 deaths per annum. Most patients are over 50 years at diagnosis; the peak incidence being over the age of 80 years. It is relatively rare in Asian populations.

AETIOLOGY

It is estimated that around one-third of cases are preventable:

- Smoking tobacco increases the risk of pancreatic cancer by more than 50%.
- High dietary fat and red meat consumption.
- Alcohol consumption; pancreatic cancer is 20% greater in people who consume more than 6 units per day.
- Obesity increases pancreatic cancer risk by 10% per 5-unit increase in the body mass index (BMI).
- The risk is three-fold greater in patients with chronic pancreatitis and doubled in diabetics. Gallstones are also associated with a 25% increase and metabolic syndrome patients have over 50% greater risk of pancreatic cancer.
- Previous surgery for peptic ulcer disease.
- Industrial exposure to the insecticide DDT.
- Familial cancer syndromes, e.g. Peutz–Jeghers syndrome, familial atypical multiple mole melanoma (FAMMM), Lynch syndrome and both BRCA 1 and BRCA 2 mutations. Risk is increased by over 70% in those with a first degree relative having pancreatic cancer and 45% in those with a first degree relative with prostate cancer.

PATHOLOGY

The tumour is well circumscribed or may diffusely infiltrate the pancreas; 30% arise in the head and are often associated with a dilated common bile duct, and 20% in the body or tail, the remainder being more diffuse in origin. Carcinoma arises from the ducts (90%) and glandular elements (10%) rather than the hormone-producing cells and is invariably a mucin-producing adenocarcinoma. There might be evidence of a chronic pancreatitis distal to any blocked pancreatic ducts and the majority stain for carcinoembryonic antigen (CEA).

NATURAL HISTORY

The tumour infiltrates diffusely through the gland, or might grow along the pancreatic duct system, eventually reaching the common bile duct and ampulla of Vater. The capsule can be breached leading to invasion of the stomach, duodenum, spleen, aorta and retroperitoneal tissues, and transcoelomic spread can occur with diffuse peritoneal involvement and ascites. Regional lymph nodes are frequently involved and include the pancreaticoduodenal, gastroduodenal, hepatic, superior mesenteric and coeliac groups. The majority have distant metastases by the time of diagnosis at sites including the liver, lungs, skin and brain.

SYMPTOMS

Pancreatic cancer is notorious for presenting late in the natural history of the disease, reflecting the deep-seated anatomical position of the pancreas and high prevalence of non-specific upper gastrointestinal symptoms in the population. Tumours of the head of the pancreas most frequently present with obstructive jaundice (progressive jaundice, dark urine, pale stools and itching) due to occlusion of the common bile duct. Tumours of the body and tail of the pancreas are more likely to present with pain, usually epigastric with radiation to the back. Extensive pancreatic infiltration or blockage of the major ducts will lead to malabsorption owing to exocrine dysfunction, which results in pale, fatty, offensive stools (steatorrhoea) which float on water and are difficult to flush away. Pancreatic endocrine dysfunction will lead to impaired glucose tolerance or diabetes mellitus in 20%, causing thirst, polyuria, nocturia and weight loss.

SIGNS

The patient often has jaundice, and the gallbladder may be palpable in the right upper quadrant of the abdomen, suggesting extrahepatic biliary obstruction that is not due to chronic gallstone disease (positive Courvoisier's sign). There will be pale stools on rectal examination and dark urine. Scratch marks on the trunk are a sign of pruritus owing to bile salt retention. A mass might be palpable in the epigastrium, fixed owing to its retroperitoneal location. Weight loss is common and can lead to profound cachexia. The liver might be enlarged and knobbly, consistent with metastatic infiltration. Petechiae, purpura and bruising are seen in advanced disease from disseminated intravascular coagulation (DIC).

DIFFERENTIAL DIAGNOSIS

Gallstones are a common cause of obstructive jaundice and abdominal pain, although they are not commonly associated with systemic symptoms and are not a cause of glucose intolerance. Benign tumours such as a glucagonoma, gastrinoma or VIPoma should also be considered.

INVESTIGATIONS

COMPUTED TOMOGRAPHY (CT) OF THE ABDOMEN

This characteristically shows dilatation of the common bile duct associated with a mass lesion in the head of the pancreas, a discrete mass in the body or tail of the pancreas, or diffuse enlargement of the pancreas as shown in Figure 9.6. All patients presenting with suspected pancreatic cancer should undergo this investigation as it is the best way of defining the extent of local invasion, the presence of enlarged regional lymph nodes and liver metastases. It also facilitates a fine needle biopsy when a definitive diagnosis cannot be made by less invasive procedures.

ENDOSCOPIC ULTRASOUND (EUS)

EUS is indicated if the CT is inconclusive and at the same time an ultrasound-guided biopsy can be taken if a pancreatic mass is identified.

FDG CT POSITRON EMISSION TOMOGRAPHY (CT-PET)

CT-PET will give additional information to CT alone not only in assessing the primary tumour for operability but also in identifying lymph node and distant metastases.

MAGNETIC RESONANCE IMAGING (MRI)

The superior soft-tissue resolution of MRI is best exploited when curative surgery is contemplated. It is useful for clarifying the local extent of tumour infiltration with regards to adjacent anatomical

Gastrointestinal cancer

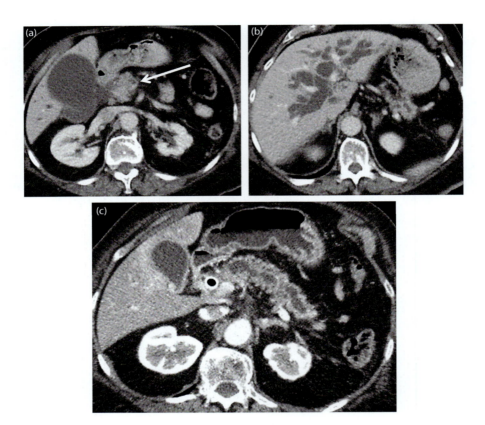

Figure 9.6 CT scans showing pancreatic carcinoma (a) and associated gross dilatation of hepatic bile ducts (b). Following stenting (c) there has been decompression of the bilary tract and a reduction in size of the gall bladder.

structures that cannot be sacrificed, and may be of use in surgical planning. It is also more sensitive for liver metastases.

Magnetic resonance cholangiopancreatography (MRI/MRCP) is particularly of value in evaluating cystic lesions.

BLOOD TESTS

Routine blood tests including full blood count, renal and hepatic function are taken. Liver function tests are particularly important in this setting to demonstrate the degree of obstructive jaundice, characterized by raised total serum bilirubin, elevated alkaline phosphatase and γ-glutamyltransferase with normal or slightly elevated liver transferases (ALT):

Clotting profile is important prior to any biopsy since clotting may be impaired in liver dysfunction

Serum CA19-9 is a tumour marker most frequently raised in upper gastrointestinal malignancies including pancreatic cancer. *Serum CEA* may also be raised and if so it is a useful marker of disease activity.

LAPAROSCOPY

When resection is possible on the basis of radiological evaluation, laparoscopy may be indicated to exclude small volume peritoneal metastases and liver metastases.

STAGING

The TNM system is widely used:

- Tis: Carcinoma *in situ*
- T0: No evidence of primary

- TX: Primary cannot be assessed
- T1: Limited to pancreas, 2 cm or less in greatest dimension
- T2: Limited to pancreas, >2 cm in greatest dimension
- T3: Extends beyond the pancreas but without involving coeliac axis or superior mesenteric artery
- T4: Tumour involves coeliac axis or superior mesenteric artery
- N0: No regional lymphadenopathy
- N1: Regional lymph nodes involved
- M0: No distant metastases
- M1: Distant metastases

TREATMENT

RADICAL TREATMENT

Surgery

This is the only potentially curative option. Patients must be carefully selected for radical surgery as only 10%–20% will be suitable candidates. The operation of choice was originally described by Whipple and comprises a pancreaticoduodenectomy; modern surgery uses a pylorus-preserving approach where it is possible to reduce postoperative morbidity. Lymphadenectomy is also performed in this procedure.

Radiotherapy

Carcinoma of the pancreas is incurable using current radiotherapy techniques and doses owing to the high incidence of metastases at diagnosis, and the proximity of radiation dose-limiting normal tissues such as the spinal cord, small bowel and kidneys. Some of these issues can be overcome by delivering radiotherapy intraoperatively but even this has not made a significant impact on curability and survival. Newer radiotherapy techniques such as intensity-modulated radiotherapy (IMRT) could allow a higher dose delivery in the future. For the present, local recurrence remains a major problem with recurrence rates varying between 50% and 80%. The only treatment that has been shown to reduce this is postoperative chemoradiotherapy (CRT) using 5FU, which is more effective than radiotherapy alone, but the problem of occult liver metastases is not adequately addressed with this approach and the start of treatment is invariably delayed by the recovery period after surgery. Preoperative CRT has the advantage of starting immediately following diagnosis and allowing greater selection for surgery pending the results of restaging of the local disease and liver after CRT. The optimum use of multimodality treatment is still a matter of debate and controversy.

Chemotherapy

Adjuvant chemotherapy using gemcitabine and capecitabine after surgery with curative intent should be considered for all patients. A total of six cycles is recommended which nearly doubles the median disease-free survival to 13 months compared with 7 months for observation alone and overall median survival at 5 years to 21% compared with 9% for observation alone.

Palliative treatment

Surgery

Many patients are found to be inoperable at laparotomy. Rather than going on to perform an operation that stands no chance of prolonging the patient's survival, if the patient has obstructive jaundice or is at risk of developing it in the near future, surgeons should consider a bypass procedure (gastrojejunostomy) to allow free drainage of bile. Gastroenterostomy will relieve duodenal obstruction by a large periampullary carcinoma.

Obstructive jaundice may also be relieved by endoscopically placed self-expanding metal stents which may be more appropriate in those presenting with advanced disease.

Radiotherapy

Patients with locally advanced pancreatic cancer may benefit from consolidation chemoradiation using capecitabine with radiotherapy. Radiation may also be used palliatively for relieving pain from retroperitoneal tumour extension.

Chemotherapy

Combination chemotherapy is more effective than single-agent chemotherapy. FOLFIRINOX (5FU, folinic acid and oxaliplatin) or gemcitabine and capecitabine are most commonly used. Gemcitabine and albumin-bound paclitaxel and gemcitabine with erlotinib also have activity in pancreatic cancer. In patients who cannot tolerate combination chemotherapy then single-agent gemcitabine should be considered.

Medical treatment for symptomatic relief

Cholestyramine can relieve the pruritus of intractable obstructive jaundice, while pancreatic enzyme supplements will relieve the steatorrhoea associated with the malabsorption of fats. Vitamin K administered intravenously is indicated if there is a symptomatic coagulopathy related to a deficiency of the vitamin K-dependent clotting factors. Coeliac axis nerve blocks can alleviate intractable pain.

CASE HISTORY

PANCREATIC CANCER

A previously fit 55-year-old man presents with dark urine, pale stools and jaundice. Liver function tests indicate a γ-glutamyltransferase (GGT) of 670 U/L (normal <42) and alkaline phosphatase (ALP) of 725 U/L (normal range 38–126). The bilirubin is elevated at 90 μmol/L (normal range <17). Liver ultrasound suggests dilatation of the extrahepatic biliary tree, with enlargement of the head of the pancreas. An ERCP is performed and washings from the pancreatic duct confirm adenocarcinoma cells. CT imaging confirms a mass in the head of the pancreas with no evidence of metastatic disease elsewhere. This is confirmed by PET imaging. The CA19-9 is not elevated. He is referred to a hepatobiliary surgeon and undergoes a radical pancreaticoduodenectomy. Pathological examination of the surgical specimen confirms complete excision of a pancreatic adenocarcinoma. He is started on insulin for iatrogenic diabetes mellitus and pancreatic enzyme supplements. He expresses a wish to be treated as actively as possible so receives six cycles of postoperative adjuvant chemotherapy using single-agent gemcitabine and capecitabine.

Two years later, he develops pain in the right upper quadrant of the abdomen. Liver ultrasound confirms multiple liver metastases. During this time, he develops swelling of the left leg and a Doppler ultrasound confirms a deep vein thrombosis. Despite anticoagulation with warfarin, 2 weeks later the toes on the right foot become painful, cold and discoloured. Arteriography confirms a popliteal artery thrombosis. This is managed conservatively; 24 hours later, before he can be considered for salvage chemotherapy, he dies of a sudden, massive pulmonary embolus from the coagulopathy induced by his cancer.

TUMOUR-RELATED COMPLICATIONS

There are a number of recognized vascular complications:

- Renal vein thrombosis
- Portal vein thrombosis
- Splenic vein thrombosis
- Thrombophlebitis migrans
- Disseminated intravascular coagulation

Renal vein thrombosis results in renal congestion and a nephrotic syndrome. Portal vein thrombosis leads to a Budd–Chiari syndrome, characterized by the rapid accumulation of ascites and hepatic congestion, while splenic vein thrombosis leads to portal hypertension and oesophageal varices. Thrombophlebitis migrans is characterized by intermittent bouts of tenderness, erythema and induration of superficial veins. Disseminated intravascular coagulation is due to mucin production by the tumour, which leads to an inappropriate activation of the clotting cascade (see Chapter 8).

Non-metastatic manifestations include:

- Profound depression
- Migratory thrombophlebitis
- Hypercalcaemia (production of parathyroid hormone-like peptides)
- Cushing syndrome (ACTH production)
- Carcinoid syndrome (5-HT production)
- Marantic endocarditis
- Syndrome of metastatic fat necrosis

TREATMENT-RELATED COMPLICATIONS

SURGERY

Radical pancreaticoduodenectomy can be complicated by biliary leakage, pancreatic fistula, delayed gastric emptying and ileus, infection and haemorrhage. Significant morbidity is experienced by one-third to one-half of patients. Mortality is around 2%.

The loss of exocrine and endocrine pancreatic secretions leads to permanent diabetes mellitus requiring insulin and malabsorption of fat requiring enzyme supplements with each meal.

RADIOTHERAPY

Radiotherapy to the pancreatic bed will result in temporary anorexia, nausea, vomiting, gastritis, colic and diarrhoea. Late complications are infrequently encountered owing to the extremely poor prognosis of the disease.

CHEMOTHERAPY

Drug-specific toxicity.

PROGNOSIS

Pancreatic cancer accounts for 6% of all cancer deaths in the United Kingdom with little change in the past 40 years. Around 20% will be alive 1 year after diagnosis falling to 3%–4% after 5 years. Of those undergoing radical surgery, 5-year survival is about 20%.

RARE TUMOURS

GASTROENTEROPANCREATIC (GEP) NEUROENDOCRINE TUMOURS

These comprise:

- Carcinoid
- Gastrinoma insulinoma
- Glucagonoma
- VIPoma

The pancreas is a rare site for *carcinoid* (see Chapter 14). Partial pancreatectomy will be curative unless there has been metastasis to the liver.

Gastrinoma is a gastrin-secreting tumour which leads to Zollinger–Ellison syndrome, characterized by hypersecretion of acid in the stomach leading to intractable peptic ulceration. An elevated serum gastrin level is diagnostic and about two-thirds are malignant. It is sometimes associated with adenomata of the pituitary and parathyroid as part of multiple endocrine neoplasia type 1 (MEN 1). After detailed staging with a CT scan and selective venous angiography, the treatment of choice is a partial pancreatectomy.

Insulinoma arises from the beta cells of the islets and secretes insulin, leading to fasting hypoglycaemia. There is an association with MEN 1. Ninety percent are benign and 10% multiple. Treatment is surgical as for gastrinoma. Historically, diazoxide (a beta cell toxin) has been used to relieve the unremitting hypoglycaemia of advanced disease.

Glucagonoma from the alpha cells of the pancreas secretes glucagon, leading to a syndrome of diabetes mellitus, a migratory necrolytic erythema of the skin and stomatitis. Approximately half are malignant with metastases in the liver. Surgery is the treatment of choice.

VIPoma leads to Werner–Morrison syndrome characterized by severe watery diarrhoea and hypokalaemia. The majority are benign.

The somatostatin analogue octreotide can be radiolabelled and used as a useful tracer for whole-body imaging. It therefore contributes to staging and predicts for response to octreotide when used therapeutically. Octreotide has shown considerable activity in GEP tumours and therefore has an important role in symptom relief and disease stabilization in advanced stages of disease.

HEPATOCELLULAR CANCER

EPIDEMIOLOGY

Worldwide this is the fourth commonest cancer. In the United Kingdom the incidence has increased by 2.5 times in the past 25 years with a continued increase projected over the next 20 years. Currently each year in the United Kingdom there are over 5500 cases of liver cancer, 1700 cases in men and 1200 cases in women, accounting for 2% of all cancer cases and leading to a total of 5400 deaths per annum.

There is a particularly high incidence in areas where hepatitis B is endemic such as West Africa and China.

AETIOLOGY

Around one-half of all cases of liver cancer are preventable:

- Smoking causes 20%.
- Infections, in particular hepatitis B and C viruses account for 10% in the United Kingdom but 90% in low income developing countries. Liver cancer is 5–6 times more common in people with HIV/AIDS.
- Obesity accounts for 23%.
- Alcohol causes 7% doubling of the risk in carriers of hepatitis B and C.
- Cirrhosis carries a high risk of hepatocellular cancer, especially in those with hepatitis B- and C-related cirrhosis. It is 19 times higher in people with primary biliary cirrhosis and four times greater in those with non-alcoholic fatty liver disease.
- Haemochromatosis carries an 11 times greater risk of hepatocellular carcinoma.
- Diabetes and gallstones also increase the risk.
- Occupational exposure to arsenic, polychlorinated biphenyls and trichloroethylene are also related but all together account for only 1% of cases.

PATHOLOGY

The tumour grows rapidly, is usually large, arises from the liver parenchyma or a cirrhotic nodule and may be multifocal. In cut section there is bile staining, haemorrhage and necrosis. It invades through the liver capsule, along the hepatic ducts and blood vessels. Intrahepatic ducts proximal to the tumour will be obstructed and therefore dilated. The tumour is composed of hepatocytes which have lost the characteristic architecture of the portal tracts and frequently stain for α-fetoprotein (AFP). Other important stains in confirming the diagnosis of hepatocellular carcinoma are reticulin, CD34 and a high Ki67 index.

A number of rarer subtypes are recognized including clear cell, steatohepatic, scirrhous, cirrhotomimetic, sarcomatoid and fibrolamellar.

NATURAL HISTORY

The tumour may remain confined to the liver, invading along the intrahepatic bile ducts and hepatic veins, or breach the liver capsule, leading to invasion of adjacent structures such as the hepatic veins, portal vein, inferior vena cava, right hemidiaphragm, right kidney, right adrenal, stomach and transverse colon. The hilar lymph nodes at the base of the liver and portal nodes are frequently involved.

The lungs are the most common site of distant metastases, although bone, skin and brain can also be involved. Spread beyond the liver capsule sometimes leads to diffuse peritoneal involvement which in turn can cause malignant ascites.

SYMPTOMS

There is often a long history of increasing ill-health with hepatic pain owing to distension of the liver capsule which contains many stretch receptors. The onset of pain can be acute and severe if precipitated by a sudden haemorrhage into the tumour, which leads to its rapid enlargement. Swollen legs are a common complaint in advanced cases owing to a combination of hypoalbuminaemia and compression of the inferior vena cava. Systemic symptoms such as anorexia, nausea, weight loss, fever and malaise are frequent.

SIGNS

There might be evidence of an underlying cirrhosis such as clubbing, leuconychia, palmar erythema, jaundice, spider naevi, gynaecomastia, testicular atrophy, ascites, ankle oedema, dilated superficial abdominal wall veins and splenomegaly. Signs of hepatic encephalopathy are rare. The liver can be diffusely enlarged owing to cirrhosis, focally enlarged owing to the hepatoma or both. An arterial bruit and hepatic rub might be heard over the tumour owing to its rich vascular supply and capsular invasion, respectively.

DIFFERENTIAL DIAGNOSIS

It is important to distinguish a well differentiated hepatocellular carcinoma from an adenoma and a poorly differentiated hepatoma from poorly differentiated cholangiocarcinoma and metastases. A high serum AFP or positive staining for AFP within a biopsy supports the diagnosis of hepatoma. An immunohistochemical panel including HepPar-1, arginase and glypican-3 which are hepatocellular markers will help distinguish hepatocellular carcinoma from other histologies.

INVESTIGATIONS

COMPUTED TOMOGRAPHY (CT) OF THE CHEST, ABDOMEN AND PELVIS

This will give full staging information with respect to possible sites of metastases. It is mandatory if surgery or radiotherapy is planned (Figure 9.7).

MAGNETIC RESONANCE IMAGING (MRI) OF LIVER

This will provide the most accurate picture of the primary tumour and its distribution within the liver.

There are now consensus criteria for making a diagnosis of hepatocellular carcinoma on imaging alone without the need for biopsy; the Liver Imaging Reporting and Data System (LI-RADS) is now widely used to standardize reporting of liver lesions and their likelihood of representing hepatocellular carcinoma based on size and contrast enhancing characteristics. Only in equivocal cases or where contrast enhanced imaging is not possible a biopsy will be indicated.

LIVER FUNCTION TESTS, CLOTTING PARAMETERS

Liver function derangement is common but more likely to be due to an underlying cirrhosis than the hepatoma itself. Assessment of clotting is necessary prior to a liver biopsy or any invasive procedure.

HEPATITIS SEROLOGY

Serology for types A, B, C and D should be performed.

SERUM α-FETOPROTEIN

This is elevated in 70% of cases. It is a useful diagnostic test and of value in monitoring response to therapy (especially surgery) and in predicting relapse.

STAGING

The TNM system is widely used:

- Tis: Carcinoma *in situ*
- T0: No evidence of primary
- TX: Primary cannot be assessed
- T1: Solitary tumour 2 cm or less in greatest dimension without vascular invasion
- T2: Solitary tumour 2 cm or less in greatest dimension with vascular invasion; or multiple tumours limited to one lobe, none >2 cm without vascular invasion; or solitary tumour >2 cm without vascular invasion
- T3: Solitary tumour >2 cm in greatest dimension with vascular invasion; or multiple tumours limited to one lobe, none >2 cm with vascular invasion; or multiple tumours limited to one lobe, any >2 cm with or without vascular invasion
- T4: Multiple tumours in more than one lobe; or tumour(s) involving a major branch of the portal or hepatic vein(s); or tumour(s) with direct invasion of adjacent organs other than gallbladder or tumour(s) with perforation of visceral peritoneum

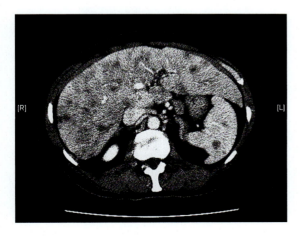

Figure 9.7 Hepatocellular carcinoma. CT image of the upper abdomen showing a large, round, necrotic tumour arising from the substance of the liver.

- N0: No regional lymphadenopathy
- N1: Regional lymph nodes involved
- M0: No distant metastases
- M1: Distant metastases

TREATMENT

RADICAL TREATMENT

Surgery

Patients with early stage (single lesion) tumours preserved liver function and without significant comorbidities should undergo resection.

Liver transplantation can be considered in patients with cirrhosis and end stage liver disease with solitary tumours of up to 5 cm or three separate lesions up to 3 cm without evidence of metastases.

Radiofrequency ablation (RFA)

RFA should be considered for patients with early stage disease, tumours up to 5 cm, who have impaired liver function or comorbidities. It is contraindicated if the tumour is close to a major vessel, another organ such as the gallbladder or the dome of the diaphragm.

Transarterial chemo-embolization (TACE)

TACE involves infusion of chemotherapy, usually cisplatin, doxorubicin or mitomycin C, through the hepatic artery directly into the tumour vasculature. It is contraindicated in portal vein thrombosis and decompensated liver disease. It is an alternative to RFA for smaller tumours in patients who have comorbidities or impaired hepatic function and can also be used for larger or multinodular lesions. Whilst not curative it can produce a period of remission.

Radiotherapy

Modern radiotherapy techniques using stereotactic radiotherapy (SBRT) can deliver high doses to localized tumours in the liver. This may be considered as an alternative to RFA or where RFA is contraindicated.

Percutaneous ethanol injection (PEI)

PEI can achieve local ablation in small localized tumours; complete ablation is related to size and not reliably achieved in tumours >2 cm. Repeat injections may be needed but high local control rates can be achieved.

PALLIATIVE TREATMENT

Chemotherapy

Sorafenib is a multikinase inhibitor, which decreases cell growth and angiogenesis. It increases median survival to 11 months compared with 8 months for those treated by placebo. The commonest side effects are diarrhoea, hand–foot syndrome and fatigue. Lenvatinib is a newer drug in this class which has slightly higher activity but may cause hypertension.

Regorafenib or nivolumab are both indicated for second-line systemic treatment in patients progressing after sorafenib.

Radiotherapy

Low doses of radiation can be given with the expectation of relieving hepatic pain.

TUMOUR-RELATED COMPLICATIONS

A number of non-metastatic manifestations are recognized including:

- Hypoglycaemia (insulin-like peptides)
- Polycythaemia (erythropoietin-like peptides)
- Hypercalcaemia (parathyroid hormone-like peptides)
- Feminization (oestrogens)
- Pyrexia of unknown origin (pyrogens)
- Porphyria cutanea tarda (porphyrins)

Tumour pressure may cause obstructive jaundice. Portal vein thrombosis leads to splenomegaly, ascites and oesophageal varices, while hepatic vein thrombosis leads to Budd–Chiari syndrome with ascites, hepatomegaly and leg oedema. Inferior vena cava obstruction will lead to oedema below the umbilicus. Sudden haemorrhage can occur into the tumour causing acute right upper abdominal pain, or into the abdomen causing abdominal pain and distension, which may lead to death.

TREATMENT-RELATED COMPLICATIONS

SURGERY

Partial hepatectomy can lead to hepatic decompensation if the function of the remaining liver is poor. Transplant patients will also have the problems of rejection and chronic immunosuppression to overcome.

RADIOTHERAPY

Hepatic irradiation may cause anorexia, nausea and vomiting during treatment, and radiation hepatitis can result when a large volume of liver has been irradiated. Modern techniques using SBRT are associated with relatively few side effects.

CHEMOTHERAPY

Drug-specific toxicity.

PROGNOSIS

The important tumour-related prognostic factors are tumour size, surgical margin status, the presence of vascular invasion, absence of a tumour capsule and poor histological grade of differentiation. Liver resection for small tumours produces superior results.

The 5-year survival for symptomatic hepatocellular carcinoma is 0%–10%; resection or transplantation results in up to 75% of patients surviving for 5 years or more. Metastatic patients receiving systemic therapy such as sorafenib will have a median survival of 12 months.

PREVENTION

Vaccination against hepatitis B in all children and adults at risk of infection is important. Screening of blood products for hepatitis C, treatment of pre-existing chronic liver disease and avoidance of excessive alcohol consumption will reduce the risk of cirrhosis and consequent HCC developments.

SCREENING

Measurements of α-fetoprotein and liver ultrasound are the most sensitive investigations for screening and detecting hepatoma while it is operable although new tests based on proteomics are under evaluation which may increase sensitivity.

Screening should be offered to high risk individuals including hepatitis B virus (HBV) carriers, hepatitis C virus-related cirrhosis, alcoholic cirrhosis, primary biliary cirrhosis, non-alcoholic steatohepatitis-related cirrhosis and genetic haemochromatosis.

RARE TUMOURS

ANGIOSARCOMA

This is very rare and associated with medical exposure to thorotrast and industrial exposure to vinyl chloride monomer.

CHOLANGIOCARCINOMA

This is a malignant tumour arising from the epithelium lining the extrahepatic biliary tract.

EPIDEMIOLOGY

This is rare in the developed countries. For example, in the United Kingdom there are fewer than 1000 new cases and 300 deaths registered per annum. It is about half as common as carcinoma of the gallbladder. The peak age incidence is 50–70 years and there is a slight male predominance. The highest incidence is found in Thailand and it is more common in areas where liver flukes are endemic, e.g. South East Asia.

AETIOLOGY

Recognized associations include:

- Chronic liver disease
- High alcohol intake
- Oral contraceptive use
- Chemical and drug exposure, e.g. isoniazid and polychlorinated biphenyls
- Liver flukes, e.g. *Clonorchis sinensis*

- Primary sclerosing cholangitis – a rare complication of chronic ulcerative colitis
- Chronic infective cholangitis secondary to gallstones
- Radiation – previous use of thorotrast contrast medium (of historical significance only)
- Congenital biliary abnormalities, e.g. choledochal cyst

PATHOLOGY

Tumours of the upper third of the extrahepatic biliary tree tend to be diffusely sclerosing leading to a malignant stricture. Tumours in the middle third tend to be nodular while those in the lower third tend to be papillary. The tumour is usually a well-differentiated mucin secreting adenocarcinoma with about half staining for carcinoembryonic antigen (CEA).

NATURAL HISTORY

Tumours of the upper third can infiltrate the liver, while those of the lower third can infiltrate the duodenum and pancreas. Tumours also spread to the hilar, superior mesenteric and coeliac lymph nodes. The liver is the most common site of distant metastases, although lung and bone may also be involved.

SYMPTOMS

The most common presentation is with obstructive jaundice, pruritus, dark urine and pale stools. Recurrent cholangitis from subacute biliary tract obstruction also occurs.

SIGNS

The patient will be jaundiced, the gallbladder may be palpable (positive Courvoisier's sign) and the liver congested and therefore smoothly enlarged.

DIFFERENTIAL DIAGNOSIS

Other causes of obstructive jaundice include:

- Gallstones
- Carcinoma of the head of the pancreas
- Carcinoma of the ampulla of Vater
- Benign biliary tract stricture following surgical trauma
- Sclerosing cholangitis
- Lymph node metastases at the porta hepatis

INVESTIGATIONS

BLOOD TESTS

There will be evidence of biliary obstruction with raised levels of bilirubin, alkaline phosphatase and γ-glutamyltransferase.

Important serum markers are CA 19-9 and CA 125. Serum CEA may also be raised.

ULTRASOUND OF THE BILIARY TRACT

This is the most sensitive test with a high discriminatory ability to distinguish benign from malignant biliary disease.

CT SCAN OF THE UPPER ABDOMEN

This will show the degree of local invasion, any enlarged regional lymph nodes and exclude liver metastases.

MR SCAN OF THE UPPER ABDOMEN

This has a similar sensitivity to CT but shows a biliary architecture and small liver metastases in more detail. MR angiography will be helpful in determining operability. MRCP has a similar sensitivity to ERCP but is non-invasive.

ENDOSCOPIC RETROGRADE CHOLEPANCREATICOGRAM (ERCP)

This is the investigation of choice to obtain a tissue diagnosis by biopsy or cytology from brushings and biliary aspirates. It may also be combined with therapeutic manoeuvres such as passage of a stent to relieve jaundice.

PERCUTANEOUS TRANSHEPATIC CHOLANGIOGRAPHY (PTC)

This is indicated when ERCP has failed to opacify the biliary tree or adequately display the tumour because of its position.

STAGING

The TNM staging is used for tumours of the extrahepatic ducts:

TX: Primary tumour cannot be assessed
T0: No evidence of primary tumour
Tis: Carcinoma *in situ*
T1: Tumour confined to the bile duct, with extension up to the muscle layer or fibrous tissue
T2a: Tumour invades beyond the wall of the bile duct to surrounding adipose tissue
T2b: Tumour invades adjacent hepatic parenchyma
T3: Tumour invades unilateral branches of the portal vein or hepatic artery
T4: Tumour invades main portal vein or its branches bilaterally; or the common hepatic artery; or the second-order biliary radicles bilaterally; or unilateral second-order biliary radicles with contralateral portal vein or hepatic artery involvement
NX: Regional lymph nodes cannot be assessed
N0: No regional lymph node metastasis
N1: Regional lymph node metastasis
N2: Metastasis to periaortic, pericaval, superior mesenteric artery and/or coeliac artery lymph nodes
M0: No distant metastasis
M1: Distant metastasis

TREATMENT

RADICAL TREATMENT

Surgery

This offers the best chance of cure although only 10%–20% will be resectable. The optimum surgical procedure for carcinoma of the extrahepatic bile duct will vary according to its location along the biliary tree, the extent of hepatic parenchymal involvement, and the proximity of the tumour to major blood vessels in this region. Distal tumours are more likely to be resectable than proximal ones. Tumours of the lower third require pancreaticoduodenectomy, while those with more proximal lesions may be carefully staged and selected for hepatic lobectomy or liver transplantation.

PALLIATIVE TREATMENT

Surgery

Choledochojejunostomy will relieve obstructive jaundice in cases not amenable to endoscopic or percutaneous stenting. Cholecystectomy should be considered to prevent the possibility of an acute cholecystitis.

Radiotherapy

Radiotherapy alone or chemoradiation may be considered for inoperable but localized tumours. Newer stereotactic techniques enable a high dose to be delivered to localized lesions but the added benefit of this approach over conventional techniques has yet to be proven.

Radiotherapy in palliative doses may improve pain from local infiltration.

Chemotherapy

Gemcitabine with cis- or carboplatin is currently the most active drug combination. This may be given alongside radiotherapy. Intra-arterial chemotherapy may have added advantages.

TUMOUR-RELATED COMPLICATIONS

These include:

- Acute cholangitis, which presents with fever, rigours and right upper abdominal pain and usually responds to broad-spectrum antibiotics
- Secondary biliary cirrhosis, which is caused by chronic cholestasis

TREATMENT-RELATED COMPLICATIONS

SURGERY

The bile duct is a delicate structure prone to stricturing after handling. Biliary fistulae are also a problem after anastomosis.

RADIOTHERAPY

External beam irradiation carries the same morbidity as outlined for stomach cancer.

PROGNOSIS

In operable cases the 5-year survival is between 25% and 45%; around 50% of patients undergoing liver transplant are long-term survivors.

Response rates to chemotherapy and radiotherapy are however poor and mean survival in untreated cases is only 3 months.

CARCINOMA OF THE GALLBLADDER

This is the commonest biliary tract tumour but a rare tumour in the developed countries. Each year in the United Kingdom there are 600 cases of gallbladder cancer, 400 cases in women and 200 cases in men, accounting for 0.2% of all cancer cases and leading to a total of 400 deaths per annum. In developed countries, it has a peak age incidence of 60–80 years. Aetiological factors include:

- Gallstones – 0.5%–1% of cholecystectomies performed for cholelithiasis will yield an occult carcinoma of the gallbladder
- Typhoid carriage – there is a greatly increased risk owing to carriage of the *Salmonella typhi* bacterium in the gallbladder, which in turn leads to a chronic cholecystitis
- Working in rubber plants
- Large gallbladder polyps
- Choledochal cysts and other biliary tract anatomical anomalies
- Primary sclerosing cholangitis

Many patients are diagnosed incidentally at cholecystectomy and are asymptomatic with no physical signs. Otherwise the presentation resembles benign gallbladder disease with bouts of acute cholecystitis or more chronic and less severe right upper abdominal pain where a mass could be palpable. Eighty percent arise at the fundus or neck of the gallbladder and 90% are adenocarcinomas. The adjacent liver capsule and parenchyma are involved early and there can be lymphatic spread to the hilar nodes around the liver. The liver and lungs are the most common sites for blood-borne metastases.

Staging investigations include liver function tests, chest x-ray, liver ultrasound and a CT/MRI scan of the upper abdomen.

Treatment comprises cholecystectomy with a wide excision of the surrounding liver, excision of the extrahepatic bile duct and regional lymph node dissection. Low-dose radiotherapy can be of value in relieving pain from local infiltration, and a biliary drainage procedure will palliate biliary obstruction. In those with superficial involvement of the mucosa, the disease might be cured with cholecystectomy alone. Of those with liver involvement, 50% die within 3 months of diagnosis and less than 5% survive for 1 year.

Epidemiological studies suggest a survival advantage for adjuvant chemotherapy using 5FU-based schedules in early stage disease after complete resection.

CARCINOMA OF THE COLON AND RECTUM

The colon and rectum are parts of the large bowel located in the abdomen and pelvis and are in continuity with each other. The colon acts as a site of water absorption, turning the liquid effluent from the small bowel into solid stool. The more distal rectum acts as a reservoir for this stool prior to its evacuation through the anus.

EPIDEMIOLOGY

Each year in the United Kingdom there are over 40,000 cases of colorectal cancer; it is the fourth most common cancer, accounting for 12% of all new cancer cases. The majority occur in the rectum. It is most common in white males, particularly those in deprived areas with the highest prevalence in the 65–75 age group. It is relatively less common in Asian and black people. It is predominantly a disease of the developed world, being most common in New Zealand, Canada, United States and United Kingdom while rare in Africa and Asia. Incidence rates in the United Kingdom have remained approximately steady over the past 10 years but a fall of 11% is predicted in the next decade reflecting the introduction of screening programmes.

AETIOLOGY

Diet could account for the marked geographical variation in incidence. This is presumed to be due to changes in the bowel flora, which produce carcinogens from ingested food, the effect being exacerbated by the slower bowel transit time seen in people taking a low-fibre diet. The incidence has increased in Japan as a Western style diet has been adopted, and Japanese migrants to the West have subsequently acquired the risk of the indigenous population. Important factors include:

- High processed and red meat consumption.
- High total fat consumption.
- High calorific intake.
- High tobacco and alcohol intake.
- Obesity with an increase in incidence with BMI estimated at 10% for every 5 BMI units gained in adulthood.
- Inflammatory bowel disease including ulcerative colitis and Crohn colitis has a risk of up to 70% greater than the general population. There is a 5% risk in patients with irritable bowel syndrome for 20 years or more.
- Diabetes carries a 20%–30% greater risk of bowel cancer.
- Genetic factors: Around 20% of bowel cancers are associated with hereditary factors other than Familial adenomatous polyposis (FAP) and Hereditary non-polyposis colorectal cancer (HNPCC). Individuals with an affected first-degree relative have a two–three-fold increased risk of developing colorectal cancer themselves. Cancer develops around a decade earlier in such individuals. This risk is higher if the index case is diagnosed at under 45 years of age. If two first-degree relatives have had the disease, the risk rises four–five-fold to 16%.

Hereditary non-polyposis colon cancer (HNPCC) is synonymous to Lynch syndrome and accounts for up to 4% of cases. This is a dominantly inherited condition, i.e. there is a 50% chance of inheriting the mutated DNA mismatch repair gene from an affected parent. Unlike familial adenomatous polyposis (FAP), there are no characteristic extracolonic physical signs and there is no propensity to develop a multitude of polyps. Colon cancer on average develops at 40 years of age and individuals have a 70%–80% chance of developing bowel cancer by the age of 70 years. Families can be divided into Lynch syndromes I and II. In Lynch syndrome I, the cancers are mainly gastrointestinal. In Lynch syndrome II, endometrial and ovarian cancers may arise at a young age.

Familial adenomatous polyposis (FAP) accounts for 1% of bowel cancers. It is a rare, dominantly inherited condition, i.e. there is a 50% chance of inheriting the mutated *APC* tumour-suppressor gene from an affected parent. The *APC* gene is located on chromosome 5q21. It has a prevalence of 1 in 10,000 births. There are characteristic physical signs to indicate a gene carrier, e.g. congenital hypertrophy of the retinal pigment epithelium (CHRPE), osteomas of the jaw, prepuberty epidermoid cysts. Affected individuals develop multiple (>100) benign polyps from a very young age (puberty). Inevitably, over the subsequent years, one or more of these polyps will transform into a cancer, usually during the third and fourth decades, 20–30 years before the general population. The risk for colorectal cancer is estimated at 90% by age 45 years. Prophylactic surgical excision of the colon and rectum is advised in young adults. Upper gastrointestinal malignancy (usually duodenal) will also develop in 5% and benign desmoid tumours in 10%. The latter can arise within the abdomen and may prove fatal owing to relentless local spread. Gardener syndrome is similar to familial polyposis coli but characterized by skeletal and cutaneous abnormalities, e.g. osteomas of the mandible and skull, sebaceous cysts and dermoid cysts.

Carriers of the BRCA 1-mutated gene also have a higher risk of developing bowel cancer.

Peutz–Jeghers syndrome is dominantly inherited and caused by a mutation in the *STK11* tumour-suppressor gene located on chromosome 19p13. It is characterized by the development of multiple bowel hamartomas and an increased risk of colon cancer. The risk for colorectal cancer is estimated at 40% by age 70 years.

PATHOLOGY

One-third arises in the rectum or rectosigmoid, one-quarter in the sigmoid colon and one-tenth at the caecum. The rest are evenly distributed along the large bowel, two-thirds arising on the left side. Most

Gastrointestinal cancer

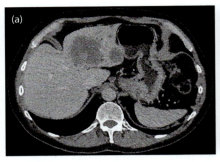
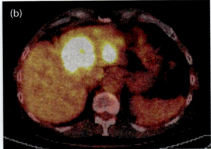

Figure 9.8 Multiple liver metastases from rectal cancer on (a) CT and (b) corresponding slice on FDG PET.

cancers represent malignant change in a benign adenomatous polyp (e.g. tubular, tubulovillous and villous), the highest risk being from villous adenomas and serrated adenomas, especially those greater than 2 cm. The tumour may be nodular, ulcerating or diffusely infiltrating, and multiple primaries are found in approximately 5%. The vast majority is adenocarcinoma (85% glandular, 15% mucinous, 2% signet ring), usually well differentiated, and may show evidence of a preceding benign adenomatous polyp. The tumour cells frequently stain for carcinoembryonic antigen (CEA) and CK20.

Hereditary cancers are characterized by mutations in mismatch repair genes characterized by the high-level microsatellite instability (MSI-H) phenotype. In contrast, sporadic cancers will have the microsatellite-stable (MSS) or low-level microsatellite instability (MSI-L) phenotypes and may have mutations in the BRAF and KRAS genes.

NATURAL HISTORY

The tumour spreads longitudinally and circumferentially along the mucosa, in some cases leading to obstruction of the bowel lumen, and invades deep to the mucosa to infiltrate the muscular wall of the bowel and serosa. Penetration of the serosa leads to direct infiltration of the surrounding abdominal and pelvic viscera, while submucosal spread in the lamina propria can lead to skip lesions well away from the primary tumour. Tumour cells have a propensity to seed in abdominal scars, perineal skin, stomas and even anal fissures. Transcoelomic spread may lead to diffuse peritoneal involvement resulting in ascites and spread to the ovaries. The regional mesenteric

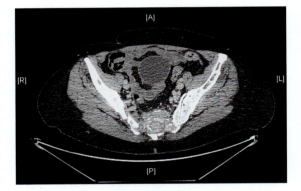

Figure 9.9 Presacral recurrence of a rectal cancer. Transverse pelvic CT image.

lymph nodes can be involved, wherein there is a likelihood of lymph node metastases increasing with the depth of bowel wall invasion. The tumour spreads to the liver (Figure 9.8) via the portal circulation, and from there to the lungs, bone, brain and skin. Rectal cancer has a particular propensity for local recurrence and often this leads to a presacral mass (Figure 9.9).

SYMPTOMS

The tumour most commonly presents with symptoms referable to the large bowel, 20% presenting as a surgical emergency with acute bowel obstruction or peritonitis owing to perforation. In the remainder, there is usually a history of one or more of the following:

- Change in bowel habit
- Blood per rectum

- Mucus per rectum
- Tenesmus
- Obstructive symptoms
- Iron-deficiency anaemia

A change in bowel habit is often the presenting symptom with an increase or decrease in frequency of defaecation or a change in stool consistency. Alternating diarrhoea and constipation is highly suspicious of cancer. Blood per rectum is another symptom that leads patients to seek medical advice. It varies in quantity depending on the degree of tumour ulceration and vascularity. The blood will be bright red and more likely streaked on the outside of the stool if the tumour arises in the rectum or sigmoid, or dark red and mixed in with the stool if the tumour arises more proximally in the colon. Mucus per rectum is more likely to be noticed with distal lesions. Tenesmus is a frequent urge to defaecate but leading to the passage of a little stool on each occasion and the lack of the feeling of complete rectal emptying. This is usually seen in rectal tumours, particularly if bulky or invading deeply and may be associated with rectal pain. Obstructive symptoms can manifest as intermittent colicky abdominal pain. They are more common in tumours of the descending colon where the faeces are more solid compared with right colon tumours where the stool is more liquid. Chronic bleeding leads to iron deficiency and in turn anaemia. It is a particular feature of right-sided colonic tumours, which may have few associated gastrointestinal symptoms.

SIGNS

The primary tumour may be palpable by digital examination of the rectum as a circumscribed area of mucosal induration, often with irregular heaped-up margins and a friable ulcer base, which bleeds on contact. Proximal tumours may be palpable in the pouch of Douglas per vaginam, and caecal tumours as a mass in the right iliac fossa.

Signs indicative of spread outside the pelvis include:

- Troisier's sign owing to enlargement of Virchow lymph node in the left supraclavicular fossa; this is uncommon at presentation and heralds a poor outcome from the disease
- Ascites indicating peritoneal involvement
- Hepatomegaly suggesting possible liver metastases

Rarely, locally advanced disease in the pelvis can lead to formation of a fistula between the adjacent bladder (colovesical – suggested by faecal debris in the urine or pneumaturia) or vagina (colovaginal – suggested by leakage of faeces per vaginam).

INVESTIGATIONS

DIGITAL EXAMINATION OF THE RECTUM AND VAGINA

This allows evaluation of the site, size and extent of local invasion of tumours of the rectum. A normal digital examination does not exclude the diagnosis of rectal cancer.

PROCTOSCOPY AND SIGMOIDOSCOPY

This will identify tumours in the distal large bowel. Assessment of the tumour size, extent and distance from the anal verge together with biopsy to obtain a tissue diagnosis should be undertaken.

COLONOSCOPY

This is the investigation of choice for suspected colorectal cancer. Even when a distal tumour has been identified colonoscopy should still be performed to exclude a synchronous primary elsewhere in the large bowel, occurring in 2%–4% of cases, and to identify polyps which will require removal to prevent development of metachronous cancers.

COMPUTED TOMOGRAPHY (CT)

CT colography is an alternative non-invasive means of viewing the entire large bowel and is an alternative to colonoscopy if a tissue biopsy has already been obtained.

Staging CT of the chest/abdomen/pelvis is mandatory to identify local extension, regional lymphadenopathy and more distant metastases in the lungs and liver.

Gastrointestinal cancer

ENDORECTAL ULTRASOUND OR MAGNETIC RESONANCE IMAGING (MRI)

These are indicated to assess the extent of a low rectal tumour in relation to the sphincters (Figure 9.10) and aid surgical planning.

STAGING

The clinicopathological staging according to Dukes is the best known staging system:

- *Stage A*: Confined to the bowel wall and has not penetrated its full thickness
- *Stage B:* Tumour has breached the bowel wall
- *Stage C*: Regional lymph node involvement
- *Stage D*: Distant metastases

There are a number of variants in clinical use. An alternative is the TNM system:

- Tis: Carcinoma *in situ*
- T0: No evidence of primary
- TX: Primary cannot be assessed
- T1: Involving submucosa
- T2: Involving muscularis propria
- T3: Involving subserosa, non-peritonealized pericolic/perirectal tissues
- T4: Other organs/structures/visceral peritoneum
- N0: No regional lymphadenopathy
- N1: Three or fewer pericolic/perirectal lymph nodes
- N2: >3 pericolic/perirectal lymph nodes
- N3: Nodes on named vascular trunk/apical node(s)
- M0: No distant metastases
- M1: Distant metastases

MANAGEMENT

RADICAL TREATMENT

Surgery

This is the only curative treatment modality; 80% of all tumours are resectable. Prior to resection of the primary tumour, a detailed inspection and palpation of the open abdomen and pelvis is performed to document the exact extent of disease, with special

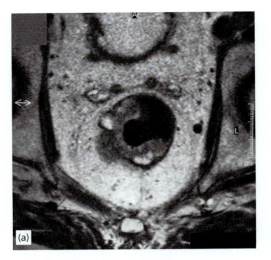
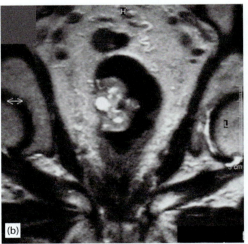
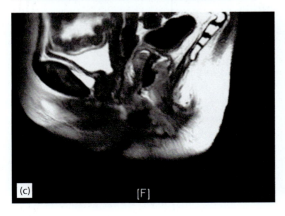

Figure 9.10 Rectal carcinoma. Staging MRIs. (a) Transverse view. (b) Coronal view. (c) Sagittal view.

reference to the liver, and suspicious tissues should be biopsied if not part of the main resection. The ovaries should be checked in women as they represent a potential site of spread.

Tumours of the colon are treated by hemicolectomy with either immediate reanastomosis (usual) or formation of a temporary colostomy, which can be closed at a later date. En bloc removal of regional lymph nodes should be included with a minimum of 12 nodes to achieve accurate staging information. Some surgeons ligate the vascular pedicle prior to mobilization of the tumour to try to prevent vascular dissemination of tumour. Laparoscopic-assisted colectomy is associated with more rapid recovery and reduced hospital stays.

Rectal cancer surgery is total mesorectal excision. In stage II and III tumours preoperative chemoradiation is taken. In selected cases total mesorectal excision (TME) alone may be sufficient; low risk cases suitable for this are defined by T1N0 tumours, <3 cm diameter occupying <30% of the circumference and with well or moderately differentiated histology.

Abdominoperineal resection may be required for the lowest rectal tumours, but in many cases it can be avoided with current surgical techniques. In each case, the mesentery containing the regional lymph nodes is also resected.

Advances in laparoscopic techniques and robotic surgery have made such refinements available to patients with colorectal cancer. Although more costly with prolonged operating times, they offer the advantage of less perioperative blood loss, reduced postoperative pain and ileus and more rapid postoperative recovery times. The long-term surgical oncology outcomes are awaited.

Patients presenting with synchronous oligometastases (<4 metastases in liver or lung) may still be considered for radical local surgery and excision of the metastasis. Of patients undergoing potentially curative excisions of all tumour-bearing liver, approximately one in three will survive for 5 years and one in four will survive for 10 years. This contrasts with a 5-year survival of not more than 5% for inoperable cases.

Radiotherapy

Radiotherapy has a little role in the curative treatment of colon cancer. This is due to:

- Local recurrence not being a major cause of relapse
- The difficulty in accurately determining the volume to be irradiated
- The proximity of a number of organs at risk limits the dose of radiation that can be delivered

Conversely, rectal cancer has a higher risk of recurrence and neoadjuvant radiotherapy or chemoradiation has been shown to increase the number of complete resections with clear histological margin resections and improve local control. A short course of 25 Gy in five fractions on consecutive days may be given and this has been shown to reduce the absolute risk of recurrence from 20% down to less than 10%. A meta-analysis of individual studies suggests a significant survival advantage with a reduction in the odds of dying of rectal cancer of approximately 20%, equivalent approximately to 7% in absolute survival benefit. Chemoradiation delivering 40–50 Gy in 5 weeks with 5FU chemotherapy is an alternative approach.

In inoperable fixed tumours chemoradiotherapy may be given to enable tumour regression and surgery to become feasible or as a radical option if the tumour does not become operable. However there is a high incidence of occult metastases in this group, which limits the treatment outcome.

Patients presenting with oligometastases may still be considered for radical treatment; stereotactic radiotherapy is an alternative to surgery for localized deposits in the liver or lungs.

Chemotherapy

Despite an 80% resection rate, almost half Dukes' C stage patients will have a relapse of their disease in the liver, usually within 2 years of surgery. Therefore adjuvant chemotherapy to eradicate the micrometastases shed from the tumour prior to or during its resection is important. Chemotherapy has a role in the adjuvant therapy of both colonic and rectal cancers.

Chemotherapy using 5FU and oxaliplatin (FOLFOX) or capecitabine and oxaliplatin (XELOX) is recommended for all patients with stage III cancers. This may also be offered to some high risk stage II cancers, e.g. those with T4 cancers, presentation with obstruction or perforation, venous invasion, inadequate lymph node sampling.

PALLIATIVE TREATMENT

Meta-analysis of the randomized trials addressing active treatment versus best supportive care shows an unequivocal advantage to a proactive approach. Active treatment yields a 35% mortality reduction, equivalent to a 16% 1-year absolute improvement in survival, and improvement in median survival from 8 months for best supportive care to around 30 months for active treatment. These benefits are independent of the age of the patient.

Surgery

If the tumour is inoperable, a bypass procedure or defunctioning colostomy may be of value in alleviating symptoms; however, the procedure of choice for low tumours will be stenting to overcome obstruction before considering appropriate management.

Radiotherapy

This is of benefit in inoperable disease, local recurrence after surgery and symptomatic metastases. It is very effective at relieving bleeding, mucorrhoea and local pain, with response rates of about 75%. Symptomatic pre-sacral recurrence is a particular problem after surgery and can be treated by radiotherapy. In an era where more patients will have received preoperative radiotherapy, re-treatment of the pelvis may be limited by radiation tolerance of surrounding organs.

Chemotherapy

Those developing metastatic disease are best treated actively. Comparisons of best supportive care versus immediate 5FU chemotherapy indicate a doubling in survival for the more proactive approach.

First-line chemotherapy is based on a two-drug combination, usually 5FU with folinic acid and oxaliplatin (FOLFOX) or irinotecan (FOLFIRI). Capecitabine may be used in place of 5FU/folinic acid. In addition, biological agents have been shown to enhance the response to chemotherapy using either a VEGF inhibitor (bevacizumab or regorafenib) or EGFR inhibitor (cetuximab or panitumumab). The EGFR inhibitor combinations are indicated in patients with NRAS or KRAS wild-type mutations.

PROGNOSIS

Dukes' staging and operability are the most important prognostic factors. The 5-year survivals are 93%–97% for stage I disease, 72%–85% for stage II disease, 44%–83% (depending on nodal involvement) for stage III disease and <8% for stage IV disease.

Unfavourable histopathological features include:

- Increasing anatomical extent of tumour – depth of local invasion, lymph gland involvement (increasing number and proximal location are poor features) and distant metastases
- Incomplete surgical excision of tumour, e.g. circumferential resection margin (CRM) positivity following total mesorectal excision (TME)
- Infiltrative tumour margins rather than expansile
- No peritumoral lymphoid reaction at deepest point of invasion and absence of lymphoid aggregates in the surrounding tissue
- Increasing tumour grade (decreasing differentiation)
- Venous invasion
- Lymphatic invasion
- Perineural invasion
- Signet-ring and small cell types

Mutations in KRAS, PIC3CA and BRAF are associated with a worse prognosis than tumours exhibiting the wild-type of these genes. The presence of deficient mismatch repair status (dMMR) is associated with a better prognosis in patients who receive chemotherapy.

CASE HISTORY

COLON CANCER

A 60-year-old man presents to his GP with a 6-week history of intermittent bright red blood per rectum associated with some perianal irritation. His bowels are regular and he has no other symptoms of note. Visual inspection shows a prolapsed haemorrhoid and he declines digital examination of the rectum as he has had similar symptoms over the preceding 5 years. A diagnosis of haemorrhoids is made and the symptoms settle by the time he returns for a prescription of antihypertensive medicines 2 weeks later.

Eight weeks later, he returns with a 4-week history of more frequent and profuse passage of fresh blood per rectum. This is associated with mucoid discharge per rectum and a feeling of incomplete rectal evacuation. He consents to rectal examination and this reveals an ulcerating tumour of the mid-rectum. He is referred to a colorectal surgeon for further investigation. Sigmoidoscopy confirms the tumour and shows no other mucosal abnormality and biopsies confirm a moderately differentiated adenocarcinoma. Colonoscopy confirms no other mucosal abnormality elsewhere in the large bowel. CT scan of the chest, abdomen and pelvis shows no evidence of lung or liver metastases, no pelvic lymphadenopathy and no evidence of direct invasion of the adjacent pelvic viscera. The serum CEA is twice the upper limit of normal (normal range <4 μg/L) and the liver function tests normal. After discussion at the multidisciplinary team meeting, he is referred to a clinical oncologist and receives five fractions of preoperative radiotherapy using fields encompassing the rectum and immediate lymphatic drainage. One week later, he undergoes a total mesorectal excision with immediate re-anastomosis. Histopathological review confirms a moderate/poorly differentiated adenocarcinoma, which penetrates through the full thickness of the rectal wall but has a clear circumferential resection margin and clear margins of excision proximally and distally. There is no involvement of the perirectal or other pelvic lymph nodes but prominent venous invasion is noted. The CEA returns to normal during the immediate postoperative period. His tumour is therefore designated as Dukes B and he receives 6 months of adjuvant FOLFOX chemotherapy because of the vascular invasion and poorly differentiated elements of the tumour.

He remains completely well on a routine follow-up until 18 months later when a routine pre-clinic CEA estimation is found to be 12 times the upper limit of normal at 48 μg/L. There are no adverse physical signs. This triggers restaging investigations. CT reveals two metastases in the left lobe of the liver and no evidence of locoregional recurrence of the original primary tumour. The chest is clear. There is no radiological abnormality elsewhere. MRI of the liver confirms a smaller third metastasis in the left lobe close to the other two and no involvement of the major hepatic vessels. He is referred to a hepatobiliary surgeon and is deemed medically fit for salvage surgery. A segmental resection of the left lobe of the liver is performed. The CEA returns to normal postoperatively. He remains well and disease-free 4 years later.

SCREENING

For asymptomatic individuals, screening results in diagnosis of colorectal cancer at an early stage, as evidenced by an increase in the proportion of Dukes A and B tumours in the screened population. This in turn leads to an improved survival in the screened population. Meta-analysis of four randomized controlled trials has shown that FOBT screening reduced the risk of death from colorectal cancer by 25% with an estimated one in six deaths from colorectal cancer prevented.

Digital rectal examination (DRE) is cheap and simple to apply to a population. However, it is only going to screen the most distal large bowel. It has not been shown to be an effective screening strategy.

The most cost-effective and socially acceptable method of screening is faecal occult blood testing (FOBT). A tiny sample of stool is obtained non-invasively and chemically tested for the presence of blood. The specimen collection can be undertaken in the patient's own home and can be mailed back to the laboratory; 95% will be negative at the first screen, whilst 3%–4% will be weakly positive. Most of these will re-test as negative after dietary restriction (no vitamin C, no iron supplements, no NSAIDs, no red meat, no fresh fruit). This leaves approximately 2% with a positive FOBT who will require further investigation (e.g. colonoscopy, sigmoidoscopy/double contrast barium enema): less than 10% of these individuals will be found to have a bowel cancer. As with any screening method, a very small proportion of patients will have a false-negative result.

Immunochemical FOBT has replaced older methods based on guaiac detection of haem with increased sensitivity and specificity.

Current screening in the United Kingdom offers FOBT to all ages between 60 and 70 years. An alternative approach used in Canada recommends a single colonoscopy to asymptomatic people over 50 years.

In the United Kingdom colonoscopy is recommended for asymptomatic people with two or more first-degree relatives with colorectal cancer or a single first-degree relative with colon cancer or adenomatous polyps diagnosed when the patient was younger than 60 years from the age of 50 years.

More intensive screening and genetic testing is indicated for those with known syndromes, inflammatory bowel disease and acromegaly.

PREVENTION

Dietary interventions such as increasing fibre and reducing consumption of meat and animal fats can be a useful strategy. Low dose aspirin is recommended for those with a high risk of colorectal cancer such as people with Lynch syndrome. There is some evidence that COX-2 inhibitors (e.g. celecoxib and rofecoxib) reduce the odds of developing metachronous colorectal cancer in people diagnosed with KRAS wild-type cancers.

Prompt diagnosis and excision of large bowel benign polyps, particularly villous adenomata, will prevent subsequent transformation into a cancer.

In those with FAP, Lynch syndrome with a proven large bowel polyposis and selected cases of chronic, extensive ulcerative colitis, risk-reducing colectomy may be considered.

CARCINOMA OF THE ANUS

EPIDEMIOLOGY

In the United Kingdom there are almost 1500 new cases of anal cancer each year and the incidence has been increasing over the past two decades, particularly in women where there has been a doubling of incidence in the past 10 years. Each year it results in the death of over 350 people with a projection that this will increase by 50% over the next 20 years. The incidence increases with age, the peak incidence being >85 years. The male:female ratio of cases is 1:2; anal margin tumours are more common in men, whilst anal canal tumours are more common in women.

AETIOLOGY

Incidence and mortality is highest in the lower socioeconomic groups. It is one of the HPV-related cancers and therefore related to receptive anal intercourse which may also cause local trauma, another related aetiological factor. Human papilloma virus types 16 and 18 account for 90% of cases; it is also more prevalent in the HIV-positive populations.

PATHOLOGY

Invasive cancers are usually preceded by asymptomatic anal intraepithelial neoplasia (AIN), which is comparable to cervical intraepithelial neoplasia (CIN).

The tumour can arise from skin at the anal margin or from the anal canal, appearing as a nodule, polyp or ulcer with everted edges; 90% are squamous carcinomas, most of the remainder adenocarcinomas arising from mucous glands. Anal margin tumours are well differentiated as they are akin to squamous carcinomas of the skin, whereas 75% of anal canal tumours are poorly differentiated. There may be *in situ* carcinoma in the surrounding epithelium.

NATURAL HISTORY

The tumour will spread circumferentially and longitudinally within the anus and can invade the lower rectum or perianal skin. Deeper infiltration leads to involvement of the sphincters, ischiorectal fossae, vagina and urethra. Lymphatic spread occurs in 10% and is more common with anal canal tumours. The first station lymph nodes are inguinal, from which there can be spread to the iliac nodes. Involvement of the distal rectum can lead to infiltration of the inferior mesenteric nodes. Haematogenous spread is very uncommon at presentation. Sites of distant metastases include the liver, lungs and skeleton.

SYMPTOMS

Patients present with anal symptoms such as:

- Discharge
- Irritation/discomfort
- Bleeding
- Tenesmus

Minor symptoms are frequently neglected by both patients and physicians alike as they resemble those from haemorrhoids, which are far more prevalent.

SIGNS

Tumours of the anal verge or most distal part of the anal canal should be easily seen on clinical examination (Figure 9.11). The tumour should be palpable as an indurated ulcer or nodule on digital examination.

The groynes must be examined to assess the inguinal nodes which may be involved in up to one-third of patients at presentation.

In 10% features of liver or lung metastases are present at presentation.

DIFFERENTIAL DIAGNOSIS

This includes:

- Genital warts – these may be confused with a papilliform, well-differentiated carcinoma
- Crohn disease of the anus
- Syphilis
- Other less common malignant tumours, e.g. basal cell carcinoma or melanoma

INVESTIGATIONS

PROCTOSCOPY

This is an essential investigation, allowing direct visualization and biopsy of the tumour, and complements the findings of a digital rectal examination. Anal ultrasound will also aid staging and assessment of the depth of the tumour.

EXAMINATION UNDER ANAESTHETIC (EUA)

This is the best staging investigation in an anxious or uncooperative patient. In a woman, a full bimanual examination is mandatory to assess the extent of local spread. An EUA will also allow a biopsy to be taken if not possible on proctoscopy.

FINE NEEDLE ASPIRATION (FNA) OF ANY ENLARGED INGUINAL LYMPH NODES

This will help to distinguish reactive lymph nodes from malignant ones, which is important in planning treatment.

COMPUTED TOMOGRAPHY (CT) OF THE CHEST, ABDOMEN AND PELVIS

This provides full staging to assess regional and distant lymph nodes as well as metastatic sites in particular liver and lungs.

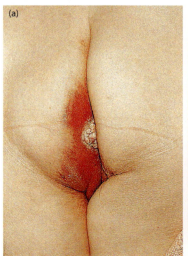 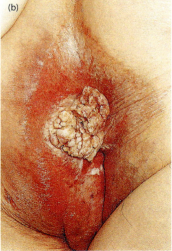

Figure 9.11 Anal margin carcinoma. Papilliform tumour arising from skin at anal verge. (a) Distant view. (b) Close view with buttocks parted.

Gastrointestinal cancer

MAGNETIC RESONANCE (MR) OF THE PELVIS

This can offer more precise information regarding the local extent of the tumour.

STAGING

The TNM staging system is used:

- Tis: Carcinoma *in situ*
- T0: No evidence of primary tumour
- TX: Primary tumour cannot be assessed
- T1: Tumour 2 cm or less in greatest dimension
- T2: Tumour more than 2 cm but not more than 5 cm in greatest dimension
- T3: Tumour more than 5 cm in greatest dimension
- T4: Tumour of any size that invades adjacent organ(s), e.g. vagina, urethra, bladder (involvement of the sphincter muscle(s) alone is not classified as T4)
- NX: Regional lymph nodes cannot be assessed
- N0: No regional lymph node metastasis
- N1: Metastasis in perirectal lymph node(s)
- N2: Metastasis in unilateral internal iliac and/or inguinal lymph node(s)
- N3: Metastasis in perirectal and inguinal lymph nodes and/or bilateral internal iliac and/or inguinal lymph nodes
- MX: Distant metastasis cannot be assessed
- M0: No distant metastasis
- M1: Distant metastasis

TREATMENT

RADICAL TREATMENT

Surgery

In general, surgery is reserved for salvage after relapse following chemoradiation. In selected cases anal margin tumours can be treated by sphincter-sparing wide local excision alone, but most cases will require an abdominoperineal resection (APR), which will result in the patient having a permanent colostomy. Preoperative counselling by a stomatherapist should be arranged for all patients for whom an APR is planned. Patients with cytologically positive inguinal nodes should undergo a block dissection of the groines.

Chemoradiotherapy (CRT)

Non-surgical treatment has the advantage of allowing sphincter preservation and modern chemoradiation will achieve local control in 80%–90% of cases. CRT has therefore become the standard of care for this disease. With CRT, 5FU is delivered continuously during the first and fifth weeks of radiotherapy with bolus mitomycin C on the first day of radiotherapy. Radiotherapy is delivered to the pelvis and inguinal nodes bilaterally, typically to a dose of 45 Gy in 25 fractions over 5 weeks. This is followed, after a short break, by a boost dose of 15–20 Gy to the anal tumour alone, either by external beam radiation over 1.5 weeks or by interstitial brachytherapy. A poor objective response after the initial phase of CRT is an indication to proceed immediately to APR. CRT is associated with an increased severity of acute treatment reactions, particularly with respect to perineal skin reactions and diarrhoea (Figure 9.12).

Most local recurrences occur within 1 year of completing treatment and can still be salvaged by an APR.

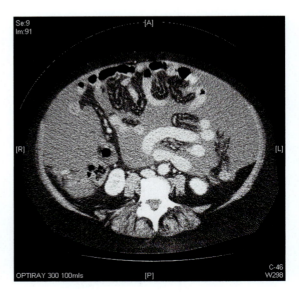

Figure 9.12 Pseudomyxoma peritonei. The CT image shows the abdomen is filled with mucoid material.

PALLIATIVE TREATMENT

Surgery

In the exceptional case of a very advanced inoperable tumour leading to anal occlusion, a defunctioning colostomy may be justified.

Radiotherapy

Pelvic/perineal radiotherapy can be used to palliate symptomatic local recurrence after radical surgery.

TUMOUR-RELATED COMPLICATIONS

An advanced tumour can lead to a fistula between the anal canal and the perineum, vagina or urethra leading to faecal incontinence. The ischiorectal fossae are anatomically close to the anus and particularly prone to secondary infection and abscess formation.

TREATMENT-RELATED COMPLICATIONS

RADIOTHERAPY

The perianal region does not tolerate radiotherapy well as the skin is constantly subjected to friction when sitting or walking, trauma when patients are having to defaecate frequently, moisture owing to sweating and perhaps discharge from the anus. During radiotherapy the patient can be expected to experience diarrhoea, tenesmus and perianal irritation/soreness. These symptoms will begin 1–2 weeks after starting radiotherapy and persist for 4–8 weeks after it has finished.

In the longer term, chronic proctocolitis might manifest as diarrhoea, tenesmus, bleeding and mucus per rectum, which can be treated conservatively with topical steroids. Small bowel stricture, intestinal obstruction and bladder contracture occur in 5%–10% of cases. Infertility is inevitable for both males and females and sexual difficulty can occur due to erectile dysfunction in males and vaginal narrowing and drying in females.

High doses of radiation to the groines can lead to occlusion of the lymphatics, then leading to chronic lymphoedema best managed with pressure garments.

SURGERY

The main morbidity in the short term is from dehiscence of the perineal wound and pelvic infection. Extensive pelvic surgery such as an abdominoperineal resection might damage autonomic nerves leading to urinary incontinence and impotence in men. The psychosexual trauma and effect on body image can be considerable.

CHEMOTHERAPY

Apart from the usual complications from these chemotherapy drugs, CRT leads to added gastrointestinal toxicity causing anorexia, diarrhoea and enhanced radiation skin reaction.

PROGNOSIS

The overall 5-year survival is 70%–80%. In patients with T1 and T2 tumours cure rates are 80%–90%. Adverse features include anal canal versus margin tumours, increasing TNM stage at presentation, and poorly differentiated tumours.

SCREENING/PREVENTION

The high incidence of anal intraepithelial neoplasia in STD clinics can make screening a worthwhile exercise in this small group, particularly in men who have sex with men. Health education could lead to earlier diagnosis.

Use of the quadrivalent HPV vaccine reduces the incidence of AIN in men who have sex with men and increasingly population-based vaccination programmes for both men and women are being introduced which is hoped to reduce the incidence of anal cancer in years to come.

A greater awareness of the disease could lead to earlier diagnosis rather than ad hoc prescription or purchase of proprietary haemorrhoid remedies.

TUMOURS OF THE PERITONEUM

The commonest presentation is with ascites where there is an abnormal accumulation of peritoneal fluid leading to abdominal discomfort and distension. As the peritoneum invests the gastrointestinal tract, abnormal areas of constriction of the bowel can lead to symptoms and signs of subacute or acute bowel obstruction.

The peritoneum is most frequently a site of trans-coelomic spread from abdominal or pelvic malignancies. Occasionally, extra-abdominal malignant tumours will spread to the peritoneum, e.g. lobular breast cancer or lung cancer.

Primary peritoneal mesothelioma is well described and has many features in common with pleural mesothelioma (see Chapter 7). Pseudomyxoma peritonei is a rare, low-grade malignant condition, which may have a very protracted natural history. It is characterized by the accumulation of large amounts of intra-abdominal mucin, often originating from a low-grade tumour of the appendix, ovary or pancreas. Both conditions are potentially treatable by cytoreductive radical peritonectomy (Sugarbaker procedure) and heated intraoperative intraperitoneal chemotherapy. The surgery is radical, involving:

- Removal of the right hemicolon, spleen, gallbladder, greater omentum and lesser omentum
- Stripping of peritoneum from pelvis and diaphragm
- Hepatic capsulectomy
- Hysterectomy and bilateral salpingo-oophorectomy in women
- Removal of rectum in selected cases

Not surprisingly, the procedure is associated with high morbidity and mortality. However, comparative studies suggest that it can increase median survival if performed well.

FURTHER READING

Ajani JA, D'Amico TA, Almhanna K et al. Gastric cancer, version 3.2016, NCCN clinical practice guidelines in oncology. *J Natl Compr Canc Netw.* 2016 Oct; 14(10): 1286–1312.

BMJ Best Practice: Hepatocellular carcinoma. https://bestpractice.bmj.com/topics/en-gb/369

BMJ Best Practice: Cholangiocarcinoma. https://bestpractice.bmj.com/topics/en-gb/721

BMJ Best Practice: Colorectal cancer. https://bestpractice.bmj.com/topics/en-gb/258

BMJ Best Practice: Anal cancer. https://bestpractice.bmj.com/topics/en-gb/1183

Brenner H, Kloor M, Pox CP. Colorectal cancer. *Lancet.* 2014 Apr 26; 383(9927): 1490–1502.

Oesophago-gastric cancer: Assessment and management in adults NICE guideline [NG83]. https://www.nice.org.uk/guidance/ng83/ Published date: January 2018

Waddell T, Verheij M, Allum W, Cunningham D, Cervantes A, Arnold D. Gastric cancer: ESMO-ESSO-ESTRO clinical practice guidelines for diagnosis, treatment and follow-up. *Eur J Surg Oncol.* 2014 May; 40(5): 584–591. doi: 10.1016/j.ejso.2013.09.020.

SELF-ASSESSMENT QUESTIONS

1. Which three of the following statements are true about oesophageal cancer?
   a. It is rare in Africa
   b. A family history is common
   c. Tumours of the upper third are commoner in women
   d. May be caused by chronic acid reflux
   e. There is no association with smoking tobacco
   f. May be associated with asbestos exposure
   g. May be caused by excessive alcohol consumption

2. Which one of the following is not a presenting feature of oesophageal cancer?
   a. Dysphagia
   b. Acid reflux
   c. Regurgitation of food
   d. Weight loss
   e. Pulmonary aspiration

3. Which three of the following statements are true for oesophageal cancer?
   a. Radiotherapy alone cures >10% of cases
   b. Surgery offers the best chance of cure
   c. Upper third cancers are best treated by radiotherapy
   d. Distant spread to the liver is rare

Self-assessment questions

    e. Cisplatin is a useful drug
    f. Docetaxel is a drug of choice for metastatic disease
    g. Cetuximab is a useful treatment

4. Which three of the following statements are true for stomach cancer?
    a. It is commoner in lower socioeconomic groups
    b. It is three times commoner in males than females
    c. Often presents with abdominal pain
    d. Spread outside the stomach is common
    e. May be associated with non-malignant skin eruptions
    f. Docetaxel is a drug of choice for metastatic disease
    g. Cetuximab is a useful treatment

5. Which one of the following is not true about gastrointestinal stromal tumours?
    a. They are rare tumours
    b. Commoner in older age groups
    c. A specific cytogenetic abnormality is characteristic
    d. A tyrosine kinase inhibitor is an effective treatment'
    e. They are amenable to treatment with immunotherapy

6. Which three of the following statements are true about pancreatic cancer?
    a. Commonest in 40–60 age group
    b. A family history is common
    c. Mainly arises from the ducts of the gland
    d. Most cases are caused by gallstones
    e. Commonly presents with obstructive jaundice
    f. CA125 is a useful serum tumour marker protein
    g. CEA is a useful serum tumour marker protein

7. Which one of the following is true about the treatment of pancreatic cancer?
    a. Surgery offers the best chance of cure
    b. 10%–20% will be long-term survivors
    c. Chemotherapy has no role in the management of early pancreatic cancer
    d. 5FU is the most active chemotherapy agent
    e. Tamoxifen is a useful treatment

8. Which three of the following statements are true about hepatocellular carcinoma?
    a. It is common in Africa
    b. Has a viral aetiology in some cases
    c. Human chorionic gonadotropin is a useful serum tumour marker
    d. Diarrhoea is a common symptom
    e. It is highly sensitive to chemotherapy
    f. Can be successfully treated with bevacizumab
    g. Has a very poor prognosis

9. Which one of the following is not true about cancer of the gallbladder and biliary tree?
    a. Can be associated with gallstones
    b. Can be associated with typhoid carriage
    c. They are common tumours
    d. They generally have a low probability of long-term cure
    e. Adjuvant chemotherapy has no proven role in these diseases

10. Which three of the following statements are true about the epidemiology and aetiology of colorectal cancer?
    a. It is commoner than breast cancer
    b. It causes more deaths per annum than breast cancer
    c. It is relatively common in Africa and Asia
    d. There is a strong male predominance
    e. Colon cancer is commoner than rectal cancer
    f. It is commoner in more affluent socioeconomic groups
    g. There is a strong association with HIV infection

11. Which three of the following statements are true about the presentation of colorectal cancer?
    a. Bleeding is a common symptom
    b. Vitamin B12 deficiency can occur
    c. A normal digital rectal examination excludes rectal cancer
    d. Abdominal obstruction is a sign of locally advanced disease
    e. Abdominal distension is common
    f. Many will have overt metastatic disease in the liver at diagnosis
    g. Supraclavicular lymph nodes are uncommon

12. Which one of the following is true about the treatment of colorectal cancer?
    a. Surgery alone is not curative
    b. Those having a colostomy have a worse prognosis
    c. Preoperative radiotherapy for rectal cancer substantially increases the risk of operative complications
    d. Platinum compounds have no significant activity in this disease
    e. Advanced stages of the disease responds to VEGF inhibitors

13. Which three of the following statements are not prognostic factors for colorectal cancer?
    a. Dukes' staging
    b. Presentation with rectal bleeding
    c. Previous colonic polyps
    d. Number of involved lymph nodes
    e. Normal colonoscopy in preceding 3 years
    f. Complete surgical excision of tumour
    g. Vascular invasion

14. Which one of the following is not true about anal cancer?
    a. It is associated with human papilloma virus
    b. Associated with HIV infection
    c. Nearly always treated by abdominoperineal resection
    d. Relatively sensitive to radiotherapy
    e. Has a high rate of local control

Urological cancer

RENAL CELL CARCINOMA

EPIDEMIOLOGY

Renal cell carcinoma accounts for 2% of all malignancies with over 7000 cases each year in the United Kingdom and over 3000 deaths per year. It is more common in males than females. The incidence is high in Europe, particularly Denmark, and lowest in Japan and an overall increase in incidence has been reported worldwide, much of which is attributed to increased access to investigations such as abdominal CT scan, which can identify previously occult diseases.

AETIOLOGY

There are several possible aetiological factors:

- Smoking tobacco
- Cadmium exposure
- A rare familial pattern associated with *HLABW44* and *HLA-DR8*
- Increased incidence in von Hippel–Lindau (VHL) disease, horseshoe kidneys and adult polycystic kidneys

PATHOLOGY

Tumours can arise from any part of the renal tissue: a quarter involve the whole kidney, one-third the upper pole and one-third the lower pole. Macroscopically, the tumour is usually solid, expanding the renal tissue with a central area of necrosis or cystic degeneration and other haemorrhagic areas. Occasionally, a tumour arises within the wall of a cyst. Renal cell tumours are thought to arise from the lining cells of the proximal convoluted tubule.

Microscopically, they are adenocarcinomas composed of characteristic clear cells, although the degree of differentiation can vary from a well-differentiated tumour to a highly anaplastic appearance. The most commonly used grading system is the Fuhrman grading system based predominantly on nuclear size and shape.

The majority show aberrant expression of the VHL gene and upregulation of vascular endothelial growth factor (VEGF) with prominent neoangiogenesis.

NATURAL HISTORY

The tumour invades the surrounding kidney and can grow into the renal vein and thence into the inferior vena cava (IVC).

Lymph node spread involves the renal hilar nodes and progresses to the para-aortic chain. Blood-borne metastases characteristically spread to the lung and bone, although many other sites including the skin, central nervous system and liver are also recognized. Approximately 25% of patients will present with a metastatic disease and of the remainder a further 30%–40% will eventually express distant metastases.

Spontaneous regression of metastases, typically lung deposits monitored on chest x-ray, is often referred to in the context of renal cell cancer. While such events undoubtedly occur, the true incidence is extremely low, the verified incidence being around 7% of patients with a metastatic disease.

Urological cancer

Spontaneous regression of the primary tumour is virtually unknown.

SYMPTOMS

Haematuria, typically painless, is the most common presenting symptom. Loin pain can occur acutely from haemorrhage within the tumour or chronically as the tumour enlarges.

Symptoms of metastases might be present, in particular bone pain or even pathological fracture (bone metastases) and cough with or without haemoptysis (lung metastases).

Symptoms of paraneoplastic conditions associated with renal cell cancer may be present: these include hypercalcaemia and polycythaemia. There might also be general symptoms of malignancy such as malaise, anorexia and weight loss.

SIGNS

The primary tumour can be a palpable mass in the loin, and in 10%–20% of patients there is an associated fever.

DIFFERENTIAL DIAGNOSIS

Other causes of haematuria should be considered, in particular benign renal adenomas, tumours of the renal pelvis, renal tract stones and bladder tumours.

Other causes of loin pain which should be taken into account include renal stones or hydronephrosis.

INVESTIGATIONS

BLOOD TESTS

A full blood count sometimes shows anaemia owing to chronic haematuria, or polycythaemia from tumour production of erythropoietin-like substances. Serum calcium may be raised.

RADIOGRAPHY

Chest x-ray might show typical 'cannonball' metastases.

CT SCAN

The renal tumour will be imaged using either ultrasound or CT scan. The latter also gives information on renal vein/IVC invasion and involvement of surrounding structures. Figure 10.1 shows the appearance of a renal carcinoma on CT scan.

CT of the abdomen and thorax is also essential to screen for metastases in lymph nodes, lungs and liver.

FINE NEEDLE ASPIRATE OR BIOPSY

The radiological appearances of renal carcinoma are usually typical. Fine needle aspirate cytology or biopsy is usually avoided because of the risk of tumour seeding in the biopsy tract unless there is doubt on CT scan.

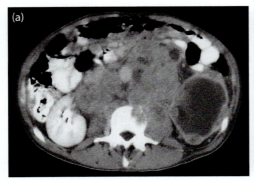 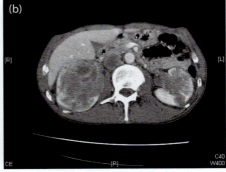

Figure 10.1 (a) CT scan demonstrating a large renal carcinoma rising from the left kidney. (b) CT scan demonstrating bilateral renal carcinomas more advanced on the right than the left.

STAGING

Important features of the TNM staging are the size of the primary tumour and involvement of surrounding structures including the renal vein, which will determine operability of the primary and the presence of distant metastases.

TNM staging for renal carcinoma is used:

- T1 – Tumour ≤7 cm limited to kidney
  - T1a – Tumour ≤4 cm
  - T1b – Tumour >4–7 cm
- T2 – Tumour >7 cm limited to kidney
- T3 – Tumour extends into major vessels, adrenal glands or surrounding tissues but not beyond Gerota fascia
  - T3a – Invasion into adrenals or perinephric tissues
  - T3b – Extension into vena cava above diaphragm
- T4 – Tumour extends beyond Gerota fascia
- N0 – No lymph node involvement
- N1 – 1 lymph node involved
- N2 – >1 lymph node involved

TREATMENT

SURGERY

Radical nephrectomy in which the perirenal fat, perirenal fascia, adrenal gland and regional nodes are removed en bloc is the operation of choice with superior local control rates to simple nephrectomy. Tumour invading the renal vein can be successfully removed and this is therefore not an absolute contraindication to radical treatment.

Small peripheral tumours can be considered for partial nephrectomy and there is an increasing use of cryotherapy and high-frequency ultrasound ablation for such lesions in patients unfit for surgery.

Tumours less than 3 cm in diameter in elderly patients have a low probability of metastases and where there are contributing comorbidities a risk from surgery may be observed.

PALLIATIVE TREATMENT

Local irradiation of painful bone metastases may be required. Brain metastases can benefit from cranial irradiation, or if it is solitary without extensive disease elsewhere, surgical excision can be considered.

Lung metastases can also be amenable to surgical excision in the occasional patients who present with a solitary lung metastasis some years after treatment of the primary tumour.

SYSTEMIC TREATMENT

Substantial advances have been made in the management of advanced and metastatic renal cancer in recent years. Renal cancer is responsive to immunomodulatory therapies and antiangiogenic agents. First-line treatment will now use sunitinib or pazopanib, both tyrosine kinase inhibitors (TKI), or nivolumab which is an immunomodulatory drug. Other active drugs which may be considered are everolimus, an mTOR inhibitor; axitinib, a tyrosine kinase inhibitor and cabozantinib, a TKI targeting c-MET and VEGF2.

Despite these advances, however, treatment with biological agents is at best palliative in the setting of widespread metastatic disease but the availability of several agents results in not only first-line therapy but also second- and third-line agents has improved survival considerably from a median of only 5 months in the era of interferon to over 2 years with current agents.

TUMOUR-RELATED COMPLICATIONS

Complications of renal cell carcinoma include hypercalcaemia and polycythaemia. Renal function is usually unaffected provided the contralateral kidney is normal.

PROGNOSIS

The prognosis for tumour localized to the kidney is good, with 5-year survival after radical nephrectomy of around 50%.

Even in the presence of metastases, renal cell cancer often has a long and indolent course so that 5%–10% of patients with lung metastases will survive for 5 years or more.

SCREENING AND FUTURE PROSPECTS

Simple urinalysis for microscopic haematuria and cytology are readily available. However, while sensitive, it is non-specific and results in unacceptably high false-positive rates for routine application.

Renal cancer has been an area of major endeavour in drug development with the use of immune modulating agents, vascular targeting and antiangiogenic agents. Current research is seeking the optimal sequencing and combinations of these agents.

PROSTATE CANCER

EPIDEMIOLOGY

Each year in the United Kingdom there are 35,000 cases of prostate cancer, making it the commonest form of cancer in men, accounting for 12% of all cancer cases and leading to a total of 10,000 deaths per annum. In the United Kingdom it is the second most common cause of death from cancer in men after lung cancer. The UK incidence of 52 in 100,000 compares with 274 in 100,000 in US black men, 171 in 100,000 in US white men and six in 100,000 men in Japan. The high rates in the United States are again attributed at least in part to the widespread prostate-specific antigen (PSA) screening that occurs there.

The incidence of prostate cancer is rising. This may reflect an increasing proportion of the population over 70 years, a greater diagnostic rate and possibly a true increase in incidence in younger men. Despite this, mortality has been stable over recent years supporting the view that the increase in diagnosis is largely due to identification of early previously undetected disease mainly through PSA screening of healthy individuals.

AETIOLOGY

- *Age*: It is rarely found in men under 45 years but increases with age, being almost universal at postmortem in men aged over 80 years.
- *Familial*: A family history of prostate cancer in a first-degree relative increases the risk in an individual by two to three times. When seen in young men under 45 years there can be a stronger genetic basis. Recently, a seven-gene signature for prostate cancer has been identified. The most frequent alteration in prostate cancer is methylation of the promoter of *GSTP1*, a gene involved in carcinogen detoxification. An association with breast cancer in female relatives has also been described linked to the *BRCA2* gene which carries a five-fold increased risk of prostate cancer and accounts for 2% of all cases.
- *Other factors*: It is more common in city dwellers than rural communities, and is associated with a high fat and meat diet, and an occupational exposure to cadmium. It is more common in married men, related to the number of sexual partners, frequency of sexual activity and a history of sexually transmitted diseases. The androgen receptor signalling pathway is thought to play an important role in the early development of prostate cancer.

It is important to note that benign prostatic hypertrophy can coexist with prostate cancer but is not causally related.

PATHOLOGY

Cancer of the prostate develops most commonly in the peripheral part of the gland, accounting for 70%, while only 10% arise centrally. The remainder arises in the transitional zone. Eighty-five percent are diffuse multifocal tumours. *In situ* cancer (prostate intraepithelial neoplasia – PIN) is now a recognized precursor to invasive disease and may be seen in adjacent parts of a gland containing invasive cancer.

Microscopically, prostate cancer is typically an adenocarcinoma of varying differentiation. Various grading systems based on morphological appearances have been described, all of which correlate with outcomes. The commonly used system is the Gleason score, which is based on the pattern of growth of the tumour and is recorded as the sum of primary and secondary grades giving a summed score from 2 to 10. A Gleason score of 8 or above correlates with a relatively poor outcome. Another poor prognostic feature is perineural invasion.

Where there is doubt as to the primary origin of a tumour deposit, a prostatic primary will be characterized by staining for acid phosphatase and

Prostate cancer

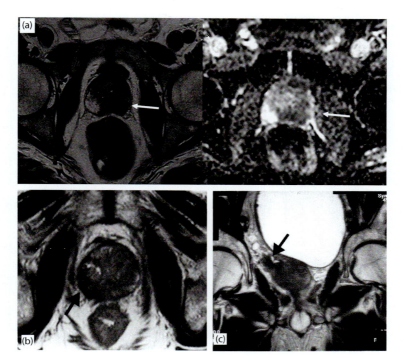

Figure 10.2 MR scan of prostate demonstrating (a) large tumour arising in left peripheral zone on T2 and confirmed on diffusion weighted images (DWI); (b) early extracapsular invasion; and (c) seminal vesicle invasion.

prostate-specific antigen. Androgen and progestogen receptors have been demonstrated on the surface of prostate cancer cells, although the value of this in routine clinical use remains uncertain.

NATURAL HISTORY

Local growth results in infiltration of the prostate gland and surrounding tissues, particularly into the seminal vesicles, bladder and rectum as shown in Figure 10.2. Predictive tables (the Partin tables) are available that correlate the risk of extracapsular extension and seminal vesicle invasion with PSA, T stage and Gleason score. A patient with a PSA of 4.1–6.0 ng/mL, Gleason score of 5–6 and stage T2a has a 19% risk of capsular penetration and zero risk of seminal vesicle invasion. In contrast, when the PSA is 6.1–10.0 ng/mL and Gleason score 7 (4+3) with the same stage, the risk of capsular penetration is 58% and seminal vesicle invasion is 11%.

Lymph node metastases occur with initial involvement of pelvic nodes, which increases with clinical stage, presenting PSA and Gleason score. The probability of lymph node metastases can be calculated from the Roach score; the percentage risk is given by the formula $(PSA/3) + 10(Gleason\ Score - 6)$.

Distant spread is usually blood-borne, typically by retrograde venous spread through the vertebral plexus of veins, so that bone metastases to the spine are common, although all parts of the skeleton may be affected (Figure 10.3).

Soft-tissue metastases, e.g. lungs or liver, although well recognized are relatively uncommon in prostatic cancer.

SYMPTOMS

Prostate cancer is often asymptomatic and found either at postmortem or incidentally during the investigation of another condition. The following symptoms may be present:

- Prostatic outflow obstructive symptoms, with frequency, hesitancy, poor stream, nocturia and terminal dribble
- Haematospermia

Urological cancer

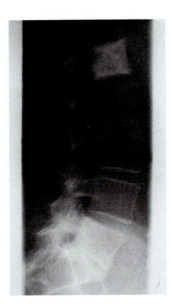

Figure 10.3 Lateral x-ray of the lumbar spine showing metastases in L1 causing extensive sclerotic changes compared with surrounding normal vertebrae.

- Erectile dysfunction
- Bone pain or, less often, spinal cord compression, owing to bone metastases
- Hypercalcaemia
- General symptoms of malignancy, including malaise, anorexia and weight loss

SIGNS

The tumour may be palpable per rectum as a hard nodule or diffusely infiltrating abnormality, which in more advanced cases might be invading surrounding pelvic tissues. Typically there is loss of the midline sulcus of the gland, which is present in the normal or hypertrophied prostate.

Bone metastases might be clinically apparent when complicated by pain, pathological fracture or neurological signs.

DIFFERENTIAL DIAGNOSIS

Benign prostatic hypertrophy can produce the same symptoms of bladder outflow obstruction and indeed can coexist with prostatic cancer.

The most common cause of a raised PSA is prostatitis.

INVESTIGATIONS

ROUTINE BLOOD TESTS

A full blood count might show a reduction of haemoglobin, white cells or platelets with widespread bone metastases. Hypercalcaemia and impaired renal function should be excluded from routine biochemistry.

PROSTATE-SPECIFIC ANTIGEN

PSA is the most common means of diagnosing prostate cancer; however, whilst very sensitive, it is relatively non-specific for prostate cancer distinct from benign prostate pathology. Up to two-thirds of men with a modestly raised PSA will not have prostate cancer and around 20% of patients with prostate cancer can have a PSA in the normal range. As a sole screening test for prostate cancer it is therefore relatively poor and has to be supplemented by further investigations, in particular digital rectal examination and transrectal biopsy before a diagnosis can be confirmed. Exceptions to this are patients presenting with radiology showing typical bone metastases and a PSA of >100 µg/L.

PSA also has an important role in monitoring patients once a diagnosis has been confirmed. Prognosis is related to the rate of PSA change measured by the PSA doubling time.

MAGNETIC RESONANCE SCANNING

MRI gives excellent views of the prostate gland and its relation to surrounding normal soft tissue structures such as bladder and rectum. Best definition is obtained using specific rectal coils. It is now the investigation of choice for staging prostate cancer and it is now a routine to perform multiparametric MR sequences in which, in addition to the standard T1 and T2 anatomical images, functional imaging with diffusion weighted images (DWI) and dynamic contrast enhanced (DCE) images are taken improving the sensitivity and specificity of the test; examples are shown in Figure 10.2.

MRI can also be used where there is uncertainty over the presence of bone metastases, particularly in

Prostate cancer

the spine where, in an ageing population, degenerative disease is common and might cause uptake on an isotope scan, although in many cases plain x-rays will be sufficient to diagnose characteristic osteoblastic metastases (Figure 10.3).

Whole body MR including diffusion weighted images (DWI) are increasingly used in staging to exclude the presence of small volume metastases.

ULTRASOUND

Transrectal ultrasound is used routinely to provide real-time images and is used to direct needle biopsy towards the suspicious areas of the gland and also in brachytherapy to direct accurate placement of radioactive sources. Doppler flow studies can give even greater detail of the internal structure of the gland and highlight abnormal areas.

CT SCAN

This may give more detail of distal lymph node changes in the common iliac and para-aortic regions but will only be used for staging of the primary tumour in the prostate where MRI is contraindicated, e.g. a patient with a pacemaker.

ISOTOPE BONE SCAN

Isotope bone scan is the most widespread screening test for bone metastases but is not as sensitive as MR or PET. A positive scan is shown in Figure 10.4.

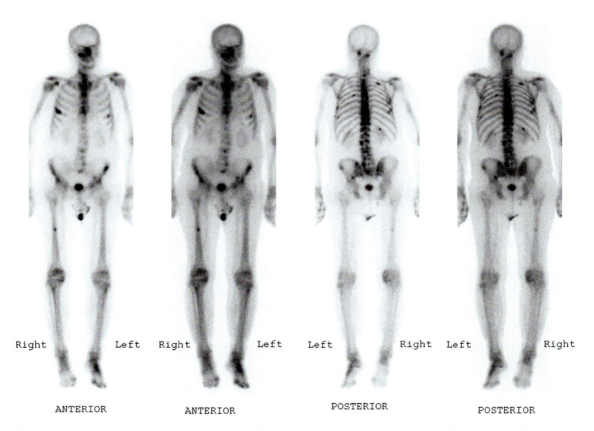

Figure 10.4 Isotope bone scan demonstrating multiple areas of increased uptake in spine, ribs, pelvis and right femur due to bone metastases from carcinoma of the prostate. Anterior view is on the left and posterior view on the right.

COMPUTED TOMOGRAPHY-POSITRON EMISSION TOMOGRAPHY

PET scanning is increasingly being used for prostate cancer. Choline PET is currently the most widely used tracer but more sensitive and specific ligands such as PSMA PET are now available and appear to give even better identification of early metastatic disease.

BIOPSY OR RESECTION

Histological confirmation is made either at transurethral resection of the prostate (TURP) or on transrectal ultrasound-guided needle biopsy per rectum. Wide sampling of the gland from all four quadrants should be undertaken with a minimum of 12 samples for a representative result. Previous fears that TURP could cause dissemination of cancer cells are unfounded but, in the absence of major bladder outflow symptoms, a needle biopsy is to be preferred.

The widespread adoption of multiparametric MR with which index lesions of significant prostate cancer can be identified radiologically has shown that in some men the cancer will be predominately anterior and often not accessible by a transrectal biopsy. For this reason, transperineal biopsy is often undertaken enabling more widespread sampling of the entire gland.

STAGING

Staging of cancer of the prostate is defined in the TNM system as shown as follows. The important principles are to distinguish early localized carcinoma of the prostate from locally extensive disease from that which has already metastasized.

- T0 – No evidence of primary tumour
- T1 – Asymptomatic or incidental finding
  - T1a – Incidental finding in ≤5% resected tissue
  - T1b – Incidental finding in >5% resected tissue
  - T1c – Diagnosis at needle biopsy because of asymptomatic raised PSA
- T2 – Tumour confined within the capsule of gland
  - T2a – Tumour involves one half of a lobe or less
  - T2b – Tumour involves more than one half of a lobe but not both lobes
  - T2c – Tumour involves both lobes
- T3 – Tumour extension beyond the capsule of gland
  - T3a – Tumour extends beyond capsule unilaterally or bilaterally
  - T3b – Tumour involves seminal vesicles
- T4 – Invasion of rectum or other pelvic structures
- N1, N2, N3 – Involvement of regional nodes
- M1 – Distant metastases

TREATMENT

Radical treatment is indicated for prostatic cancer localized to the prostate gland with no evidence on the basis of MRI or isotope bone scan of distant metastases. A PSA level of under 20 ng/mL virtually excludes the possibility of bone metastases, whilst a level of >50 ng/mL carries a very high probability of distant spread even if the bone scan is 'normal', and such levels will usually exclude radical treatment approaches.

ACTIVE SURVEILLANCE

It is clear that many men who are diagnosed with early low-risk disease, with a PSA <10 ng/mL and a Gleason score <7, have indolent disease, which may never compromise their survival; this is evident in the large proportion of men dying from other causes who, as their age increases, have an increasing likelihood of harbouring asymptomatic undiagnosed prostate cancer. The ever-increasing use of PSA screening has amplified the problem of managing this group of patients in whom it is clearly important to identify those who have the potential to develop more aggressive prostate cancer and equally to enable those with indolent disease to avoid potentially morbid treatment. At present there is no reliable marker to separate out these two populations.

Many patients over 70 years with low PSA and Gleason scores at diagnosis will be offered active surveillance as a treatment option. This requires a regular monitoring of the serum PSA, typically every 3 months, with repeat biopsies after 2 years to ensure there has been no change in the nature of the cancer. Treatment can be introduced if the PSA rises above 10 µg/L or if the calculated PSA doubling time is <2 years, or if the patient indicates that he wishes to do so. Whilst this approach suits some patients, who are only too pleased to avoid major treatment intervention, many find the associated anxiety and uncertainty unacceptable.

RADICAL PROSTATECTOMY

This is indicated for disease that is localized to the gland, i.e. stages T1 and T2. The operation is usually a robotic laparoscopic procedure and involves removal of the entire prostate and adjacent bladder neck, both seminal vesicles, the vasa deferentia and surrounding fascia. A pelvic lymph node dissection may also be included. It requires considerable surgical expertise. Complications include erectile dysfunction and occasional urinary incontinence. 'Nerve sparing' techniques to preserve the neurovascular bundle responsible for penile erection are used but may not be possible where there is tumour infiltration close to these critical structures.

Postoperative radiotherapy may play a role where excision margins are close to or involved with tumour or when pelvic lymph nodes are involved. After prostatectomy the PSA should be undetectable; any presence of PSA even at very low levels suggests residual prostatic tissue and is an indication for postoperative radiotherapy. There is evidence that this is most effective when the PSA remains <0.2 ng/mL. The role of antiandrogen treatment in this setting remains under investigation.

RADICAL RADIOTHERAPY

This is a treatment option for all patients with disease localized to the pelvis. A small treatment volume encompassing known disease in the prostate and seminal vesicles is adequate, although there are advocates of prophylactic treatment of pelvic lymph nodes in patients with higher PSA levels and high Gleason scores (>7). CT and MR scanning to enable intensity modulated radiotherapy (IMRT) is now routine to deliver a standard dose of 78 Gy in 39 fractions or the equivalent dose of 60 Gy in 20 fractions; external beam radiotherapy is associated with bowel frequency and urgency and may alter bladder function. Minor long-term bowel frequency and rectal bleeding are seen in about one-third of patients but major changes which would affect the lifestyle of the patients are seen in less than 5%. Erectile dysfunction is seen in up to 40% of patients.

There is some evidence from the biological response of prostate cancer to radiation that larger single doses might be more effective and this approach is currently under investigation using brachytherapy or stereotactic body radiotherapy (SBRT).

Brachytherapy with permanent implants of radioactive iodine-125 or palladium-103 offers an alternative approach to external beam radiotherapy in patients with early localized disease. A permanent iodine seed implant is shown in Figure 10.5. Combined treatments using external beam with a brachytherapy boost, usually by a temporary implant using an iridium afterloading technique, are also advocated as a means of increasing radiation dose without additional side effects. This has been shown to prolong biochemical control rates compared to external beam alone.

Principle side effects from brachytherapy are mainly related to urethral and bladder irritation. In the majority of patients potency is preserved and brachytherapy is associated with very few bowel effects although acute prostatitis and urethritis immediately following the procedure might be more pronounced than with external beam treatment.

HORMONE THERAPY

'Hormone therapy' refers to the use of androgen deprivation or blockade. It is effective when first introduced in most patients (see Chapter 6). It may be used as:

- *Primary treatment* in frail or medically compromised patients.

Urological cancer

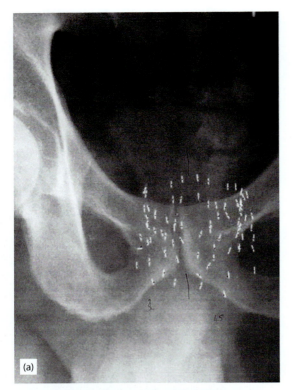

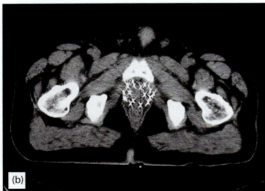

Figure 10.5 (a) Plain x-ray showing iodine seeds after implantation into prostate gland and (b) CT scan showing position taken 1 month after the implant procedure.

- Metastatic disease treatment at presentation.
- *Neoadjuvant or adjuvant treatment*. It has a role in primary treatment for locally advanced tumours prior to definitive radiotherapy by allowing initial reduction of tumour bulk and early control of local symptoms. When used as an adjuvant treatment for 3 years after definitive radiotherapy or surgery for stage T3 prostate cancer an improvement in survival has been demonstrated. There is also an advantage for at least 6 months from adjuvant antiandrogen treatment in 'intermediate risk' disease defined by a PSA >10 ng/mL, a Gleason score of 7 or above and stage T2a or b.
- *Relapse* after definitive primary treatment.

PALLIATIVE TREATMENT

For metastatic disease, hormone therapy will receive a response in most patients, although eventually resistance to this approach will be seen. Hormone therapy can be given in a number of forms as shown in Table 10.1. All of these are equally effective and the choice will in general be based on patient acceptability and availability.

Antiandrogen drugs include cyproterone acetate, flutamide and bicalutamide. Gonadotrophin-releasing hormone (GnRH) analogue drugs include goserelin and leuprorelin.

First-line treatment for a patient presenting with metastatic prostate cancer will generally be either a GnRH analogue or an oral antiandrogen such as flutamide or bicalutamide. Over 80% of patients will respond to this manoeuvre. When a GnRH analogue drug is started, the initial exposure should be covered by a period of 10–14 days oral antiandrogen

Table 10.1 Hormone therapy for prostate cancer: relative clinical merits

Bilateral orchidectomy	Antiandrogen drugs	GnRH analogue
Surgical procedure	Oral medication	Monthly or 3-monthly injection
Permanent	Reversible	Reversible (but may take several months for recovery)
Compliance guaranteed	Tablets may be missed	Compliance guaranteed
Patient acceptance variable	Readily accepted	Readily accepted

administration to block the initial flare seen with these agents. There is no evidence that continuing combination therapy, sometimes referred to as MAB (maximal androgen blockade) has major advantages over single-agent therapy. Permanent androgen deprivation by orchidectomy may be offered to responders with the alternative of continuing with medical treatment.

There is good evidence that chemotherapy involving six cycles of docetaxel with initiation of hormone therapy in patients presenting with metastatic disease is beneficial and extends survival by 1–2 years when used in this way.

Patients will inevitably relapse despite an initial response, the median duration of response being around 24 months. There are now several options for patients who reach this 'castrate-resistant' state. New drugs having a different action on the androgen receptor pathway can be very successful in achieving a further period of response. Abiraterone inhibits an enzyme in androgen synthesis and enzalutamide works both at the androgen receptor and inhibits translocation of the androgen receptor into the cell and its binding to DNA.

Chemotherapy should be considered for selected patients with relapse after hormone treatment. Docetaxel with prednisolone is now the schedule of choice having been shown to be superior to mitoxantrone. It will achieve an improvement in quality of life scores and a median improvement in survival of 2 months has been demonstrated. Toxicity can counterbalance this, however, with many patients experience fatigue, neuromuscular symptoms, skin and nail changes and bone marrow depression.

Radium 223 is a bone-seeking radioisotope which emits alpha particles. These have a short range in tissue and thus the radiation dose can be concentrated at sites of radium uptake, typically sites of osteoblastic response to metastases. It is given as an intravenous injection every 4 weeks for a course of six injections and has been shown to have similar effects on chemotherapy or second-line hormone therapy such as abiraterone or enzalutamide. Because of its short range there is limited toxicity which may include fatigue and mild reductions in blood indices.

CASE HISTORY

PROSTATE CANCER

MJ, a 68-year-old man, had been noticing for some weeks a nagging pain in the back with some local tenderness over the lumbar spine. The pain was worse on standing and walking but never went away completely. He had done no recent heavy work to provoke it. For several years he had noted that he passed water more frequently and had started having to get up at night two or three times to pass water. He consulted his GP who confirmed some local tenderness in the lumbar spine and in view of his urinary symptoms performed a rectal examination. This revealed an enlarged hard irregular prostate gland.

His GP arranged for x-rays of the spine and some blood tests including a serum PSA. This returned with an elevated level at 385 ng/mL and the x-rays showed scattered sclerotic changes compatible with metastatic disease. He was referred to a specialist oncology clinic where it was confirmed that the findings were compatible with a diagnosis of metastatic prostate cancer. The raised PSA level was considered sufficient to confirm the diagnosis and no biopsy of the prostate gland was recommended. Treatment was started with cyproterone acetate tablets for 2 weeks and a goserelin subcutaneous implant was given. He was also advised to consider chemotherapy in view of his metastatic disease at presentation. When reviewed 6 weeks later MJ reported a considerable improvement in his back pain but was complaining of intermittent hot flushes. It was explained that these were a common side effect of the goserelin injections. A repeat PSA had fallen to 26 ng/mL and he was recommended to continue with the goserelin at 3-monthly intervals. He agreed to start chemotherapy and received six cycles of docetaxel and prednisolone. During his chemotherapy he had complete alopecia and some mild numbness of his fingers and toes. He also noted that his fingernails developed a purplish discoloration. These recovered during the following 3 months.

MJ remained well for the next 2 years, the hot flushes regressing and his pain remaining well controlled. He then noted over a period of a few days increasing difficulty in climbing stairs accompanied by a return of his backache. The following day he was unable to pass water and reported a loss of feeling in his legs. His GP referred him for an urgent assessment to his local casualty department. There he was found to be in urinary retention, with a grade 3–4 weakness of the lower limbs and a reduction in pin prick and light touch sensation to the level of the umbilicus. A urinary catheter was inserted and an urgent MR scan was performed. This showed extensive spinal metastases with involvement of the spinal canal at T10. Urgent transfer to the local cancer centre was arranged. He was started on dexamethasone and immediate local radiotherapy to the lower thoracic spine was given over the next week. A repeat PSA level was found to be 376 ng/mL. Following completion of radiotherapy his pain settled once more. The power in his lower limbs improved and he was able to walk independently with the aid of a stick. He also regained control of his bladder function.

In view of his rising PSA despite taking goserelin he was recommended to start an additional peripheral anti-androgen using bicalutamide tablets. When reviewed 2 months later his PSA had fallen to 230 ng/mL but he was complaining of discomfort and swelling in his breasts; it was explained that this was a recognized side effect of the bicalutamide tablets.

He remained well for the next few months slowly becoming more active but 6 months later he started complaining of scattered pains in the spine, pelvis and ribs despite increasing his analgesia. His PSA had risen to 416 ng/mL. It was recommended that he start enzalutamide in place of the bicalutamide tablets. He was also started on zoledronic acid injections every 4 weeks to reduce the effects from his bone metastases. Three months later he returned to the clinic for review; his PSA had fallen to 37 ng/mL and his pain had settled. He had noted more hot flushes returning after starting the enzalutamide but otherwise no additional side effects. He continued on the combination of goserelin and enzalutamide for the next 18 months, his PSA settling to a range of 6–8 ng/mL. It was then noted that there was a slow rise in his PSA month by month with a PSA doubling time of only 3 months. The option of further chemotherapy using docetaxel again or carbazetaxel was discussed and he agreed to discontinue the enzalutamide and receive carbazetaxel with prednisolone. When he attended his second chemotherapy he mentioned that he was having more difficulty in walking and felt his legs were getting weaker. An urgent MRI showed recurrence of his spinal canal compression. The risks of further radiotherapy to the spine were discussed and he felt that he was willing to take the chance of radiation damage to the spinal cord from further radiotherapy rather than allow the cancer to cause progressive spinal cord damage. Further irradiation was given but his general condition deteriorated and he became unable to mobilize himself without help. He required increasing levels of morphine to control his discomfort. He continued to deteriorate whilst remaining comfortable. A few weeks later he developed a productive cough and a chest x-ray showed patchy consolidation. His condition deteriorated further as he developed bronchopneumonia from which he died 3 days later.

Other palliative treatments that will be of value in these patients include the appropriate use of analgesics and co-analgesics including bisphosphonates such as zoledronic acid to reduce skeletal complications and bone pain. Palliative radiotherapy has an important role in bone pain. Palliative radiotherapy is also indicated for neurological complications.

Hypercalcaemia requires active management when symptomatic (see Chapter 22).

TUMOUR-RELATED COMPLICATIONS

These include:

- Obstructive hydronephrosis
- Hypercalcaemia
- Spinal cord compression
- Pathological fracture

TREATMENT-RELATED COMPLICATIONS

SURGERY

Surgery can lead to impotence and urinary incontinence.

RADIOTHERAPY

Bowel and bladder damage can result from external beam radiotherapy.

Impotence also occurs but less often than after surgery; in both settings there is good response to drugs such as sildenafil.

Brachytherapy is associated only rarely with long-term bowel or bladder problems but can be followed by an immediate period of post-implant acute urethritis.

HORMONE THERAPY

Androgen blockade is commonly associated with hot flushes, lethargy, gynaecomastia, reduced libido and varying degrees of impotence. Oral anti-androgens can cause nausea and, rarely, hepatic dysfunction.

PROGNOSIS

While aggressive forms of prostatic cancer are recognized, particularly in young men, in the majority of cases the natural history of the disease will span several years. Because of this, it is difficult to judge the results of treatment on short-term survival figures.

Untreated, localized carcinoma of the prostate will still give a 5-year survival of 80%, although many will have locally progressive disease. After radical treatment, surgical or radiotherapeutic, 10-year survivals in excess of 80% are to be expected, falling to around 50% for disease extending outside the capsule of the gland. In general, the majority of men diagnosed with early localized disease having a low PSA and Gleason score will not die from their prostate cancer.

In contrast, patients presenting with metastatic disease have a median survival of around 42 months.

SCREENING AND FUTURE PROSPECTS

Digital rectal examination, serum prostate-specific antigen and transrectal ultrasound offer a high chance of detecting preclinical prostate cancer. Extensive studies are currently underway in Europe to evaluate the effect of screening healthy men and this is already a common practice in the United States, where 50% of prostate cancers are detected while still localized to the gland, compared with smaller proportions where screening is not actively promoted such as in the United Kingdom. The impact of screening on overall survival remains unproven.

New techniques of radiotherapy using stereotactic body radiotherapy (SBRT) are looking to reduce the overall time needed for treatment and minimize toxicity by more accurate delivery of the radiation dose.

The optimal sequencing of the various new agents for metastatic disease including abiraterone, enzalutamide and radium 223 alongside conventional chemotherapy, and whether they work better sequentially or in combination is an area of current research.

RARER TUMOURS

Transitional cell tumours of the prostate arising from the urethra usually present and are managed in the same way as other urothelial tumours.

BLADDER CANCER

EPIDEMIOLOGY

Each year in the United Kingdom there are 10,000 cases of bladder cancer, 7000 cases in men and 3000 cases in women, making it the fifth commonest form of cancer, accounting for 3.5% of all cancer cases and leading to a total of 4800 deaths per annum. There is a male:female ratio of 5:2. It is unusual under the age of 50 years, being most common in people in their 70s and 80s. The UK incidence at 25.3 per 100,000 is below the European average which is 34.4 per 100,000. In contrast to prostate cancer, it is twice as common in white US males with an incidence of 40.2 per 100,000 compared with black US males at 19.8 per 100,000. This may be accounted for by genetic differences.

AETIOLOGY

- *Chemical carcinogens and smoking*: Bladder cancer is more common in industrialized societies than in agricultural areas. Specific carcinogens include aniline dyes; rubber industry by-products such as β-naphthylamine and benzidine; and drugs, e.g. exposure to excessive amounts of phenacetin or cyclophosphamide. This may be associated with genetic changes in genes that code for enzymes important in the detoxification of chemicals. Glutathione S-transferase (GST) is involved in the detoxification of polycyclic aromatic hydrocarbons found in tobacco smoke. Individuals with absent or only single copies of the *GSTM1* gene have increased bladder cancer risk compared with those having two copies of the gene. The *N*-acetyl transferase 2 (NAT2) enzyme is important in the inactivation of aromatic amines; individuals who have a 'slow' variant, particularly those who smoke, are also at increased risk of bladder cancer. There is also evidence that genetic variation in the nucleotide excision repair pathway is associated with risk of bladder cancer.

- *Chronic irritation*: This is related to bladder diverticulae and infection with schistosomiasis is also important in those areas where this is common, being associated with squamous carcinomas in younger age groups.
- *Familial cases* are rare and usually seen in the hereditary non-polyposis colon cancer (HNPCC) syndrome.

PATHOLOGY

Macroscopically, bladder cancer can appear as papillary or solid lesions and may be solitary or more usually multiple. The usual area of the bladder affected is the lateral wall and involvement of the bladder base is also common.

Microscopically, the majority of cancers are transitional CLL carcinoma (TCC) of varying differentiation graded from well to poorly differentiated using a numerical scale G1–G3. These account for 90% of all bladder cancers. Of the remainder, 7% are squamous carcinomas and 3% are adenocarcinomas.

The majority of bladder TCCs are superficial indolent tumours that do not progress beyond this stage. However, around 25% of superficial bladder cancer will progress to become muscle invasive; other than tumour grade there are no clear markers as to which tumours will undergo this change. In around 60% of both superficial and invasive TCC deletions affecting chromosome 9 are seen and in over 70% of superficial cancer mutations of fibroblast growth factor 3 gene (*FGFR3*) are seen. Numerous other genetic changes have been reported in invasive cancers including *cyclin D1*, *ERB-B2* and *TP53*, but no consistent picture has yet emerged to account for the change in behaviour between the superficial and invasive variants.

Bladder cancer may also be classified by its genetic signature into basal and luminal subtypes.

NATURAL HISTORY

Most bladder cancers probably arise as fairly indolent papillomas, which, left untreated, progress both in terms of dedifferentiation and local invasion. The primary tumour invades locally into the bladder muscle wall and thence into perivesical fat. More advanced disease can involve prostate, anterior vaginal wall or rectum.

Lymphatic spread involves pelvic lymph nodes and then para-aortic nodes. Blood-borne metastases particularly arise in lungs and bone.

In many, if not all, patients there is a generalized instability of the urothelium and a risk of further tumours developing not only elsewhere in the bladder but also throughout the ureters and renal pelvis. Biopsies of adjacent sites frequently demonstrate dysplasia and a clinical picture of multiple recurrent transitional cell tumours throughout the tract is well recognized.

SYMPTOMS

These may include:

- Painless haematuria and other urinary symptoms such as frequency, urgency and dysuria
- Cough, haemoptysis or bone pain caused by metastases are less frequent presentations of bladder cancer
- General symptoms of malaise, anorexia and weight loss

SIGNS

In most patients there will be no clinical signs of bladder cancer. Bladder tumours are rarely palpable per rectum or per vaginam and only in advanced cases a suprapubic mass will be palpable.

DIFFERENTIAL DIAGNOSIS

Other causes of haematuria should be considered, including urinary tract infection, stones and renal tumours.

INVESTIGATIONS

BLOOD TESTS

Routine blood investigations could reveal anaemia owing to chronic haematuria and renal impairment if there is obstructive hydronephrosis.

RADIOGRAPHY

Chest x-ray may demonstrate metastases if present.

URINE TESTS

Urine cytology can reveal malignant cells and is a useful screening test. Negative urinalysis, however, should not exclude further investigations.

ULTRASOUND OF KIDNEYS, URETERS AND BLADDER (KUB)

Ultrasound will detect hydronephrosis and may identify a site of obstruction or a visible tumour mass within the bladder.

CT UROGRAPHY

CT urography can demonstrate a filling defect in the bladder and renal tract obstruction if present. Typical appearances of a large bladder cancer are shown in Figure 10.6.

It is also important to exclude tumours in other parts of the urinary tract since a generalized instability of the urothelium is often present with multiple tumours developing between the renal pelvis and the urethra.

Note: It is important to ensure the patient has normal renal function before giving an intravenous contrast agent as this can cause deterioration of renal function.

CYSTOSCOPY

Cystoscopy is the definitive investigation at which mucosal abnormalities can be carefully documented and biopsies are taken. Transurethral resection of bladder tumour (TURBT) can also be performed during the course of this although more usually this is done as a definitive second procedure after a diagnostic cystoscopy.

MAGNETIC RESONANCE IMAGING

MRI will demonstrate extravesical extension of tumour and lymph node enlargement if present. It is now the imaging modality of choice for staging bladder cancer.

CT SCAN

This will be used to stage abdominal lymph nodes, liver and lungs for metastases. It also has a role in staging the primary tumour where MRI is contraindicated or not available.

ISOTOPE BONE SCAN

Since bone metastases are relatively common in bladder cancer, this is an important part of the staging for a patient newly diagnosed with invasive high-grade bladder TCC.

STAGING

The TNM staging system is commonly used:

- Tis: *In situ* carcinoma
- T1: Superficial invasive carcinoma confined to subepithelial connective tissue
- T2: Invasion of bladder muscle
    - T2a: Invasion of superficial muscle
    - T2b: Invasion of deep muscle
- T3: Invasion through muscle wall of bladder
- T4a: Invasion of surrounding pelvic structures
- T4b: Distant metastases

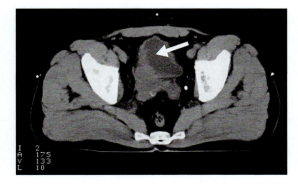

Figure 10.6 CT scan showing extensive bladder cancer filling the bladder cavity and with invasion through the bladder wall on the right side.

Urological cancer

The important features in deciding on appropriate therapy are the extent of local invasion into the bladder wall, tumour differentiation and distant spread. Bladder cancers may be considered in three subgroups of increasing likelihood of progression:

- Low-risk non-muscle invasive bladder cancer
- Intermediate (medium) risk non-muscle invasive bladder cancer
- High risk non-muscle invasive bladder cancer

TREATMENT

LOCAL RESECTION

Transurethral resection is performed for superficial (T1) bladder tumours followed by careful cystoscopic surveillance. Recurrence will occur in around 50% of cases and progression to a higher stage or worse grade will occur in around 15%. This is particularly the case in large tumours, high-grade tumours and those with multiple areas of mucosal dysplasia or frank malignancy. In patients who fail initial resection, further local resection may be attempted. Where there are multiple recurrences and when there is progression to a high-grade tumour, then alternative therapies will be required.

INTRAVESICAL CHEMOTHERAPY

This will improve local control of superficial bladder cancer. Various agents have been used, including Adriamycin, thiotepa and mitomycin C. Currently,

---

CASE HISTORY

BLADDER CANCER

A 56-year-old man has an episode of passing blood in his urine; he has no pain associated with this or other symptoms. He consults his GP who refers him to the Haematuria Clinic at his local hospital. There he undergoes an ultrasound examination of the kidney and bladder, an IVU and a flexible outpatient cystoscopy. When he returns for the results he is told that the ultrasound and IVU are clear but at cystoscopy an abnormal raised reddened area had been seen on the lateral wall of the bladder. He was advised to undergo a further cystoscopy with transurethral resection and biopsy of this area. The histology from the biopsies taken showed flat transitional cell carcinoma *in situ* (CIS). He was advised to have a course of BCG treatment. He attended the urology ward weekly for 6 weeks to have a urethral catheter passed and the BCG infusion into the bladder. He was allowed to go home the same day; he noted for the next 24 hours that he had burning when he passed urine and it was more frequent and urgent. On one occasion he had a further small amount of blood. He was reassured that this was a common side effect after BCG.

Three months after completing the BCG he had a further cystoscopy; he was delighted to learn that no abnormality was seen. It was recommended that he receive a further maintenance course of 3-weekly BCG infusions before his next cystoscopy 6 months later.

He continued with regular cystoscopies for the next 2 years. He was then told after a routine check cystoscopy that a further reddened raised area had been seen in the bladder. He returned for a repeat cystoscopy and biopsy. This showed a return of the transitional cell CIS; one or two areas of poorly differentiated cells were noted where there was early invasion; the tumour was therefore staged T1G3 with associated CIS. After discussion with his urologist and oncologist he was advised that surgery could be curative but would involve a radical cystectomy; radiotherapy was not very effective in this setting and there was no role for further BCG or chemotherapy. He agreed to proceed with surgery. Radical cystectomy with construction of a neobladder from small bowel was performed. He made a good postoperative recovery, and was discharged after 7 days with an indwelling catheter. When this was first removed he had difficulty in training his pelvic muscles to control his new bladder and was taught to pass a catheter himself at home twice a day to ensure it was empty. After a couple of months, however, he adjusted to controlling his new bladder and was able to pass water through the penis and remain continent. He had been told to expect difficulties with erectile function but was pleased to find that treatment with tadalafil enabled him to return to normal sexual activity.

He remained under review in the urology clinic with occasional x-rays of his remaining urinary tract to ensure any further tumours of the urothelium are detected at an early stage.

for low-risk superficial cancers mitomycin C is used whilst for intermediate risk superficial cancer or CIS BCG is used, which gives better results although a higher incidence of local complications with acute cystitis. A rare complication of intravesical BCG is a generalized syndrome including joint pain and pulmonary infection. Typically an initial course of weekly instillations for 6 weeks is given followed by maintenance treatment for 2 years which will reduce the incidence of relapse.

RADICAL RADIOTHERAPY

This is indicated for the treatment of T2 and T3 tumours. Paradoxically in non-invasive (stage Ta) and superficial (stage T1) tumours, radiotherapy has low response rates.

Three-dimensional CT planned conformal treatment or IMRT will be used delivering doses of up to 65 Gy. It is now a standard practice to give radiotherapy for bladder cancer with either a hypoxic sensitizer using a combination of carbogen gas (95% O_2 and 5% CO_2) and nicotinamide or chemotherapy using mitomycin C with 5FU or cisplatin.

CYSTECTOMY

This may be considered for progressive superficial bladder cancer and locally advanced muscle-invading tumours. It is also used to salvage recurrence after radical radiotherapy and involves removal of the bladder and perivesical tissues together with pelvic lymphadenectomy. For multifocal lesions, urethrectomy is also recommended. Urine is diverted via an ileal conduit to the abdominal wall or into a neobladder fashioned from the bowel, which can be retrained to void or be drained by intermittent self-catheterization.

Partial cystectomy is occasionally used for a localized superficial tumour or where there is only minimal muscle invasion.

CHEMOTHERAPY

Whilst chemotherapy is not effective alone as a primary treatment, there is now good evidence that the use of neoadjuvant chemotherapy, i.e. preceding definitive surgery or radiotherapy, will result in improved results for both local control and survival. The absolute benefit, however, is relatively modest with an overall survival advantage of 5% in favour of adding chemotherapy. It is now usual to include three cycles of chemotherapy prior to cystectomy or radical radiotherapy for locally advanced bladder cancer. The standard combinations are gemcitabine with cisplatin (GC) or methotrexate, vinblastine and cisplatin (MVC) to which may also be added Adriamycin (MVAC).

CHOICE OF RADICAL TREATMENT

There are two prevailing philosophies in the treatment of invasive bladder cancer. In many parts of Europe and the United States radical cystectomy is considered the gold standard; however, it is increasingly recognized that both radical cystectomy and a 'bladder preservation' strategy using TURBT, chemotherapy and radiotherapy are equally effective in terms of survival. It is therefore appropriate that patients should be given the choice where there is no particular indication for one over the other. Indications for cystectomy might include multifocal tumour, widespread CIS and hydronephrosis. It is also important to include with the bladder preservation option a subsequent policy of close surveillance with 6 monthly cystoscopies for 5 years and the prospect of a salvage cystectomy if there is recurrence.

PALLIATIVE TREATMENT

Palliative local treatment might be required for advanced tumours or in the frail and elderly who cannot tolerate radical treatment. Local radiotherapy will help haematuria and local pain, given in short, low-dose schedules over 1 or 2 weeks.

Bladder cancer is sensitive to chemotherapy using the GC, MVC or MVAC combinations. Response rates of 50%–60% can be achieved, some of which are complete responses resulting in useful palliation in selected patients with symptoms related to uncontrolled local tumour or soft-tissue metastases.

Palliative radiotherapy for bone metastases, a relatively common feature of advanced bladder cancer, should also be available.

TUMOUR-RELATED COMPLICATIONS

Haematuria leading to clot retention and clot colic may occur as well as ureteric obstruction leading to hydronephrosis and renal failure.

TREATMENT-RELATED COMPLICATIONS

SURGERY

Cystectomy has an operative mortality particularly in the elderly. Stoma problems (e.g. prolapse, bleeding or stricture) can arise and impotence occurs.

RADIOTHERAPY

This can result in both bowel and bladder damage.

PROGNOSIS

Ten-year cause-specific survival ranges from around 70% for T1 bladder cancer to 40% for T3 and <5% for T4 tumours. Tumours which are basal-type have a worse prognosis than non-basal tumours.

SCREENING AND FUTURE DEVELOPMENTS

Urine cytology is currently in use for patients at high risk by virtue of industrial exposure to known bladder carcinogens.

Because the bladder size and shape can change from day to day and a course of radical radiotherapy may span 4–6 weeks a new approach uses adaptive radiotherapy in which the radiation plan is chosen depending upon the 'best fit' for each day from a library of plans prepared beforehand.

Molecular signatures to select those patients who may have more or less radiocurable tumours are under evaluation to better identify those patients in whom radical surgery should not be deferred.

RARER TUMOURS

The squamous and adenocarcinomas of the bladder are treated in the same way as the transitional cell tumours. Generally, their prognosis is worse and they respond less well to non-surgical treatments.

CANCER OF THE TESTIS

EPIDEMIOLOGY

Each year in the United Kingdom there are 2000 cases of testicular cancer, accounting for 0.7% of all cancer cases and leading to a total of 80 deaths per annum. Testicular tumours occur most commonly in men aged between 20 and 40. The UK incidence of 57 per million is five times the incidence in Japan. In the United States it is more common in white people than in black people. A slow but steady increase in incidence has been observed over recent years. The success of treatment, however, is reflected in the very low mortality rates with around only 70 deaths per year in the United Kingdom.

AETIOLOGY

Many testicular tumours are thought to arise as a developmental abnormality in those with maldescent, which increases the likelihood of a testicular tumour by up to 40-fold. Other factors are a contralateral testicular tumour (the incidence of second malignancy in the other testis being around 3%) and possibly previous orchitis, although this remains speculative.

Men with a first-degree relative having testicular cancer have an increased risk with a relative risk of 8–10 amongst siblings and 4–6 between father and son. Genetic changes in the region of the short arm of chromosome 12 are thought to be relevant to the development of testicular cancer.

PATHOLOGY

There are two main types of testicular tumour: seminoma and teratoma. Around 40% are seminomas and 32% teratomas, with a further 14% containing components of both seminoma and teratoma.

Macroscopically, seminomas are solid tumours, well-circumscribed, often lobulated and pale in appearance. In contrast, teratomas are often haemorrhagic and contain cystic areas.

Microscopically, seminoma is composed of sheets of uniform rounded cells and may contain granulomata. Particularly well-differentiated variants are recognized (spermatocytic seminoma) as are more aggressive types (anaplastic seminoma). In contrast, teratoma can contain a range of cell types with varying differentiation. Undifferentiated teratoma contains no recognizable mature elements. Trophoblastic elements may predominate and there might be recognizable yolk sac elements.

NATURAL HISTORY

Testicular tumours invade locally into the tunica vaginalis and along the spermatic cord. Lymph node spread occurs relatively early to para-aortic nodes and thence to mediastinal nodes. Blood-borne spread is most common to the lungs and liver.

SYMPTOMS

These include:
- Testicular swelling or discomfort, particularly with a past history of maldescent
- Gynaecomastia owing to excess HCG secretion from the tumour
- Backache from enlarged para-aortic nodes
- Cough, haemoptysis or dyspnoea from lung metastases

SIGNS

These may include:
- Testicular swelling which may have an associated hydrocele
- Central abdominal mass owing to palpable para-aortic nodes
- Pleural effusion
- Gynaecomastia owing to stimulation by high levels of HCG

DIFFERENTIAL DIAGNOSIS

The following conditions need to be ruled out:
- Benign hydrocele
- Testicular torsion
- Other causes of backache such as degenerative spinal disease
- Other causes of lymphadenopathy, e.g. lymphoma

INVESTIGATIONS

Routine investigations may demonstrate renal impairment owing to ureteric obstruction by enlarged para-aortic nodes. Abnormal liver function tests could reflect liver metastases. Chest x-ray can also demonstrate metastases as either lung deposits or pleural effusion.

ULTRASOUND

Testicular ultrasound will demonstrate a solid mass, sometimes with cystic elements in the testis.

SERUM MARKERS

There are specific serum markers for germ cell tumours. These are serum α-fetoprotein (AFP) and β-human chorionic gonadotrophin (HCG) and should be measured both prior to any surgical intervention and serially thereafter. Their value in monitoring response to treatment is shown in Figure 10.7. Placental alkaline phosphatase is of value for seminoma but is also affected by cigarette smoking and may therefore be misleading in smokers; lactate dehydrogenase (LDH) is a further marker of use in seminoma.

Around 90% of patients with teratoma will have either AFP or HCG elevated and 40%–50% will have both markers raised. The absolute level and rate of fall after treatment are useful prognostic features.

CT SCAN

CT scan of the pelvis and abdomen is essential to evaluate pelvic nodes and liver, and CT scan of the lungs will give accurate assessment of lung metastases. Figure 10.8 demonstrates the appearances of para-aortic lymph involvement and lung metastases on CT scan.

STAGING

The TNM staging system is sometimes used to describe the extent of the primary tumour but for the overall disease the Royal Marsden Hospital staging system is more widely applied. These are shown as follows:

Urological cancer

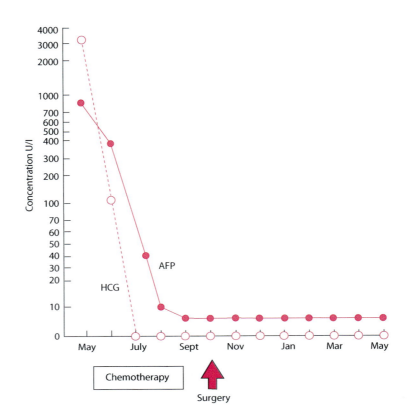

Figure 10.7 Changes in serum AFP and HCG from diagnosis through treatment with chemotherapy and later surgical removal of a residual tumour mass in a patient presenting with advanced testicular germ cell tumour.

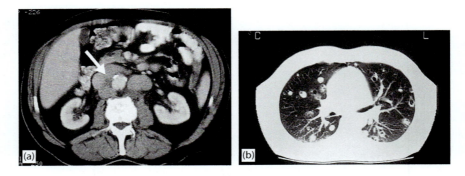

Figure 10.8 CT scans demonstrating (a) enlarged para-aortic lymph nodes and (b) lung metastases from testicular teratoma.

TNM STAGE

- T1: Limited to testis
- T2: Involving tunica albuginea or epididymis
- T3: Invading spermatic cord
- T4: Invading scrotum
- N1: Single node <2 cm max diameter
- N2: Single node 2–5 cm max diameter or multiple nodes <5 cm max diameter
- N3: Any node >5 cm max diameter
- M1: Distant metastases

ROYAL MARSDEN STAGE

- I: Limited to testis
- II: Involving nodes below diaphragm
- III: Involving nodes both sides of diaphragm
- IV: Distant metastases
  - IVL: Lungs
  - IVH: Liver

TREATMENT

All patients will proceed to inguinal orchidectomy with removal of the affected testis. Scrotal interference should be avoided at all costs because of the risk of tumour implantation in the scrotal wound and subsequent relapse.

STAGE 1 TUMOURS

If there is no evidence of residual tumour after surgery, then the prognosis is extremely good and around 85% of patients will be cured with no further treatment.

Patients with seminomas can be offered surveillance, radiotherapy to the para-aortic nodes or a single dose of carboplatin. Surveillance is less popular in seminoma than teratoma as the absence of detectable serum markers means that there is greater dependence on radiology. Current evidence suggests that both low-dose para-aortic node radiotherapy delivering only 20 Gy and a single dose of carboplatin are equivalent in preventing subsequent relapse.

Patients with teratomas are entered into a programme of intensive surveillance with monthly measurement of serum markers and regular abdominal and chest CT scans. Those with adverse features such as anaplastic tumour and vascular invasion will receive a short course of chemotherapy.

STAGE 2, 3 OR 4 TUMOURS

Patients with seminomas will proceed to chemotherapy except for those with very small para-aortic nodes. The drugs used are usually cisplatin or carboplatin with the possible addition of etoposide. Small volume disease can be treated by radiotherapy alone to the para-aortic and pelvic nodes, and radiotherapy can also be given following chemotherapy in other patients if there is concern regarding residual disease.

Patients with teratomas will proceed to chemotherapy. For good prognosis tumours, standard chemotherapy will be 3-weekly cycles of BEP (bleomycin, etoposide and cisplatin). High-risk patients with extensive disease or very high markers (AFP >1000, HCG >10,000) will receive more intensive regimens with weekly administration of alternating drug schedules containing bleomycin, vincristine, cisplatin, methotrexate and etoposide (BOPP or POMBACE).

In recurrent or resistant cases high-dose chemotherapy is increasingly used with peripheral blood progenitor cell or autologous bone marrow support.

PELVIC SURGERY

Pelvic lymphadenectomy is advocated as part of the primary treatment of germ cell tumours in some centres, particularly in the United States. In the United Kingdom and Europe it is more usual to give initial treatment with chemotherapy and use surgery electively for those patients with primary teratomas who have residual tumour masses after full chemotherapy. This occurs in around 20% of patients and excision of these masses is important to remove not only residual malignant teratoma but also benign differentiated teratoma since this retains the potential to develop into a malignant form at a later date. At surgery approximately 20% are malignant teratoma, 50% differentiated teratoma and the remainder are necrotic with no viable tumour.

TUMOUR-RELATED COMPLICATIONS

Gynaecomastia owing to high levels of HCG sometimes occurs.

TREATMENT-RELATED COMPLICATIONS

- Unilateral orchidectomy has no physiological effect on potency but this may be affected after pelvic lymphadenectomy.
- Abdominal radiotherapy can be related to subsequent peptic ulceration and an increased rate of second malignancies in later life.

Urological cancer

- Chemotherapy causes alopecia which is reversible.
- Cisplatin can result in peripheral neuropathy and ototoxicity. Renal impairment which is usually reversible also occurs and an increased incidence of hypertension in later life has been reported.
- Bleomycin can cause skin changes and pneumonitis in high dose.
- Fertility is impaired after chemotherapy but recovery usually occurs after standard BEP chemotherapy, and there are increasing reports of success in fathering children after treatment for testicular cancer. Despite this, semen storage is routinely advised for patients undergoing this type of chemotherapy. Potency is not affected.

PROGNOSIS

Few patients die from testicular cancer today. Cure is virtually guaranteed for stage 1 tumours and is expected in around 85% of those with more advanced stages. However, relapse after primary chemotherapy heralds a poor outlook with only 20%–30% of patients surviving long term with salvage treatment.

SCREENING

Health education programmes aimed at self-examination are the main form of population screening.

RARER TUMOURS

The remaining tumours that occur in the testis are lymphomas (7%) and the rare pure yolk sac tumours, Sertoli cell tumours and interstitial cell tumours. Mesotheliomas arising from the tunica vaginalis have also been described. Lymphomas are managed as for any extranodal lymphoma while other rare tumours are managed by surgical excision.

CANCER OF THE PENIS

EPIDEMIOLOGY

Each year in the United Kingdom there are 400 cases of penis cancer, accounting for 0.3% of all cancer cases and leading to a total of 100 deaths per annum. It accounts for less than 1% of deaths from cancer in men. It is more common in other parts of the world, in particular Africa and China where it accounts for around 15% of male cancers.

AETIOLOGY

It is virtually unknown in populations who practise circumcision. A relationship with papilloma virus has been proposed.

PATHOLOGY

Macroscopically, the tumour may be a papilliferous or solid growth on the shaft or glans of the penis. Ulceration can occur. It may develop insidiously beneath the foreskin.

Microscopically, penile cancer is a squamous carcinoma often well or moderately differentiated.

NATURAL HISTORY

The tumour will invade the shaft of the penis as shown in Figure 10.9 and spread to inguinal lymph nodes (Figure 10.10). Blood-borne spread occurs relatively late to lungs and liver.

SYMPTOMS

Tumours are usually asymptomatic but there might be local discharge and odour.

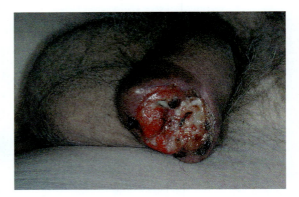

Figure 10.9 Locally advanced primary squamous carcinoma of the penis with destruction of the glans.

Cancer of the penis

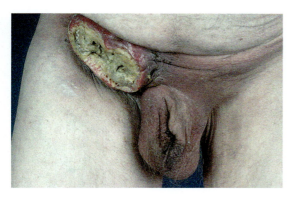

Figure 10.10 Advanced right inguinal node disease owing to metastases from a carcinoma of the penis. The primary tumour was treated some months earlier when no metastases were apparent by amputation.

SIGNS

The primary tumour is usually obvious on clinical examination. Palpable inguinal nodes are present in up to half of patients.

DIFFERENTIAL DIAGNOSIS

Other penile skin lesions should be considered, including lymphogranuloma venereum, condylomata acuminata, chancroid, traumatic ulceration, leucoplakia, Bowen disease, erythroplasia of Queyrat and giant penile condylomata (Buschke–Lowenstein tumour).

Other causes of inguinal lymphadenopathy need to be taken into account, in particular chronic infection, which accounts for around 50% of the associated lymphadenopathy.

INVESTIGATIONS

Routine investigations are rarely helpful although a chest x-ray will be necessary to exclude lung metastases.

BIOPSY

A biopsy or cytological scrapings will confirm the diagnosis.

FINE-NEEDLE ASPIRATION

FNA of enlarged nodes should be used to distinguish metastatic nodes from infected and inflammatory nodes.

CT SCAN

Where inguinal nodes are involved, a pelvic CT scan is of value to assess further lymphatic spread.

STAGING

The commonly used staging system is the Jackson staging, which is shown as follows as well as the formal TNM staging:

T stage

- T1: Superficial subepithelial
- T2: Invading corpus cavernosa
- T3: Invading urethra or prostate
- T4: Invading adjacent structures

Jackson stage

- I: Limited to glans or prepuce
- II: Invading shaft; no nodes
- III: Invading shaft; node positive
- IV: Fixed inoperable nodes or distant metastases

TREATMENT

SURGERY

This will usually involve partial or complete amputation as shown in Figure 10.10, unless the tumour is small and confined to the prepuce when local excision by circumcision may be adequate. Penile reconstruction can be offered after surgery.

RADIOTHERAPY

This can be delivered by either external beam or by the use of brachytherapy with an interstitial implant or penile mould. The penis is preserved, with surgery reserved for salvage.

Treatment of involved nodes should be by block dissection of the groyne. In the case of fixed inoperable nodes local irradiation can be performed. Advanced fixed fungating nodes are shown in Figure 10.10.

PALLIATIVE TREATMENT

This might be indicated for locally advanced disease or where there are distant metastases. Usually, a short palliative course of radiotherapy to the primary site, nodes or local recurrence will help prevent local pain and fungation.

There is no recognized chemotherapy for penile cancer although responses are seen in advanced disease using schedules containing drugs such as cisplatin, methotrexate, 5FU and mitomycin C.

TUMOUR-RELATED COMPLICATIONS

Interference with micturition and potency is seen.

TREATMENT-RELATED COMPLICATIONS

Radiotherapy can result in urethral stricture in about 10% of cases.

PROGNOSIS

Survival with stage 1 disease is over 85% at 5 years falling to 35% for stage 3 tumours. Long-term survival with stage 4 disease is unusual.

FURTHER READING

Cheng L, Albers P, Berney DM, Feldman DR, Daugaard G, Gilligan T, Looijenga LHJ. Testicular cancer. *Nat Rev Dis Primers*. 2018 Oct 5; 4(1): 29.

Clinical guideline [CG175] 2014: Prostate cancer: diagnosis and management. https://www.nice.org.uk/guidance/cg175

European Association of Urology Guidelines on Renal Cell Carcinoma: The 2019 Update. *Eur Urol*. 2019 May; 75(5):799–810. doi: 10.1016/j.eururo.2019.02.011.

Hakenberg O, Compérat E, Minhas S, Necchi A, Protzel C, Watkin N. EAU guidelines on penile cancer: 2014 update. *Eur Urol*. 2015 Jan; 67(1): 142–150. doi: 10.1016/j.eururo.2014.10.017.

NICE guideline [NG2] 2015: Bladder cancer: Diagnosis and management. https://www.nice.org.uk/guidance/ng2

Prostate Cancer, Version 2.2019, NCCN Clinical Practice Guidelines in Oncology. *J Natl Compr Canc Netw*. 2019 May 1;17(5):479–505.

Woldu SL, Bagrodia A, Lotan Y. Guideline of guidelines – Non-muscle invasive bladder cancer. *BJU Int*. 2017 Mar; 119(3): 371–380.

SELF-ASSESSMENT QUESTIONS

1. Which of the following applies to renal cell cancer?
    a. There are approximately 12,000 cases per year in the United Kingdom
    b. It occurs equally in males and females
    c. It is related to smoking
    d. It is common in Japan
    e. The mortality is similar to the incidence

2. Which of the following is correct in renal cell cancer?
    a. It arises from cells in the glomerulus
    b. Characteristically the cells are adenocarcinoma clear cells
    c. There is often detection of the retinoblastoma gene
    d. Lymph node spread is rare
    e. Most patients have metastases at presentation

3. Which three of the following are commonly presenting features of renal cell cancer?
    a. Dysuria
    b. Haematuria
    c. Urinary retention
    d. Loin pain
    e. Paraneoplastic neuropathy
    f. Renal failure
    g. Weight loss

4. Which of the following is true regarding prostate cancer?
    a. It is rare under 60 years
    b. Most cases have a family history

Self-assessment questions

   c. It is related to smoking
   d. It is the most commonly diagnosed cancer in males in the United Kingdom
   e. It is more common where there is benign prostatic enlargement

5. Which three of the following are important in determining the prognosis from prostate cancer?
   a. PSA level
   b. Haemoglobin
   c. Urinary function
   d. Gleason grade
   e. Seminal vesicle involvement
   f. Bilateral tumour
   g. Urethral involvement

6. Which three of the following are recognized presenting features of prostate cancer?
   a. Weight loss
   b. Dysuria
   c. Erectile impotence
   d. Leg oedema
   e. Constipation
   f. Haematospermia
   g. Urinary retention

7. In the treatment of prostate cancer which of the following is true?
   a. Surgery with transurethral resection is adequate for localized tumour
   b. Radiotherapy is rarely used for localized disease
   c. Hormone manipulation is aimed at reducing levels of oestrogen
   d. Urinary incontinence is common after radiotherapy
   e. Goserelin works through the pituitary gland

8. Which of the following applies to bladder cancer?
   a. In men it is more common than prostate cancer
   b. The most common form is not life-threatening
   c. It is related to alcohol consumption
   d. It is related to diet
   e. It is most common in the 50–60-year-old group

9. Which of the following is true in relation to bladder cancer?
   a. The common form is muscle-invasive squamous carcinoma
   b. Exposure to schistosomiasis results in squamous carcinoma
   c. Primary stage is related to extent of bladder surface involved
   d. Carcinoma *in situ* is more dangerous than superficial tumour
   e. Adenocarcinoma might be due to aniline dye exposure

10. In the treatment of bladder cancer which of the following is true?
    a. Intravesical therapy can be used for muscle-invasive tumour
    b. Chemotherapy has no role in primary treatment
    c. Metastases may respond to hormone therapy
    d. Radical radiotherapy may be used for superficial invasive cancer
    e. Cystectomy can be successful after radiotherapy

11. Which of the following is true regarding testicular tumours?
    a. They increase in frequency with age
    b. They typically have a rapidly fatal course
    c. They are related to previous measles infection
    d. There is an increased risk of a contralateral second testicular tumour
    e. They are most common in Asia

12. Which three of the following are characteristic of testicular tumours?
    a. Gynaecomastia
    b. Haematuria
    c. Impotence
    d. A family history of testicular tumour
    e. Raised blood levels of CEA
    f. Haematospermia
    g. A positive pregnancy test

13. Which is true of the treatment of testicular cancer?
    a. Biopsy of the testicular mass confirms the diagnosis

Urological cancer

b. Early cases may need no treatment after removal of the testis
c. Seminoma will require more intensive treatment than teratoma
d. Most patients will be impotent after treatment
e. Maintenance chemotherapy will improve long-term prognosis

14. Which of the following applies to cancer of the penis?
   a. Circumcision protects against its development
   b. The common type is an adenocarcinoma
   c. It is most common in South America
   d. Early spread to the prostate and bladder occurs
   e. Local excision is usually adequate treatment for localized tumour

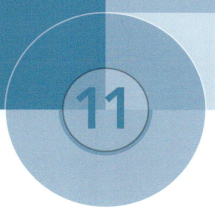

Gynaecological cancer

CERVICAL CANCER

EPIDEMIOLOGY

Each year in the United Kingdom there are around 3200 cases of cervical cancer, accounting for 1% of all cancer cases and leading to a total of 900 deaths per annum. It has an annual incidence of 8 per 100,000. In contrast, largely as a result of effective screening, there are over 30,000 cases of carcinoma *in situ* (CIN III) each year. Invasive cervical cancer is predominantly a disease of women in their 40s and 50s but is showing increasing trend in younger age groups. It is common in lower socioeconomic groups and there is a wide geographical variation, highest levels of the disease being in South America with incidence figures of up to 80 in 100,000.

AETIOLOGY

Persistent human papilloma virus (HPV) is now thought to be a feature of all cervical cancers, although only a small proportion of women acquiring HPV infection will develop cervical intraepithelial neoplasia (CIN). Prevalence rates of HPV in the population are up to 48% and around half of all infections clear within 12 months. It is the subtypes HPV 16 and 18 that are most clearly linked to CIN accounting for 58% and 16% of cases, respectively.

Cervical cancer is associated with sexual activity, being higher in women starting intercourse at an early age and having multiple partners. It is more common in women who are or who have been married than in single women. There is some evidence that the male partner is implicated, being associated with partners of lower socioeconomic groups and those high-risk males who have more than one partner who develops cervical cancer. Other recognized aetiological factors include smoking, miscarriage, use of oral contraceptives, parity and co-infection with sexually transmitted diseases. It is a recognized HIV-related malignancy.

PATHOLOGY

Macroscopically, there are two common presentations:

- Proliferative growth at the cervix with surface ulceration.
- Diffusely infiltrating tumour with the mucosa intact owing to tumour arising in the endocervical canal. The latter is sometimes described as a 'barrel cervix'.

Microscopically, the majority of cervical cancers are squamous carcinomas of varying differentiation but in recent years the proportion of adenocarcinomas arising from the external os or endocervix has increased particularly in younger women. The relative incidences are now 3:1 with overall 75% squamous and 25% adenocarcinomas.

Other tumour types arising in the cervix include unspecified poorly differentiated cancers, small-cell cancers and rarely melanoma or lymphoma.

Gynaecological cancer

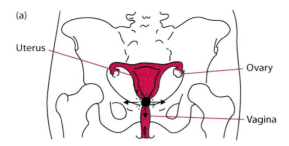

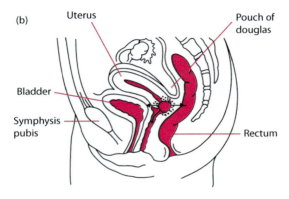

Figure 11.1 Patterns of local spread from cervical carcinoma: (a) lateral and (b) anteroposterior spread.

NATURAL HISTORY

Local spread in all directions occurs predominantly laterally and anteroposteriorly as shown in Figure 11.1. Lymph node spread occurs relatively early, being identified in around 15% of stage 1 tumours.

From paracervical nodes there is spread to internal and external iliac nodes, presacral and obturator nodes. Subsequent spread is then up the para-aortic node chain.

Blood-borne metastases occur, affecting in particular the lungs, liver and bone.

SYMPTOMS

Frequently, presentation is asymptomatic as a result of an abnormal cervical smear test. Local pain is unusual unless there is extensive pelvic infiltration.

If symptoms are present they may include:

- Vaginal bleeding, particularly after intercourse
- Vaginal discharge
- Renal failure owing to bilateral ureteric obstruction
- Haematuria or rectal bleeding owing to local spread
- Low back and sacral pain owing to pelvic and para-aortic lymphadenopathy
- General symptoms of malignancy, including anorexia, malaise and weight loss

SIGNS

Pelvic examination is mandatory; the tumour will usually be apparent at the cervix as a proliferative or ulcerative growth or a diffuse infiltration. It is important to note extension onto the vaginal mucosa and, on rectal examination, any evidence of spread into the parametrium or rectal mucosa.

DIFFERENTIAL DIAGNOSIS

Other cervical lesions should be considered, such as a cervical erosion.

Where bladder or rectal involvement is diagnosed it may be difficult to distinguish clinically between primary tumours of these sites invading the cervix, although this is usually apparent on histology.

INVESTIGATIONS

Routine investigations can reveal anaemia owing to bleeding and a raised white cell count where there has been chronic infection. Renal failure will be apparent on routine biochemical tests and a chest, abdomen and pelvis CT will be needed to exclude metastases.

CERVICAL CYTOLOGY

This is performed to diagnose malignancy and vaginal swabs taken at the same time can demonstrate the nature of an infective discharge.

BIOPSY

A full examination under anaesthetic including a cystoscopy should be performed in all cases, at which time biopsies can also be taken.

CT SCAN

A CT scan of the abdomen and pelvis will help assess local extension and enlargement of pelvic and para-aortic lymph nodes as well as hydronephrosis. CT is also used to assess liver and lungs to exclude metastases.

MAGNETIC RESONANCE IMAGING

For definition of soft tissue changes around the cervix and assessment of the primary tumour, MRI is superior to CT, as shown in Figure 11.2.

STAGING

The FIGO (International Federation of Gynaecology and Obstetrics) staging system is generally accepted in clinical assessment of cervical cancer:

- *Stage 1*
  - *1A*: Microinvasive disease limited to the cervix
  - *1B*: Confined to the cervix with invasion >5 mm depth from surface or >7 mm spread in a horizontal direction
- *Stage 2*
  - *2A*: Extension to vaginal mucosa but not into lower third of vagina
  - *2B*: Extension to parametrium but not reaching pelvic side wall
- *Stage 3*
  - *3A*: Extension to lower third of vagina
  - *3B*: Extension to pelvic side wall
- *Stage 4*
  - *4A*: Involvement of bladder and rectal mucosa
  - *4B*: Distant metastases

TREATMENT

Radical treatment will be considered for all patients except those with widespread metastatic disease or gross bladder or rectal involvement. Presentation with renal failure is not an absolute contraindication to radical treatment and in selected cases percutaneous nephrostomies to re-establish renal drainage should be performed prior to treatment as shown in Figure 11.3.

LOCALIZED TO THE CERVIX (STAGE 1)

Surgery

Radical surgery is the treatment of choice in the form of a radical hysterectomy (Wertheim's hysterectomy) during which, in addition to the removal of the uterus, tubes and ovaries, the upper vagina, parametrium and pelvic lymph nodes are also included in the resection.

Chemoradiotherapy

Radical chemoradiation can be given for early stage cancer of the cervix and the results in terms of survival are no worse than those after radical surgery, although there might be a greater incidence of long-term morbidity. It is usually therefore reserved for those with bulky primary tumours (>4 cm), radiologically positive lymph nodes, elderly patients and those medically unfit for surgery. It is also an acceptable option for younger women who refuse surgery.

Post-operative radiotherapy can be given following Wertheim's hysterectomy where the excision margins are not clear of tumour and where there is involvement of the removed pelvic lymph nodes in the resection.

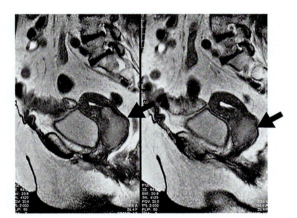

Figure 11.2 MR scan demonstrating locally advanced carcinoma of the cervix.

Gynaecological cancer

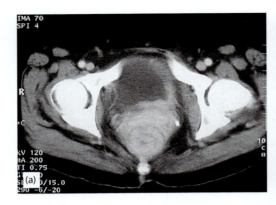
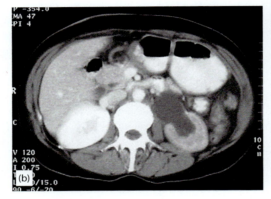
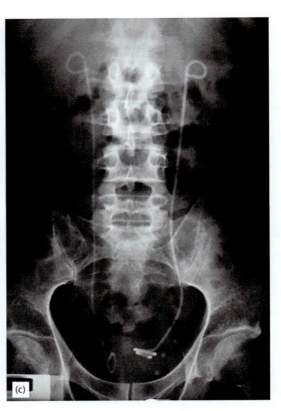

Figure 11.3 CT scan demonstrating (a) extensive local infiltration from cervical cancer into the bladder base and (b) with associated hydronephrosis. Insertion of ureteric stents is necessary in this situation if renal function is to be preserved as shown in the plain x-ray (c).

CASE HISTORY

CERVICAL CANCER

A 38-year-old woman presents with a 3-month history of post-coital bleeding. One year earlier she had a normal cervical smear report when she saw her GP for family planning advice. The GP has referred her to a consultant gynaecologist having performed a pelvic examination at which he found a hard irregular cervix and considered the likely cause of bleeding to be a cervical carcinoma. The gynaecologist confirmed the clinical history and on examination found a hard ulcerating tumour at the cervix with no obvious extension beyond this site. He subsequently performed examination under anaesthesia confirming a stage Ib carcinoma of the cervix with no parametrial or vaginal extension. A biopsy showed moderately differentiated squamous carcinoma. A cystoscopy was normal.

Further investigations included a normal full blood count and chest x-ray; an MR scan confirmed a 3 cm mass at the cervix but no extension beyond that and a CT scan showed no hydronephrosis and no signs of metastatic disease in lymph nodes, liver or lungs. Treatment was recommended with radical hysterectomy at which the uterus and cervix with an upper cuff of vagina and parametrial tissue was removed together with a pelvic lymph node dissection. Histological examination of the specimen confirmed a moderately differentiated carcinoma of the cervix but three out of five left-sided pelvic lymph nodes were positive and two out of eight right-sided pelvic lymph nodes were positive. As a result of this finding post-operative radiotherapy was recommended. The patient received a standard 5-week course of post-operative chemoradiation to the pelvis. During this time she experienced some diarrhoea and urinary frequency.

Three months later she was well but complained of some bowel frequency attributed to the radiotherapy. When seen 6 months later she complained of some persistent low back pain. Clinical examination was normal but a CT scan showed large lymph nodes in the para-aortic region. The chest x-ray showed three small volume metastasis in the left lung field and five metastasis in the right lung.

Chemotherapy was recommended. The patient received a course of carboplatin, paclitaxel and bevacizumab. During chemotherapy administration she suffered nausea and vomiting and during the following week had some nausea but otherwise tolerated the treatment well. She returned 3 weeks later for a second course of treatment which was given with similar side effects. Two weeks later she returned to the hospital earlier than planned with persistent nausea and vomiting. She was drowsy and slightly confused. Urgent investigations revealed a serum creatinine of 800. Abdominal ultrasound showed bilateral hydronephrosis and a CT scan identified enlarged common iliac and para-aortic lymph nodes obstructing both ureters. Bilateral nephrostomies were inserted; over the subsequent 3 days as urine drainage was re-established her creatinine fell to 260. At this point she developed a high fever and her full blood count had fallen with a profound neutropenia, with a total neutrophil count of 0.3. She was treated with intravenous antibiotics using ceftazidime but continued to have a high fever. The culture from her urine draining through the nephrostomy showed a staphylococcal infection. Flucloxacillin was added to an antibiotic regimen and her fever settled. Two days later she complained of acute chest pain and shortness of breath. She became acutely hypotensive and despite active resuscitation died from a presumed pulmonary embolus.

Preoperative radiotherapy has been advocated in the past but it has no proven value and, with the use of the aforementioned criteria, only 20% of women will require irradiation in addition to surgery.

TUMOUR BEYOND CERVIX (STAGES 2 AND 3)

Chemoradiotherapy

Radical chemoradiation will be the treatment of choice. This will involve a course of external beam treatment to the whole pelvis covering the major node chains up to the bifurcation of the aorta, delivering a dose of 45–50 Gy over 5 weeks with weekly cisplatin. Intracavitary brachytherapy treatment to the cervix will follow this using an intrauterine tube and vaginal source to administer a further 25–30 Gy to the cervix and surrounding tissues. A typical arrangement of intracavitary applicators is shown in Figure 11.4. Bulky tumours may require more complex implants.

A total dose of >90 Gy is associated with a better rate of local control than lower doses.

Chemotherapy

The results of radical radiotherapy for cervical cancer are improved if chemotherapy is given during radiotherapy and the usual schedule includes weekly cisplatin during external beam radiotherapy.

In contrast, the use of adjuvant chemotherapy usually given prior to radiotherapy in locally advanced disease has been disappointing and to date no proven advantage has emerged in clinical trials.

PALLIATIVE TREATMENT

If there are distant metastases or locally advanced pelvic disease, then radical local treatment is inappropriate. Chemotherapy for advanced and recurrent disease has only limited activity and complete response is extremely rare. The most effective drug

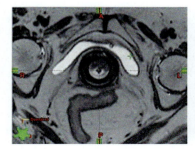
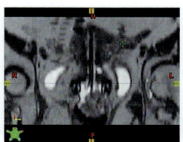
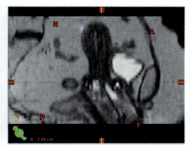

Figure 11.4 MR scan demonstrating intrauterine tube and vaginal ring source in position for the treatment of carcinoma of the cervix using brachytherapy.

Gynaecological cancer

schedule is carboplatin, paclitaxel and bevacizumab or cisplatin with topotecan. These can be associated with considerable toxicity.

Palliative radiotherapy for advanced local disease could be worthwhile and is particularly indicated for the control of local bleeding and pelvic pain. Other procedures such as a palliative colostomy might be required where there is rectal involvement, or fistulae develop.

HORMONE REPLACEMENT

Cervical cancer is not hormone dependent. This means that hormone manipulation is not a useful approach to treatment but also that, following radical treatment, in young women particularly, hormone replacement therapy should be offered.

TUMOUR-RELATED COMPLICATIONS

These include:

- Renal failure owing to bilateral ureteric obstruction
- Acute haemorrhage from the tumour occasionally resulting in hypovolaemic shock
- Fistulae between bladder or rectum and vagina
- Pyometra owing to obstruction of the cervical canal by tumour

TREATMENT-RELATED COMPLICATIONS

Radical surgery can result in urinary urgency and urge or stress incontinence. Lower limb lymphoedema following pelvic node dissection may also be seen. It can also result acutely in bowel and bladder toxicity with radiation cystitis and diarrhoea.

Chemoradiation schedules sometimes enhance the previously mentioned toxicities of radiotherapy and in addition cause pancytopenia with the risk of neutropenic sepsis.

Long-term sequelae from radiotherapy can include reduced bladder volume, telangiectasia causing haematuria or rectal bleeding, chronic diarrhoea and vaginal stenosis. Rarely bowel or bladder fistulae occur, although subsequent investigations often reveal recurrent disease in this setting.

PROGNOSIS

Outcome is closely related to stage at presentation with a 5-year survival of over 80% for stage 1 and 2A tumours, falling to only 30%–40% for stage 3 and less than 5% for stage 4. Within stage 1 tumours, prognosis is related to tumour bulk and differentiation.

For microinvasive and *in situ* carcinoma of the cervix, surgery is almost always curative, emphasizing the importance of early diagnosis in this condition where curative treatment is readily available for early-stage disease.

SCREENING

Screening for cervical neoplasia by cervical smear testing is widespread and there is good evidence that in the United States and Scandinavia the rate of decline in cervical cancer can be related to intensity of screening.

Currently, around 3 million cervical smears are performed in the United Kingdom each year, and it has been estimated that this has reduced the incidence of invasive cancers by around 30%. This accounts for around 80% of all eligible women. Current recommendations in the United Kingdom are that a first smear is to be taken by the age of 25 and repeated every 3 years till the age of 49 and then every 5 years till 64 years of age. In some countries there is a younger threshold age. A major problem with this, as with any screening programme, is to achieve good rates of compliance, particularly in those groups at high risk. It is also important to recognize the limitation of smear screening since a number of women will still be diagnosed having a normal smear. Overall, the accuracy of cervical smear cytology is only around 80% despite technically good smears and accurate interpretation. The use of high-risk HPV (HR_HPV) triage for women with borderline or mild dyskaryosis smears is now used to improve the accuracy of screening.

FUTURE PROSPECTS

The greatest impact is likely to be made by extending the current screening programmes to reach all those women at risk with high rates of compliance in order to detect early curable disease.

Vaccines are now available against HPV 16 and 18, and currently in the United Kingdom and many other countries this is administered to all girls at around the age of 14 years. Despite this in the immediate future a 40% increase in the incidence of cervical cancer in the United Kingdom is forecast up to 2035.

RARER TUMOURS

Small-cell cancers are treated in the same way as these tumours elsewhere with chemotherapy such as carboplatin and etoposide and radical local treatment either surgery or radiotherapy. Other rare tumours such as melanoma are treated as in other sites.

ENDOMETRIAL CANCER

EPIDEMIOLOGY

Each year in the United Kingdom there are over 9000 cases of endometrial cancer, accounting for 3% of all cancer cases and leading to a total of 2360 deaths per annum. Compared with cancer of the cervix, cancer of the endometrium affects the older, predominantly those in the postmenopausal age group, the median age at presentation being 61 years. There has been a substantial increase in incidence in recent years with an increase in incidence of 21% in the last decade; incidence in the United Kingdom is 16 per 100,000. There is far less geographical variation than with cervical cancer, although it is relatively rare in Japan where the incidence is about one-tenth of that in Europe and the United States.

AETIOLOGY

Endometrial carcinoma occurs typically in obese nulliparous women who have a tendency to develop diabetes and cardiovascular disease. Early menarche and late menopause increase the risk.

High levels of circulating oestrogens are a known cause and it is a recognized but rare complication of an oestrogen-secreting granulosa cell tumour of the ovary. There is an increased incidence associated with oestrogen only replacement therapy but a reduction with continuous oestrogen—progesterone replacement therapy.

Endometrial cancer can occur as part of the hereditary non-polyposis colorectal cancer (HNPCC) syndrome and daughters of women with endometrial cancer have approximately double the risk of developing endometrial cancer themselves.

PATHOLOGY

Macroscopically, the tumour arises within the uterine cavity and can be polypoid or a more diffuse multifocal growth arising from the endometrium.

Microscopically, the tumour is an adenocarcinoma, which may be of varying grade, usually designated from G1 (well differentiated) to G3 (poorly differentiated).

Mutations in the *PTEN* tumour-suppressor gene are relatively common. Cancers associated with Lynch syndrome will have mutations in mismatch repair genes (MMR).

NATURAL HISTORY

There is local invasion into the myometrium and cervix. The tubes and ovaries are sometimes also involved and the tumour occasionally extends into parametrial tissues or involves the bladder or the rectum. This is far less common than in cancer of the cervix.

Lymph node spread can occur, involving pelvic lymph nodes, and submucosal lymphatic permeation along the vaginal walls is well recognized.

Distant metastases by blood-borne spread most frequently involve lungs and bone.

SYMPTOMS

The classic presentation of endometrial cancer is with postmenopausal bleeding. In the premenopausal woman heavy or irregular periods may be the only symptom. There might be an associated vaginal discharge.

General symptoms of malaise, anorexia and weight loss are usually mild and symptoms from metastatic disease are unusual at presentation.

SIGNS

On pelvic examination the uterus may feel bulky and a vaginal discharge or bleeding from the os may be apparent. Often no physical signs can be detected.

DIFFERENTIAL DIAGNOSIS

Other causes of postmenopausal bleeding should be considered such as atrophic vaginitis and in premenopausal women other causes of irregular menstrual bleeding such as fibroids.

INVESTIGATIONS

Routine investigations can reveal anaemia owing to chronic blood loss. Other abnormalities are unusual.

BIOPSY

Cytological sampling using a pipelle will usually confirm the presence of malignancy. This should be followed by hysteroscopy and endometrial biopsy under direct vision.

RADIOLOGY

MRI scanning is now used routinely pre-operatively and accurate estimates of the extent of myometrial invasion can be obtained together with information on spread beyond the body of the uterus. An example is shown in Figure 11.5.

For more advanced cases (stage 2, 3 or 4) a CT scan will be used to assess abdominal lymph node status and lungs.

STAGING

Carcinoma of the endometrium is staged using the FIGO system:

- *Stage 1*:
  - *1A*: Confined to the endometrium; invasion <50% of myometrium
  - *1B*: Confined to the endometrium; invasion >50% of myometrium
- *Stage 2*: Invasion of cervical stroma
- *Stage 3*: Spread to pelvic tissues or pelvic nodes
- *Stage 4*:
  - *4A*: Spread to bladder or rectum
  - *4B*: Distant metastases.

A further subclassification into Type I and Type II endometrial cancer has been described.

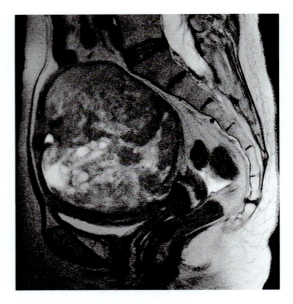

Figure 11.5 MR scan demonstrating extensive endometrial carcinoma expanding the uterine cavity and invading the muscle wall of the uterus; note bladder is flattened anteriorly from massive uterine enlargement with tumour.

- Type I are favourable tumours, usually stage 1A, moderately differentiated and sensitive to progestogen.
- Type II are less favourable tumours, more often in elderly and associated with tamoxifen use. They are deeply invasive, poorly differentiated and have a high metastatic potential.

TREATMENT

A major feature of endometrial cancer is the predominance of stage 1 tumours at presentation, accounting for 70%–80% of patients.

SURGERY

Total abdominal hysterectomy and bilateral salpingo-oophorectomy is the treatment of choice for disease localized to the endometrium. Lymph node sampling may be considered for high-grade tumours.

A radical hysterectomy (see the cervix surgery section) is indicated when there is cervical involvement (stage 2).

RADIOTHERAPY

Post-operative radiotherapy is considered for patients following hysterectomy for stage 1 disease who have poor risk features, in particular high-grade tumours and deep myometrial invasion (stage 1B).

Radical radiotherapy can on occasions be given to elderly unfit patients with stage 1 disease and is the treatment of choice for those with bulky stage 2 and stage 3 tumours. This will take the form of external beam treatment to the pelvis followed by intracavitary treatment to the uterine cavity and upper vagina. Chemoradiation has been shown to be more effective when used with adjuvant chemotherapy than radiotherapy alone in stage 3 endometrial cancer.

CHEMOTHERAPY

In stage III endometrial cancer, improved outcome is seen when additional chemotherapy is given following hysterectomy and chemoradiation; carboplatin with paclitaxel is the standard combination.

PALLIATIVE TREATMENT

Palliative radiotherapy can be given for locally advanced tumours and for painful bone metastases.

Endometrial cancer is a hormone-dependent tumour and metastatic disease will respond to progestogens such as medroxyprogesterone acetate or megestrol. Response rates are between 20% and 30% and useful palliation of symptomatic metastases can be achieved. Responses to gonadotrophin-releasing hormone analogues such as leuprorelin are also recognized. There is no good evidence to support the use of these agents as adjuvant treatment.

Chemotherapy using carboplatin and paclitaxel or docetaxel can be offered to younger fit patients with advanced disease; objective tumour responses are seen in 20%–30% of patients.

TUMOUR-RELATED COMPLICATIONS

Pyometra or haematometra can occur owing to obstruction of the uterine cavity.

TREATMENT-RELATED COMPLICATIONS

Hysterectomy can result in urinary urgency and urge or stress incontinence. Pelvic radiotherapy is sometimes associated with late bowel and bladder toxicity, causing frequency, haematuria, rectal bleeding and rectal or vaginal stenosis. Sexual dysfunction is also common after both hysterectomy and radiotherapy.

PROGNOSIS

The prognosis for endometrial carcinoma is good since the majority of patients present with stage 1 disease for which there are cure rates in excess of 85%. Prognosis for more advanced stages falls, as would be anticipated, with 5-year survival rates of around 65% for stage 2% and 35% for stage 3. Survival stage for stage is worse for women over 60 years than for younger women and also for those with the papillary serous and clear cell types of cancer.

PREVENTION

The early diagnosis of endometrial cancer is helped by its early presentation with postmenopausal bleeding. It is therefore vital that all women with this symptom are investigated appropriately to exclude endometrial cancer.

RARER TUMOURS

Sarcomas of the endometrium can arise, presenting in the same way as endometrial cancer. They may be pure sarcomas such as a leiomyosarcoma arising from a fibroid or mixed tumours, such as the mixed mesodermal tumour, which contains both epithelial and stromal components, the latter in the form of malignant sarcomatous cells.

The prognosis for endometrial sarcomas is poor. Treatment is surgical removal at hysterectomy. There is no proven role for radiotherapy or chemotherapy, although regional and distant metastases are a common problem with these tumours.

OVARIAN CANCER

EPIDEMIOLOGY

Each year in the United Kingdom there are almost 7500 cases of ovarian cancer, accounting for 2% of all cancer cases and leading to a total of 4400 deaths per annum. There is a 1 in 50 chance of a woman in the United Kingdom developing ovarian cancer in her lifetime with little change in the incidence of ovarian cancer over recent years. There is a similar incidence in the United States but a low incidence in Japan, which approaches that of American women and Japanese immigrants to the United States.

AETIOLOGY

Ovarian cancer tends to occur in women over the age of 40 years who are nulliparous and of higher socioeconomic groups. Compared with women who have had more than four pregnancies, the relative risk for nulliparous women is 2.4. Paradoxically there appears to be a protective effect from oral contraceptive use, particularly for those using it for over 5 years, while a modest increase in risk is seen in women taking hormone replacement therapy for more than 10 years. Ovarian cancer is increased in women with endometriosis and in diabetics.

Genetic factors are important in the development of around 10% of ovarian cancers. It is around three times more common in women with a first degree relative who has had ovarian cancer. A link with the breast cancer-associated genes *BRCA1* and *BRCA2*, as well as with HNPCC, is recognized. The lifetime risk in a carrier of *BRCA1* is 65% and in BRCA2 35%. Women with Lynch syndrome have a 7% risk and those with Peutz–Jeghers syndrome have a 21% risk of developing ovarian cancer.

No specific environmental agents have been identified as directly contributing to the development of ovarian cancer.

PATHOLOGY

The common appearance of ovarian cancer is that of a cystic enlargement of the ovary. Two common types are recognized macroscopically:

- The pseudomucinous cyst, characteristically a large, multiloculated tumour mass containing mucinous material
- The serous cyst, containing clear fluid within a thin-walled cyst containing papillary structures

Other tumours may form solid masses (typical of a Brenner tumour) or characteristic teratomas.

The microscopic appearances of ovarian cancer are variable and the classification often complex.

Epithelial adenocarcinomas are the common ovarian cancers with several variants recognized, such as serous, clear cell and endometrioid carcinomas.

Germ cell tumours are the other major group of tumours of the ovary but, in contrast to the testis, the majority are benign teratomas.

Rarer tumours include those derived from gonadal stroma such as the *granulosa cell* and *Sertoli cell tumours*, which are oestrogen- and androgen-secreting tumours, respectively, *mixed mesodermal tumours* analogous to those that grow in the uterus, and lymphomas.

Metastases may also present in the ovary, typically from carcinoma of the breast or stomach (Krukenberg tumours).

NATURAL HISTORY

Local growth occurs within the ovary, spreading through the cyst wall onto the surface. Transcoelomic spread across the peritoneal cavity results in the classic appearance of multiple seedlings visible throughout the pelvic and abdominal cavities studding the peritoneal surfaces. Involvement of the omentum is also common and ascites is frequently found at operation.

Lymph node spread occurs to para-aortic nodes in the first instance.

Blood-borne metastases to liver and lungs are seen in more advanced disease. Meig's syndrome is the presence of a pleural effusion accompanying an ovarian tumour and has the features of a transudate, cytologically negative for carcinoma cells.

SYMPTOMS

Ovarian cancer can remain asymptomatic for some time and often presents with vague symptoms of abdominal discomfort and pelvic pain. In more

Ovarian cancer

advanced cases this may be associated with abdominal swelling owing to either tumour or ascites, and urinary and bowel disturbance owing to local pressure.

General symptoms of malignancy including malaise, anorexia and weight loss may also be present, and metastases can cause dyspnoea or bone pain.

SIGNS

Abdominal swelling and distension with a palpable mass or clinical signs of free fluid (shifting dullness to percussion and a fluid thrill) might be present. An ovarian mass may be palpable per vaginam or per rectum and a pleural effusion detectable clinically by dullness to percussion and absent breath sounds. A left supraclavicular node may be palpable in advanced cases.

DIFFERENTIAL DIAGNOSIS

Other causes of abdominal swelling should be considered, including ascites from other causes, hepatomegaly or splenomegaly, benign ovarian masses and intestinal obstruction.

INVESTIGATIONS

Routine investigations will often be unremarkable, although in advanced cases there might be electrolyte disturbance from intestinal obstruction or ureteric obstruction causing renal failure.

RADIOGRAPHY

Chest x-ray may demonstrate metastases or a pleural effusion.

ULTRASOUND

This will image the ovaries and give information regarding the nature of ovarian cysts. Liver ultrasound will evaluate the presence or absence of liver metastases.

CT SCAN

CT scan of the abdomen and pelvis will demonstrate the primary tumour and also pelvic and

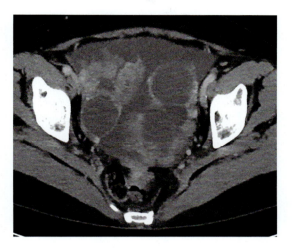

Figure 11.6 CT scan demonstrating extensive intra-abdominal tumour from carcinoma of the ovary.

para-aortic lymph node enlargement together with liver metastases if present. An example of a massive intra-abdominal tumour mass from carcinoma of the ovary is shown in Figure 11.6.

SERUM MARKERS

Serum CA125 is a valuable blood marker for ovarian cancer and is a useful monitor of response to treatment as demonstrated in Figure 11.7. A 'Risk of Malignancy' index (RMI) has been described based

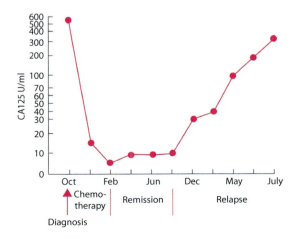

Figure 11.7 Changes in serum CA125 from high levels at diagnosis, falling through chemotherapy and later rising at relapse.

on the findings on transvaginal ultrasound, serum CA125 and menopausal status.

STAGING

The FIGO staging system for ovarian cancer is in common use:

- *Stage 1*: Confined to the ovary
  - *1a*: One ovary involved
  - *1b*: Both ovaries involved
- *Stage 2*: Spread to the pelvis
- *Stage 3*: Spread to the abdominal cavity
- *Stage 4*: Blood-borne metastases

TREATMENT

SURGERY

All patients with operable disease will proceed to laparotomy at which total abdominal hysterectomy, bilateral salpingo-oophorectomy and omentectomy are performed, together with careful examination of the para-aortic nodes, liver and peritoneal surfaces, including the sub-diaphragmatic regions and biopsy of any suspicious areas. Prognosis is directly related to the residual bulk of tumour and so maximum tumour debulking should be attempted in all patients, even where complete clearance is not possible.

For patients with stage 1a or 1b tumours that are well or moderately differentiated and with normal post-operative CA125 levels, no further treatment is indicated and close observation with serial pelvic ultrasounds and serum CA125 levels will be undertaken.

Surgery can have a role to remove persisting disease after chemotherapy, the 'second look laparotomy', at which residual tumour is removed to achieve macroscopic complete remission.

CHEMOTHERAPY

Primary chemotherapy should be given where patients present with inoperable disease which, in those who achieve a good response, will be followed by surgical removal of residual tumour.

Post-operatively, for high-grade stage 1 tumours, stage 1c tumours and more advanced disease localized to the abdominopelvic cavity, i.e. stages 2 and 3, chemotherapy is indicated. The drugs of choice are currently cisplatin or its analogue carboplatin, given for six cycles at monthly intervals together with paclitaxel.

For stage 4 disease with soft tissue metastases the outlook is poor and treatment might not influence the outcome. In patients with good general status, chemotherapy could be considered as for earlier stage disease.

PALLIATIVE TREATMENT

Chemotherapy is of value where relapse occurs after a long period of remission (>1 year) with many patients responding to re-exposure to cisplatin-based schedules. Relapse within the first year responds less well to further chemotherapy and heralds a particularly poor prognosis. Alternative drugs to be considered include liposomal daunorubicin, etoposide containing schedules or topotecan. Inclusion of bevacizumab in rechallenge with carboplatin and paclitaxel is also recommended.

Radiotherapy might be of value for symptomatic pelvic masses, vaginal bleeding from disease invading the vagina and bone metastases.

TUMOUR-RELATED COMPLICATIONS

Ascites and pleural effusions can occur. Intestinal obstruction is common in the advanced phases of the disease.

TREATMENT-RELATED COMPLICATIONS

Cisplatin and paclitaxel can both cause neurotoxicity with peripheral neuropathy or less frequently spinal cord damage. Ototoxicity can result in tinnitus and high tone deafness. Reduced renal function is common but overt renal failure need not occur provided the patient is well hydrated and renal function is properly monitored.

Both paclitaxel and carboplatin can cause significant bone marrow depression. Paclitaxel will in addition cause alopecia. Bevacizumab can cause hypertension, bleeding, thromboembolism, gastric perforation and proteinuria.

PROGNOSIS

The outlook for stage 1 ovarian cancer is good, with 10-year survival figures of over 80%. For more advanced disease the results of current chemotherapy give 5-year survival figures of 35%–50%. The survival of patients with stage 4 disease is usually only a few months.

SCREENING

Screening programmes for ovarian cancer have been proposed using serum CA125 measurements and abdominal ultrasound. Currently, they are recommended for those with a strong positive family history and those carrying the BRCA gene but routine population screening is not justified.

RARE TUMOURS

BRENNER TUMOURS

These are fibromas of the ovary and are usually benign in nature. Treatment is surgical removal.

TERATOMAS

Arising in the ovary, these are usually benign dermoid cysts. Malignant teratomas analogous to those arising in the testis are seen and, following surgical removal, adjuvant chemotherapy is recommended using drug combinations such as BEP (bleomycin, etoposide and cisplatin).

DYSGERMINOMAS

These are germ cell tumours arising in the ovary analogous to seminomas arising in the testis. For stage 1 tumours surgery is often curative. Chemotherapy using drugs such as VAC (vincristine, actinomycin D and cyclophosphamide) can be used for more widespread disease and these tumours are usually very radiosensitive; pelvic radiotherapy could have a role in persisting and recurrent disease.

GRANULOSA CELL TUMOURS

These are usually low grade and generally cured by surgery, although local recurrence some years later

---

CASE HISTORY

OVARIAN CANCER

A 48-year-old woman presents with a 1-year history of intermittent abdominal discomfort and a 1-month history of progressive abdominal distension. An abdominal ultrasound has shown a complex mass in the left ovary. Her CA125 is measured at 3562. Other investigations including a full blood count, renal function and chest x-ray are normal. She proceeds to laparotomy at which a large clinically malignant tumour is seen in the right ovary with multiple seedlings found throughout the abdominal cavity. Five litres of ascites are drained from the abdominal cavity. A total abdominal hysterectomy with bilateral salpingo-oophorectomy is performed leaving behind multiple small nodules on the peritoneum. Post-operatively a course of chemotherapy is recommended. She proceeds to receive five courses of carboplatin and paclitaxel. During treatment she suffers alopecia and complained at the end of her course of tingling in the fingers particularly when attempting to use them for fine movements. Her CA125 at completion of chemotherapy has fallen to 23.
Following chemotherapy she makes a good recovery and returns to a normal lifestyle.
Two years later she presents to her casualty department with a 3-day history of nausea, vomiting and constipation. On clinical examination intestinal obstruction is found. An emergency laparotomy is performed, which reveals widespread multiple areas of obstruction of the small bowel secondary to scattered nodules of tumour. Biopsy confirms the recurrence of her ovarian cancer. No attempt at resection is made and post-operatively she makes a slow but steady recovery with gradual resolution of her obstructive symptoms. Second-line chemotherapy is offered but she declines. Within 2 weeks she has a further episode of abdominal obstruction, which is managed conservatively with intravenous fluids and subcutaneous diamorphine and cyclizine. The symptoms are well controlled but her general condition deteriorates and she dies peacefully 10 days later.

Gynaecological cancer

is recognized. Characteristically, they secrete oestrogens and can be associated with the synchronous development of an endometrial cancer.

SERTOLI–LEYDIG CELL TUMOURS

These are usually of low malignant potential and cured by oophorectomy.

SARCOMAS

These are rare and typically mixed mesodermal tumours having both sarcomatous and epithelial elements. Their prognosis is poor unless localized within the ovary at the time of surgery.

LYMPHOMAS

These can arise within the ovary and are typically high-grade non-Hodgkin lymphomas treated as extranodal lymphomas at any other site with adjuvant chemotherapy with or without pelvic radiotherapy.

METASTASES

These can present in the ovary, usually from stomach or breast cancer. The classic bilateral ovarian metastases from carcinoma of the stomach are sometimes referred to as Krukenberg tumours.

CANCER OF THE VAGINA

EPIDEMIOLOGY

Carcinoma of the vagina is rare accounting for only 1% of all gynaecological cancers. It is a disease predominantly of elderly women. In the past, it was seen in young women associated with maternal use of stilboestrol.

Each year in the United Kingdom there are 250 cases of vaginal cancer, accounting for 0.1% of all cancer cases and leading to a total of 100 deaths per annum.

AETIOLOGY

Cancer of the vagina is closely related to HPV infection and other sexually transmitted infection including herpes simplex. There is therefore also an association with cervical neoplasia and women with a past history of CIN or invasive cervical cancer have a 20-fold risk of vaginal cancer also.

Unlike in cervical cancer, an association with genital warts, typically associated with HPV 6 and 11, is seen.

Chronic irritation of the vaginal mucosa following long-term use of a vaginal ring pessary for vaginal prolapse is also a risk factor.

Maternal use of stilboestrol during pregnancy was associated with the development of clear cell adenocarcinoma of the vagina during adolescence, fortunately no longer seen.

PATHOLOGY

Vaginal intraepithelial neoplasia (VAIN) is a recognized epithelial change analogous to CIN at the cervix and can progress to frank carcinoma.

Macroscopically, the tumour presents as an ulcer, papilliferous growth or diffuse infiltration of the vaginal mucosa.

Microscopically, the usual histology is a squamous carcinoma. Rarely, adenocarcinomas arise and the clear cell variant related to stilboestrol can also be seen without this aetiology.

NATURAL HISTORY

Direct extension results in invasion of the parametrium, bladder or rectum. Lymph node spread is to internal iliac and pelvic nodes (from the upper two-thirds of the vagina) and to inguinal and femoral nodes (from the lower third).

Blood-borne spread to liver and lungs also occurs in advanced disease.

SYMPTOMS

These include vaginal discharge and bleeding; local pain is unusual unless there has been extensive pelvic infiltration.

SIGNS

Tumour will usually be visible and palpable on speculum and digital vaginal examination.

Inguinal nodes might be palpable with tumours of the lower vagina.

DIFFERENTIAL DIAGNOSIS

This includes atrophic vaginitis; metastases from the cervix or endometrium; and a tumour of the urethra or Bartholin's gland.

INVESTIGATIONS

The diagnosis will be confirmed at examination under anaesthetic when biopsies can be taken. Routine investigations can show chronic anaemia from blood loss and, rarely, renal failure owing to ureteric obstruction from pelvic infiltration or lung metastases on chest x-ray.

FINE-NEEDLE ASPIRATION

Palpable inguinal nodes should be investigated further by FNA to distinguish inflammatory nodes from metastases.

CT SCAN

Staging should include CT scan of the pelvis to assess pelvic lymph nodes.

MAGNETIC RESONANCE IMAGING

MRI will give most accurate details of the soft-tissue anatomy of the pelvis and identify local extension of the tumour.

STAGING

Vaginal carcinoma is staged using the FIGO classification:

- *Stage 1*: Limited to the vaginal mucosa
- *Stage 2*: Extension to submucosa and parametrium but not to pelvic side walls
- *Stage 3*: Extension to pelvic side wall
- *Stage 4*: Bladder, rectum or distant metastases

TREATMENT

SURGERY

Early disease can be treated by radical hysterectomy and total vaginectomy with pelvic lymphadenectomy. Inguinal node dissection is also undertaken for tumours in the lower third of the vagina. Vaginal reconstruction should be offered to women undergoing this procedure.

RADIOTHERAPY

Radiotherapy is indicated for stage 2 and stage 3 diseases. It should also be considered for those with early tumours who are unwilling to accept vaginectomy, reserving surgery for salvage patients whose disease recurs and for those unfit for surgery. External beam irradiation to the pelvis including the inguinal nodes for lower third tumours should be followed by intracavitary or interstitial treatment to give a high dose of radiation directly to the vaginal mucosa and surrounding local tumour extension. Chemoradiation using weekly cisplatin with radiotherapy is considered for younger patients.

PALLIATIVE TREATMENT

Radiotherapy is helpful for locally advanced or recurrent disease. This takes the form of external beam treatment where there is a major pelvic component or intracavitary treatment for bleeding or ulcerated disease locally in the vagina.

There is no recognized effective chemotherapy for vaginal carcinoma.

TUMOUR-RELATED COMPLICATIONS

These may include vaginal haemorrhage and sepsis and renal failure owing to urethral obstruction.

TREATMENT-RELATED COMPLICATIONS

Recognized acute complications of pelvic radiotherapy include radiation cystitis and diarrhoea.

Late complications include vaginal stenosis and fistulae into bladder or rectum, particularly where there has been local infiltration by tumour.

Vaginal reconstruction using large bowel is described.

Gynaecological cancer

PROGNOSIS

Over 80% of stage 1 patients can expect cure; 50% of patients with stage 2% and 30% of those with stage 3 tumours will survive 5 years.

SCREENING

VAIN seems to be related to previous cervical malignancy and therefore these patients should also receive regular vaginal smears following the treatment of a cervical cancer.

RARER TUMOURS

Adenocarcinoma and clear cell carcinoma are usually treated surgically, with radiotherapy reserved for palliation of advanced tumours.

CANCER OF THE VULVA

EPIDEMIOLOGY

Each year in the United Kingdom there are 1300 cases of vulval cancer, accounting for 0.4% of all cancer cases and 5% of all gynaecological cancers with 460 deaths each year. It is usually seen in older, postmenopausal women.

AETIOLOGY

There is an association with HPV infection, both subtypes 16 and 18 related to cervical cancer, and genital wart viruses, subtypes 6 and 11. The risk in women having previous CIN or invasive cervical cancer is 10 times that of those without. There is an association with other sexually transmitted diseases including herpes simplex and HIV. Other immunosuppressed groups are also at increased risk with a 100-fold excess risk in patients after renal transplantation.

Vulval cancer is increased in smokers and chemical carcinogenesis was seen historically in the 'mulespinners' exposed to mineral oils.

PATHOLOGY

Vulval cancer may be preceded by or coexist with dystrophic conditions of the vulval skin including

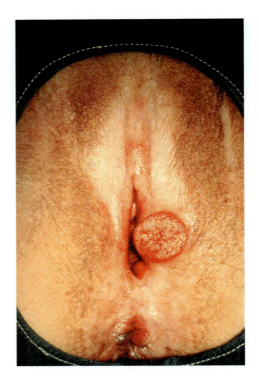

Figure 11.8 Primary squamous carcinoma of the vulva.

leucoplakia, lichen sclerosus and atrophicus and Paget disease of the vulva. True carcinoma *in situ* is also seen in the vulval skin.

Macroscopically, the invasive tumour is typically a papilliferous growth or an ulcer arising from the medial side of the labium majorum (Figure 11.8). Bilateral tumours are also seen – the so-called 'kissing cancer'.

Microscopically, vulval carcinomas are squamous carcinomas. Other rare tumours that can arise in the vulva include basal cell carcinomas, melanomas, sarcomas and tumours of the female urethra and Bartholin's gland.

NATURAL HISTORY

Local invasion of surrounding soft tissue occurs early and in advanced cases pubic bone can also become involved. Lymphatic spread is to the inguinal nodes before progressing along the pelvic node chain. Blood-borne spread to lungs can occur but is a late event.

SYMPTOMS

- There may be long-standing symptoms of skin dystrophy with local irritation.
- A lump may be obvious to the patient.
- Pain is usually a late symptom owing to bone invasion.
- Swelling of the legs can occur from inguinal nodes or femoral vein involvement.

SIGNS

- The local tumour will be apparent as an ulcer or papilliferous growth.
- Inguinal nodes can be palpable with associated leg oedema.

DIFFERENTIAL DIAGNOSIS

Vulval dystrophies can be a forerunner of invasive cancer, as discussed previously.

Infective conditions, such as condylomata, lymphogranuloma inguinale or lymphogranuloma venereum, should be considered. In the past, tuberculous or syphilitic lesions have also been described in the differential diagnosis but are rarely seen today.

INVESTIGATIONS

The tumour is usually apparent clinically and diagnosis is confirmed by a full examination under anaesthetic and biopsy.

FINE-NEEDLE ASPIRATION

Palpable nodes should be investigated with FNA for cytological confirmation of malignancy as many will be only inflammatory.

CT SCAN

In the presence of palpable nodes, CT scan of the pelvis will assess proximal spread into the iliac node chain.

MR SCAN

MR scan will give soft tissue detail to identify local infiltration and bone involvement.

RADIOGRAPHY

Chest x-ray will exclude the presence of lung metastases.

STAGING

Staging uses the FIGO classification:

- *Stage 1*: Confined to the vulva
- *Stage 2*: Extension to adjacent perineal structures (lower 1/3 urethra; lower 1/3 vagina; anus) with negative nodes
- *Stage 3*: Positive inguinofemoral nodes with or without extension to adjacent perineal structures
- *Stage 4*:
  - Invades upper urethra or vagina; bladder or rectum; fixed to pelvic bone; fixed or ulcerated inguinofemoral lymph nodes
  - Distant metastases outside pelvis

TREATMENT

SURGERY

Wide excision of the vulva (simple or radical vulvectomy) with bilateral femoral and inguinal node dissection is usually recommended.

RADIOTHERAPY

For inoperable disease, radical radiotherapy can be given using both external beam treatment, often given as chemoradiation with weekly cisplatin and interstitial implantation of the tumour. A radical dose could be given but acute reactions in this area can be severe and are often dose limiting.

PALLIATIVE TREATMENT

Local toilet surgery might be required or, where there is extensive posterior infiltration, a defunctioning colostomy. Radiotherapy is of value for local pain, discharge and bleeding.

There is no recognized chemotherapy for vulval carcinoma although responses are described following combinations effective against squamous carcinomas, such as docetaxel or mitomycin C and 5FU.

TUMOUR-RELATED COMPLICATIONS

These can include:

- Local haemorrhage and discharge
- Oedema of either or both legs from venous or lymphatic obstruction
- Urethral invasion causing difficulty with micturition
- Anal invasion possibly resulting in faecal incontinence

TREATMENT-RELATED COMPLICATIONS

Radical surgery can be complicated by delayed wound healing. Leg oedema is sometimes seen where there has been extensive dissection of the groins. Urethral stricture may develop from scarring.

PROGNOSIS

Survival is related to the extent of disease at presentation and general condition, which in the frail and elderly might preclude radical surgery.

Following radical surgery for localized disease, over 80% of patients will survive 5 years. The involvement of lymph nodes is a poor prognostic sign, reducing 5-year survival to around 40%.

RARE TUMOURS

BASAL CELL CARCINOMAS

These are usually cured by local surgery unless they have invaded deeper structures. They can also be treated by radiotherapy.

MELANOMAS

These are best treated with wide surgical excision. For more advanced local lesions or patients with distant metastases, palliative radiotherapy could be of value in obtaining local control.

SARCOMAS

These are also best treated by wide surgical excision.

CHORIOCARCINOMA

EPIDEMIOLOGY

Choriocarcinoma is a malignant tumour arising from the placental tissues. It is a rare tumour that may arise occasionally in association with a normal pregnancy, but is far more common as a complication of a hydatidiform mole.

The incidence of choriocarcinoma is around 1 in 50,000 pregnancies. There is a higher incidence in South-East Asia and Japan and in the United States it is more common in women of Asian, American Indian and African American descent. In the United Kingdom, there are around 20 cases per year.

AETIOLOGY

Hydatidiform mole is more common in pregnancies in women under 20 and over 40 of age. Past history of a mole predisposes to subsequent mole pregnancies.

PATHOLOGY

Macroscopically, choriocarcinoma arises within the uterus following normal pregnancy, ectopic pregnancy, spontaneous abortion or hydatidiform mole. It is characteristically a haemorrhagic tumour with no detectable placental remnant.

Microscopically, the distinction between a benign mole and choriocarcinoma is made by the absence of villi in the choriocarcinoma with areas of necrosis and haemorrhage. The cells of the trophoblast have malignant features with many mitoses and pleomorphic cells with multiple nucleoli. Lymphovascular invasion is common.

NATURAL HISTORY

Local invasion involves the uterine wall at an early stage. Lymph node metastases are rare. Early blood-borne dissemination occurs to lungs, liver and the central nervous system. Other common distant sites involved are skin, bowel and spleen. Bone metastases are rare.

SYMPTOMS

These include:

- Vaginal bleeding within 1 year of pregnancy
- Abdominal or pelvic discomfort

Up to one-third of patients may present with symptoms of metastatic disease such as cough, haemoptysis, weight loss, headache or fits.

SIGNS

The uterus can be enlarged and tender on pelvic examination or a pelvic mass palpable. Chest signs secondary to lung collapse or effusion might be present, the liver enlarged and palpable, and there might be focal neurological signs associated with brain metastases.

DIFFERENTIAL DIAGNOSIS

Choriocarcinoma must be distinguished from hydatidiform mole. Other causes of uterine bleeding such as fibroids and cervical or endometrial carcinoma should be considered.

INVESTIGATIONS

BLOOD TESTS

Blood levels of human chorionic gonadotrophin (HCG) are important. This is raised in normal pregnancy and also with hydatidiform mole and choriocarcinoma. It is an important indicator of tumour bulk in choriocarcinoma and an invaluable tumour marker for monitoring treatment.

ULTRASOUND

Ultrasound of the uterus gives a characteristic picture in hydatidiform mole and choriocarcinoma. It can also be used to assess the extent of local invasion through the uterine wall and fallopian tube and ovarian involvement.

CT SCAN

CT scan of the brain, chest abdomen and pelvis is required for full staging information.

MAGNETIC RESONANCE IMAGING

MRI will give further detailed evaluation of the uterus and local tumour infiltration within the pelvis.

HISTOLOGY

The diagnosis of choriocarcinoma will be confirmed histologically on examination of the uterine contents removed at examination under anaesthetic and suction evacuation.

STAGING

Choriocarcinoma is staged as follows:

- *Stage 1*: Confined to the uterus
- *Stage II*: Early spread to vagina or ovary
- *Stage III*: Lung metastases
- *Stage IV*: Metastases outside the lungs

A prognostic score has been described by which patients can be divided into those with a good, intermediate or poor prognosis. This uses a number of parameters including age, parity, preceding pregnancies, HCG level, number, site and size of metastases.

TREATMENT

Because of its rarity and the complex nature of its treatment, all patients should be referred to a major centre experienced in the management of choriocarcinoma.

SURGERY

Suction evacuation of the uterus is the initial treatment in all cases.

CHEMOTHERAPY

Subsequent chemotherapy is based on close monitoring of serum HCG levels. Indications for treatment include:

- Very high levels persisting after evacuation (>20,000 IU)
- Rising levels of HCG
- Continued uterine bleeding
- Metastatic disease

All the aforementioned are signs of active choriocarcinoma.

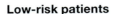
Gynaecological cancer

Low-risk patients

Low-risk patients who are young with disease restricted to the uterus and vagina or those with lung metastases account for 80%; they will receive chemotherapy with methotrexate as a single agent.

Intermediate-risk patients

Intermediate-risk patients who are over 39 years with localized disease or have spleen or liver metastases receive chemotherapy with actinomycin D, vincristine and etoposide.

High-risk patients

Those with metastases in the gastrointestinal tract or liver receive more intensive chemotherapy called EMA-CO comprising etoposide, actinomycin D, methotrexate, vincristine and cyclophosphamide. Multiple drugs are used in this context to prevent the resistance emerging in surviving cells.

Because of the high risk of CNS metastases, prophylactic treatment with intrathecal methotrexate is also recommended for high-risk patients and all those with lung metastases.

Established CNS metastases are treated with dexamethasone and multiple drug chemotherapy as for the high-risk group.

TUMOUR-RELATED COMPLICATIONS

Bleeding from the uterus or metastatic sites resulting in gastrointestinal, intracerebral or intrapulmonary haemorrhage may be seen. Respiratory failure can complicate multiple pulmonary metastases or be precipitated by their treatment owing to rapid tumour lysis.

TREATMENT-RELATED COMPLICATIONS

Rapid tumour destruction with chemotherapy of widespread metastases can cause not only respiratory failure but also extensive metabolic disturbance (tumour lysis syndrome; see Chapter 21).

Many patients have proceeded after successful treatment to have further pregnancies without complications. There is, however, some concern that oral contraceptive treatment in the immediate period after chemotherapy may provoke further relapse and oral contraception should be avoided for 6 months following completion of chemotherapy.

PROGNOSIS

The outlook for patients with choriocarcinoma is extremely good. It is only those who have high-risk disease, including those over 40 years with bulky (>5 cm) metastases, multiple sites or more than a total of eight metastases, brain metastases and very high HCG levels (>10,000 IU) in whom survival of less than 100% can be anticipated and, even in this group, over 85% will be cured.

SCREENING

Routine screening of pregnant women is not indicated but high-risk patients who have had previous trophoblastic disease (mole or choriocarcinoma) should have careful monitoring of HCG following delivery.

FURTHER READING

BMJ Best Practice: Cervical Cancer. https://best-practice.bmj.com/topics/en-gb/259/.

Matulonis UA, Sood AK, Fallowfield L, Howitt BE, Sehouli J, Karlan BY. Ovarian cancer. *Nat Rev Dis Primers*. 2016; 2, Article number: 16061 https://www.nature.com/articles/nrdp201661.

NHS Cervical Screening Programme Colposcopy and Programme Management NHSCSP, Publication Number 20. 3rd ed. March 2016.

RCOG Guidelines for the Diagnosis and Management of Vulval Carcinoma; 2014: https://www.rcog.org.uk/globalassets/documents/guidelines/vulvalcancerguideline.pdf.

Sundar S, Balega J, Crosbie E et al. BGCS uterine cancer guidelines: Recommendations for practice. *Eur J Obstet Gynecol Reprod Biol*. 2017; 213: 71–97.

SELF-ASSESSMENT QUESTIONS

1. Which of the following is true of cancer of the cervix?
   a. It increases in incidence with age

Self-assessment questions

    b. It is related to infection with the herpes zoster virus
    c. It is more common in higher socioeconomic groups
    d. It is found in most patients at screening
    e. It is falling in incidence in the United Kingdom

2. Which of the following is true of cancer of the cervix?
    a. The common form is an adenocarcinoma
    b. Squamous cancers typically arise from the endocervical canal
    c. Surface ulceration is common
    d. The usual path of spread is into the uterine cavity
    e. Lymph node spread is rare

3. Which three of the following are recognized features of cancer of the cervix?
    a. Renal failure
    b. Constipation
    c. Dysuria
    d. Amenorrhoea
    e. Post-coital bleeding
    f. Urinary incontinence
    g. Low back pain

4. In the treatment of cancer of the cervix, which of the following is true?
    a. Surgery is preferred for stages I to III diseases
    b. Chemotherapy has an important role in primary treatment
    c. Hormone replacement therapy is contraindicated
    d. Radiotherapy is indicated if lymph nodes are involved at surgery
    e. Metastatic disease may respond to anti-oestrogens

5. Which of the following is true of endometrial cancer?
    a. It is related to infection with the HPV virus
    b. It is most common in premenopausal women
    c. It can be prevented by cervical smear screening programmes
    d. It is associated with hypothyroidism
    e. It can be caused by treatment for breast cancer

6. Which three of the following are true in the treatment of endometrial cancer?
    a. Most cases are cured after radical hysterectomy
    b. Advanced disease may respond to anti-oestrogen therapy
    c. Radiotherapy is not useful as the cancer is radioresistant
    d. Chemotherapy is effective for advanced disease
    e. Hormone replacement therapy should be encouraged after treatment

7. Which of the following applies to cancer of the ovary?
    a. It is most common in women under 40 years of age
    b. It is common in Japan and the Far East
    c. It is usually diagnosed with symptoms at an early stage
    d. There is a 50% risk in patients with the *BRCA1* gene
    e. It is associated with smoking

8. In cancer of the ovary which of the following is true?
    a. Common types are cystic
    b. Teratomas are usually malignant
    c. Blood-borne spread is an early feature
    d. The common histology is a squamous carcinoma
    e. The level of CEA is used to monitor response

9. Which three of the following are usually associated with cancer of the ovary?
    a. A high level of CA125
    b. Haematuria
    c. Dysmenorrhoea
    d. Abdominal distension
    e. Renal failure
    f. Ascites
    g. Constipation

10. Which of the following is true of the treatment of ovary cancer?
    a. Radical surgery is usually curative
    b. Unilateral salpingo-oophorectomy is the usual operation for stage I
    c. Chemotherapy with cisplatin and paclitaxel is standard in stage III

Gynaecological cancer

    d. Hormone replacement therapy is contraindicated
    e. Post-operative radiotherapy is indicated for high-risk stage I disease

11. Which of the following is true of cancer of the vagina?
    a. It is more common in women who have had previous CIN
    b. It is more common than cancer of the vulva
    c. The common form is an adenocarcinoma
    d. The usual treatment when the cancer is localized is radical surgery
    e. Adjuvant chemotherapy may have a role in high-risk cases

12. Which of the following is true of cancer of the vulva?
    a. It typically spreads to iliac lymph nodes
    b. It is more common after renal transplantation
    c. Blood-borne metastases occur at an early stage
    d. Radical radiotherapy is indicated for early disease
    e. The prognosis is related to age

13. Which of the following is true of choriocarcinoma?
    a. It occurs in 1 in 5000 live pregnancies
    b. It typically occurs in women aged 20–40 years
    c. Metastases are present in a third of women at presentation
    d. Surgical excision is the best treatment
    e. Future pregnancy is contraindicated

14. Which three of the following are true of the treatment for choriocarcinoma?
    a. Chemotherapy is indicated if there is an HCG level >20,000 IU
    b. Chemotherapy response is monitored by serial levels of HCG
    c. The most useful drug is cisplatin
    d. Intrathecal chemotherapy is required by all patients
    e. Chemotherapy is not required for low-risk patients
    f. Prophylaxis against tumour lysis is required for advanced disease
    g. Infertility is a common side effect

CNS tumours

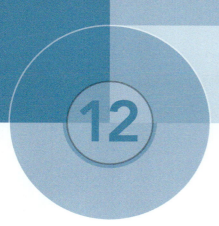

A discussion of the general principles will be followed by specific examples.

EPIDEMIOLOGY

Each year in the United Kingdom there are over 11,000 cases of CNS tumours, approximately evenly divided between men and women, accounting for 3% of all cancer cases and leading to over 5000 deaths per annum. One to two percent of autopsies performed after death from other causes reveal occult brain primary tumours. There is a bimodal age incidence with peaks at 5–9 years and over half of case diagnosed over 65 years, varying with the type of tumour, e.g. medulloblastomas are very rare beyond adolescence, glioblastomas are very rare in adolescents and children.

AETIOLOGY

Specific aetiological factors can be identified in <1% of cases. In general, brain tumours increase in incidence with age but there is a distinct profile of paediatric tumours also. Genetic predisposition to CNS tumours has been identified in the following rare syndromes:

- *Neurofibromatosis*: Neurofibroma, neurofibrosarcoma, optic nerve glioma, ependymoma and meningioma
- *Tuberose sclerosis*: Glioma and hamartoma
- *Von Hippel–Lindau syndrome*: Cerebellar haemangioblastoma
- *Li–Fraumeni syndrome*: Gliomas
- *Gorlin's syndrome*: Medulloblastoma

Industrial exposure to vinyl chloride has been associated with the development of gliomas. In HIV-positive cases, primary cerebral lymphoma is associated with infection by the Epstein–Barr virus.

PATHOLOGY

A simplified classification of tumours according to their cell of origin is outlined in Table 12.1; 80% are intracranial and 20% spinal, childhood tumours tend to be located in the cerebellum, adult tumours in the cerebral hemispheres. Highly malignant tumours will have necrosis and haemorrhage on cut section, oedema of the surrounding cerebral tissue and may not be well circumscribed. Multifocal high-grade gliomas and lymphomas are recognized. Calcification is seen in craniopharyngiomas, oligodendrogliomas and some meningiomas, making them visible on a plain skull x-ray.

Spinal tumours can be classified further according to their origin in relation to the dural/spinal cord anatomy into three groups:

- Extradural, e.g. metastases, chordoma
- Intradural extramedullary, e.g. meningiomas, neurofibromas
- Intramedullary, e.g. astrocytomas, ependymomas, haemangioblastomas, lipomas, dermoids

Tumours can be subclassified into grades according to the degree of differentiation. This grading reflects the expected behaviour of the tumour and takes into account factors such as the degree of

CNS tumours

Table 12.1 Classification of primary CNS tumours according to the tissue of origin

Tissue of origin	Tumour
Glial (50%)	Astrocytoma, oligodendroglioma, oligoastrocytoma choroid plexus tumour, ependymoma
Meninges (25%)	Meningioma, sarcoma
Pituitary (20%)	Craniopharyngioma, adenoma
Vascular (2%)	Angioma, haemangioblastoma
Pineal (<1%)	Pinealoma, pineoblastoma
Germ cells (<1%)	Teratoma, dysgerminoma
Miscellaneous	Chordoma, medulloblastoma, lymphoma, melanoma

tumour cellularity, the number and appearance of mitotic figures and the presence of necrosis.

Increasingly molecular changes are recognized as critical in distinguishing subtypes of glioma, for example changes in the IDH1 and IDH2 genes in glioblastoma, the MGMT gene which predicts for sensitivity to temozolamide in glioblastoma and the 1p19q deletion which predicts for chemosensitivity in oligodendroglioma.

NATURAL HISTORY

Direct infiltration is the main mode of spread and the cause of death of the majority of patients dying from CNS tumours. All CNS tumours, even if benign, enlarge by infiltrating adjacent neural tissue as shown in Figure 12.1, and in turn the increasing peritumoral oedema around the tumour leads to raised intracranial pressure. Raised intracranial pressure can arise from the mass effect and associated oedema and also due to hydrocephalus from compression of the ventricular system leading to impaired drainage of cerebrospinal fluid (CSF) and ventricular dilatation proximal to the block. Some tumours are prone to CSF seeding include medulloblastoma, ependymoma, pineoblastoma, germ cell tumours and lymphoma. This results in meningeal deposits anywhere from the foramen magnum down to the mid-sacrum (Figure 12.2).

Lymphatic spread is not seen as the neural tissue does not have a true lymphatic drainage system. Distant metastases are extremely rare, but are described in patients with very aggressive tumours

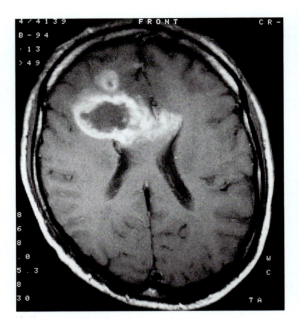

Figure 12.1 High-grade glioma. MRI of the brain showing a large tumour infiltrating across the corpus callosum.

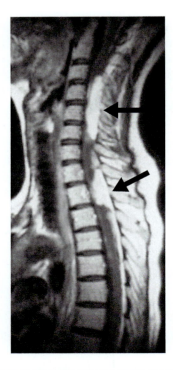

Figure 12.2 Multiple meningeal tumour deposits. Sagittal MRI of the cervicothoracic spine and spinal cord.

such as glioblastomas that have invaded the dural venous sinus system, and medulloblastomas.

SYMPTOMS AND SIGNS

CEREBRAL TUMOURS

Patients with cerebral tumours usually present with one or more of the following:

- Epilepsy
- Raised intracranial pressure
- Focal neurological deficit

The patient may present with an epileptic fit which can be generalized, affecting the whole body, or focal, or affecting a region or single part of the body related to the anatomical origin within the brain. A cerebral tumour should be considered in any patient presenting *de novo* in this manner, particularly with focal epilepsy. Raised intracranial pressure can lead to headaches with an early morning predominance, nausea, vomiting, somnolence, apathy, poor concentration, memory impairment and personality change. Clinically, there may be papilloedema, upgoing plantar responses, evidence of impaired higher mental functions and impairment of consciousness. Local pressure from a tumour will lead to dysfunction of the affected tissue which will be manifest clinically by focal neurological signs corresponding to the affected portion of the brain. These will be upper motor neurone in type, e.g. spasticity, hyperreflexia and upgoing plantar reflexes in the case of a hemi paresis.

SPINAL TUMOURS

These may present with one or more of the following:

- Back pain
- Nerve root pain
- Spinal cord compression
- Cauda equina compression

Spinal cord compression can arise when the lesion lies between the foramen magnum and the lower limit of the cord at the junction of the L1 and L2 vertebrae. There will be upper motor neurone loss of function below the level of the block, associated with a sensory level and sphincter disturbance.

Cauda equina compression arises if the lesion is somewhere below the lower limit of the spinal cord (at approximately L1/L2 level) affecting only nerve roots, and therefore the signs are those of a lower motor neurone lesion affecting the lower limbs, i.e. hypotonia, weakness, wasting, fasciculation, hyporeflexia, down-going plantar reflexes and a dermatomal sensory loss. The urethral and anal sphincters may also be impaired.

INVESTIGATIONS

MAGNETIC RESONANCE IMAGING

MRI should be considered the investigation of choice for imaging of CNS tumours. The high lipid content of neural tissue leads to high contrast and in turn a high spatial resolution. The ability to image directly in non-axial planes (rather than reconstruct non-axial planes as in CT) lends itself to high-quality images of the brain and spinal cord. These are ideal for neurosurgical planning and radiotherapy treatment planning. MRI is also superior to CT in demonstrating meningeal disease. However, MRI is not as useful as CT in showing the skeletal anatomy.

COMPUTED TOMOGRAPHY

This will give information regarding the location, size and degree of local invasion of the tumour. It is particularly good for delineating the skeletal anatomy but poor at surveying the posterior fossa owing to the thickness of the bone in this region and proximity of mastoid air cells, both of which can lead to streak artefacts. Artefacts from surgical clips and dental amalgam can also produce problems.

STEREOTACTIC NEEDLE BIOPSY OR OPEN BIOPSY

This is essential to obtain a specimen for histological diagnosis. When surgical resection is not feasible, e.g. a tumour located at a critical site such as the brainstem, a needle biopsy will be the least traumatic means of sampling a tumour. Otherwise, open biopsy and tumorectomy are performed, and have the advantages of providing a larger specimen for histological analysis and potentially being of

LUMBAR PUNCTURE

This can be of value in providing further information to assist in diagnosis and treatment, e.g. in providing CSF for cytology in carcinomatous meningitis and high-risk non-Hodgkin lymphoma, and, in the case of germ cell tumours, allowing assay of CSF α-fetoprotein and β-human chorionic gonadotrophin. However, in patients with suspected brain tumour, lumbar puncture should always be preceded by fundoscopy and a CT or MRI scan of the brain to exclude raised intracranial pressure.

TREATMENT

SURGERY

This is the treatment of choice for all brain and spinal tumours as most are relatively radioresistant, making them incurable by radiotherapy alone. Complete excision should be the goal of the neurosurgeon both to clear the tumour and to obtain adequate tissue for diagnosis. However, CNS tissue is not tolerant of trauma, is critical to normal body functioning and has no powers of regeneration, and so frequently the best that can be achieved without causing major disability is surgical debulking.

RADIOTHERAPY

Radiotherapy has a complementary role to surgery, being ideal for eradicating small volume disease left behind after attempted surgical clearance, but can also be used to treat radiosensitive tumours arising in critical areas of the brain with a high expectation of cure, e.g. a dysgerminoma arising in the pineal region. Radiotherapy to brain tumours can be challenging with a number of critical radiosensitive structures in the close vicinity including the eye, brain stem and pituitary. Focused radiotherapy techniques using stereotactic radiosurgery (SRS) enables high-dose treatment to small volumes of brain with relatively little irradiation of the surrounding normal brain. It is used for the treatment of small tumours (e.g. solitary brain metastases), boost treatments following whole brain radiotherapy (WBRT) or retreatment of recurrences after radiotherapy.

CHEMOTHERAPY

Temozolomide also has an important role in chemoradiation for high-grade gliomas; response to temozolamide can be predicted by the presence or absence of MGMT methylation, coding for a DNA repair enzyme. In oligodendroglioma, the presence of the 1p19q deletion confers chemosensitivity and a high response rate to procarbazine, CCNU and vincristine (PCV). The role of chemotherapy in other CNS tumours is mainly palliative in intent. The blood–brain barrier (BBB) acts as an obstacle to the free passage of chemotherapy drugs. Lipid-soluble drugs such as the nitrosoureas BCNU and PCV, cisplatin and very high doses of methotrexate enter the brain in sufficiently high concentrations. Methotrexate and cytosine arabinoside given intrathecally by lumbar puncture or intraventricularly via an indwelling Ommaya reservoir are of value as regional chemotherapy in the management of meningeal deposits from lymphoma, leukaemia and solid tumours.

SUPPORTIVE THERAPY

Dexamethasone 4–16 mg daily is very effective at relieving raised intracranial pressure. Prolonged usage does, however, lead to symptoms and signs of Cushing's syndrome, oral candidiasis and proximal myopathy, which may exacerbate neurological deficits. Mannitol intravenously is useful as an adjunct in an acute exacerbation of raised intracranial pressure. Anticonvulsants should be given only for documented fits. Patients with epilepsy or recent craniotomy should be advised not to drive until fit free according to national guidelines. Many patients will have problems with the activities of daily living from neurological deficits, and referral to appropriate rehabilitation services is essential.

ASTROCYTOMA

They arise from astrocytes in the brain or spinal cord, and are most common in adults but arise also during childhood. They are divided histologically

Astrocytoma

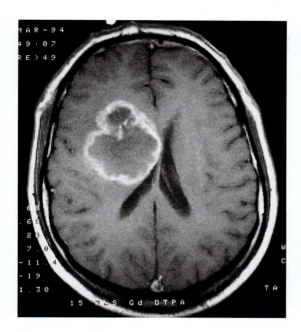

Figure 12.3 High-grade glioma. MRI of the brain showing a large tumour with a necrotic centre and compressing the adjacent ventricle.

into low grade (grades 1 and 2) and high grade (grades 3 and 4), which correlate with prognosis. Grade 4 tumours are termed glioblastoma multiforme. They constitute 50% of astrocytomas, arising in adults with a peak incidence occurring in patients over 65 years of age. They are usually found in cerebral hemispheres, especially the frontal and temporal lobes, are extensively necrotic (Figure 12.3) and haemorrhagic, and are often associated with oedema of the adjacent brain. Tumours close to the midline can spread to the contralateral hemisphere via the corpus callosum or basal ganglia. Glioblastomas are occasionally multifocal (Figure 12.4). Spinal cord astrocytomas are very rare (Figure 12.5).

Surgery should be performed with the aim of complete macroscopic and microscopic resection, although this goal is not often attained due to the diffusely infiltrative nature of the tumour and its position within the brain.

Post-operative *radiotherapy* is only given in low-grade tumours where there is a large residual tumour in older patients and in those where there is documented progression after resection. A high-grade element can become apparent which should then be treated

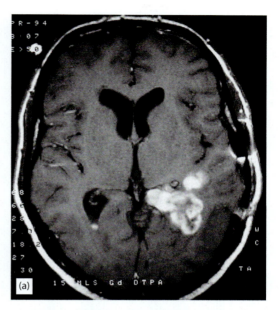

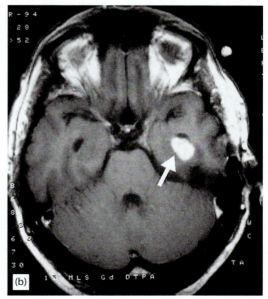

Figure 12.4 Multifocal high-grade glioma. MRI of the brain. (a) Several foci are seen in the parieto-occipital lobe. (b) Further focus in the temporal lobe.

as a high-grade tumour. Post-operative radiotherapy should be considered for all high-grade tumours; radical treatment, including temozolamide chemoradiation for grade 4 tumours, is chosen for patients under 65 years of age with good performance status.

CNS tumours

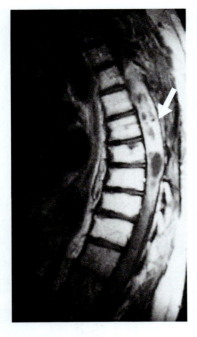

Figure 12.5 Spinal astrocytoma. Sagittal MRI of the thoracic spine. There is a part solid, part cystic mass arising from the spinal cord.

Chemotherapy is given routinely as part of the radical treatment of glioblastoma using daily temozolamide with radiotherapy followed by 6 months of adjuvant temozolamide. Response is greater in those patients with MGMT methylation in their tumour cells. Another approach where >90% tumour resection is achieved has been to use carmustine implanted biodegradable copolymer wafers (Gliadel®) into the tumour cavity at the time of surgery. Chemotherapy will also be considered for recurrent tumours in patients with good performance status to prolong symptom-free survival and overall survival. Active drugs include the nitrosoureas BCNU and CCNU, vinca alkaloids, procarbazine and cisplatin. The combination PCV is widely used, has been shown to be superior to single-agent BCNU and has been particularly active in anaplastic astrocytomas. Overall, however, the effect of chemotherapy is disappointing; meta-analysis of individual randomized trials demonstrates a 5% absolute survival advantage at 2 years for chemotherapy, equating to an increase in 2-year survival from 15% to 20%.

Poor prognostic factors include high-grade tumours, advanced age, poor neurological performance status, limited surgical resection and a presentation other than epilepsy. Five-year survival for Grade 1 tumours is about 60%, but high-grade tumours have an extremely poor prognosis, with a median survival of 3 months when biopsy alone is performed, 8 months when treated with radiotherapy alone and 14 months with chemoradiation including temozolamide.

OLIGODENDROGLIOMA

They constitute only 5% of gliomas, arising exclusively in adults with a mean age of 40 years. They are usually found in the cerebral hemispheres, particularly in the frontal lobes (50%) and adjacent to the ventricles, and 20% are bilateral. They are slow-growing, well-circumscribed tumours; 40% have foci of calcification and, unlike gliomas, there is little associated oedema for their size. Patients often have a history of epilepsy or gradual deterioration in higher mental functions. Low-grade tumours are compatible with a long survival after surgery alone, which can be curative. The principles of management mirror those for astrocytomas except that for those with the 1p19q deletion, PCV chemotherapy is indicated rather than radiotherapy.

MENINGIOMA

They constitute 15% of intracranial tumours, are most common in adults and are the only CNS tumours that are more common in females. They arise from the arachnoid mater, adjacent to the major venous sinuses, the most common sites being the parasagittal region, olfactory groove, sphenoidal ridge and suprasellar region, and sometimes arise as an intradural extramedullary spinal tumour. They are usually benign, slow growing and well circumscribed, may erode overlying skull and 20% are partly calcified. More locally invasive malignant variants are occasionally seen. Primary treatment is surgery. Radiotherapy is considered after incomplete surgical excision without which approximately 50%

of patients will recur. Radiotherapy will reduce the risk of recurrence by half in this context and is also used for inoperable cases or recurrence after surgery. The prognosis is good as the natural history is measurable in years and decades. Some cases can be managed with observation alone. Chemotherapy has no defined role in this disease.

PITUITARY TUMOURS

The vast majority are benign adenomas, with a tiny minority seen as metastases (breast and lung primary cancers) or true primary carcinomas. Pituitary adenomas can be classified according to the staining characteristics of the cell of origin into three groups:

- Chromophobe adenomas (50%) are often large, forming the bulk of non-secretory tumours but might secrete prolactin.
- Eosinophil adenomas (40%) are much smaller than chromophobe adenomas and may secrete growth hormone or prolactin.
- Basophil adenomas (10%) are usually small, and may secrete ACTH, rarely TSH, LH or FSH.

They can also be divided according to their macroscopic diameter into microadenomas (<10 mm) – the majority, or macroadenomas (>10 mm).

Adenomas present with vague symptoms such as headache or with more specific abnormalities. The optic chiasm is a close anatomical relation of the pituitary fossa below and therefore suprasellar extension can lead to chiasmal compression and visual disturbance. Testing of the visual fields to confrontation and perimetry typically reveals a bitemporal hemianopia, although occasionally lateral extension involves the cavernous sinuses resulting in a palsy of the third, fourth and sixth cranial nerves and in turn ocular palsies leading to diplopia. Examination of the fundi can reveal a pale disc consistent with optic atrophy. Hypopituitarism can result from compression of the pituitary gland adjacent to the tumour or pressure on the hypothalamus. Growth hormone secretion is the first to be impaired followed by the gonadotrophins. Diabetes insipidus indicates superior extension into the supra-optic nuclei. Pituitary apoplexy is a rare, acute presentation of pituitary failure owing to haemorrhage or infarction of the pituitary. Hypothalamic pressure can also lead to a loss of hypothalamic regulation and in turn disturbances in homeostasis such as loss of temperature regulation and disturbance of appetite and sleep.

Eighty percent of pituitary adenomas are hormonally active. Prolactin may be elevated in half of the cases from loss of the inhibitory hormone produced by the hypothalamus or direct secretion by the eosinophilic or chromophobe adenoma cells. This can present as galactorrhoea, amenorrhoea, lack of libido or erectile dysfunction. Eosinophilic adenoma can also produce growth hormone, manifest as acromegaly, and basophilic adenomas can secrete ACTH leading to Cushing's disease or Nelson's syndrome. Less than 1% secrete TSH-producing hyperthyroidism. Plurihormonal adenomas have been seen. Many of the so-called non-functioning adenomas actually produce the gonadotrophins LH and FSH but do not produce a clinically detectable syndrome until they expand the pituitary fossa and compress surrounding structures.

INVESTIGATIONS

VISUAL FIELD PERIMETRY

Objective documentation of visual field defects is important at baseline before treatment.

MAGNETIC RESONANCE IMAGING

MRI, particularly sagittal views of the pituitary fossa, provides a detailed assessment of the pituitary itself and potential sites of local tumour spread (Figure 12.6).

COMPUTED TOMOGRAPHY

Reconstructed coronal CT images can be complementary to MRI and in some cases there will be contraindications to MRI.

ENDOCRINE ASSESSMENT

Baseline pituitary function tests are important both to identify malfunction requiring intervention and to provide a baseline for evaluation following treatment.

CNS tumours

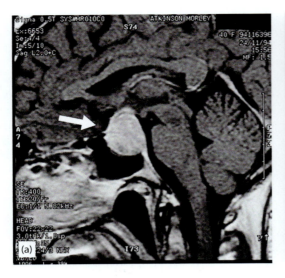
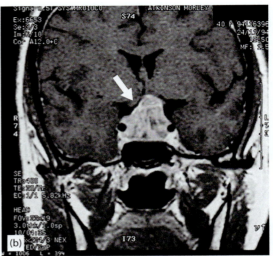

Figure 12.6 Pituitary adenoma. (a) Sagittal MRI of the brain showing an enhancing tumour that occupies the pituitary fossa and extends into the suprasellar region. (b) Coronal MRI from the same patient. Note the proximity of the tumour to the cavernous sinuses.

TREATMENT

SURGERY

Trans-sphenoidal micro-surgical hypophysectomy provides a tissue diagnosis, instant decompression of the optic chiasm and other adjacent structures and a cessation of hormone hypersecretion. Complete resection of the pituitary tumour and its extensions or substantial debulking will provide optimum long-term local control for macro-adenomas, but partial removal of the pituitary may suffice for a microadenoma. If there is much suprasellar or lateral extension of a large adenoma, a frontal (transcranial) approach will give greater access.

RADIOTHERAPY

This is only occasionally considered as primary treatment when the risks of surgery are considered high. Radiotherapy alone is successful in the long-term control of hormone hypersecretion, although the maximum benefit is expressed after some years. In acromegalics, there is a 20% per annum decline in growth hormone levels, but normalization might never occur, particularly if pre-treatment levels were very high. Similar results are seen in prolactin- and ACTH-secreting tumours. The addition of post-operative radiotherapy after surgery for macroadenomas increases 10-year disease-free survival from 10% to over 80%. There is a 30% 10-year risk of hypopituitarism after radiotherapy.

DOPAMINE AGONISTS

Bromocriptine and cabergoline mimic the prolactin inhibitory hormone produced by the hypothalamus, and are of value in the treatment of prolactinoma when they can induce dramatic tumour regression and thereby defer the need for surgery or radiotherapy.

CRANIOPHARYNGIOMA

This is relatively rare, usually arising in children, and overall constitutes 10% of pituitary tumours. It is most common in Japan but rare in the United States and Western Europe. It is a suprasellar tumour arising from nests of epidermoid cells in the pars tuberalis (Rathke's pouch), slow growing, benign, three-quarters being partly cystic and calcified (Figure 12.7).

Germ cell tumours

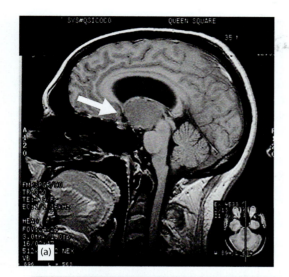

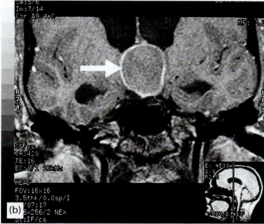

Figure 12.7 Craniopharyngioma. (a) Sagittal MRI of the brain showing a solitary, well-circumscribed, cystic mass in the suprasellar region. (b) Coronal MRI from the same patient.

Presentation is as for pituitary adenomas and surgery is the treatment of choice, with radiotherapy having the same role as for pituitary tumours, i.e. after incomplete excision or for inoperable cases. Prognosis is very good with an 80% 5-year survival and 70% 5-year disease-free survival.

PINEAL TUMOURS

These are rare tumours. Characteristically, they present with obstructive hydrocephalus owing to their proximity to the CSF ventricular outflow pathway, or ocular palsies, especially paralysis of upward gaze (Parinaud's syndrome). Surgery is particularly difficult and hazardous in this region. A ventriculoperitoneal shunt may be required. Germinomas and astrocytomas are the commonest tumours in the pineal region. Rarer, intrinsic tumours of the pineal gland include:

- *Pinealoma*: This is the most common pineal tumour with a peak incidence at 15–25 years. It is slow growing, well circumscribed, non-invasive, and treated by surgical excision.
- *Pineoblastoma*: This is much more aggressive than pinealoma, CSF dissemination being a frequent complication.

GERM CELL TUMOURS

Teratomas and dysgerminomas (analogous to seminoma) may arise from islands of ectopic germ cells in the suprasellar region (Figure 12.8) or pineal. Patients with confirmed CNS disease should be referred to a regional centre specializing in the treatment of germ cell tumours. The tumours are radiosensitive and chemosensitive but the prognosis is not as good as for their testicular counterparts. Serum and CSF α-fetoprotein and β-human chorionic gonadotrophin measurements are useful to confirm diagnosis and monitor response to treatment.

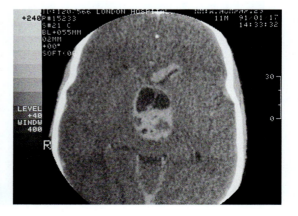

Figure 12.8 Suprasellar teratoma. Transverse CT image of the brain of a young child showing a complex cystic lesion arising in the suprasellar region.

EPENDYMOMAS

They constitute 10% of childhood intracranial tumours with a peak incidence during the first decade of life. They arise throughout the CNS from cells lining the ventricles, central canal of the spinal cord and choroid plexus, although the vast majority arise near the fourth ventricle, 40% being supratentorial and 60% infratentorial. They are well circumscribed, usually well differentiated, slow growing, and may be calcified (Figure 12.9). Spread via CSF is well recognized, particularly if high grade and infratentorial.

Combined surgery and radiotherapy give the greatest chance of local control, selected patients at high risk of CSF dissemination receiving radiotherapy to the craniospinal axis. The prognosis is a 5-year survival of about 50% falling to 40% at 10 years.

MEDULLOBLASTOMA

This is the most common intracranial tumour in children (see Chapter 18), accounting for 20% of intracranial tumours in the under 16 years with 80% arising in those under 15 years of age, most during the first decade. The cells of origin are foetal elements of the external granular layer of the cerebellum. Tumours arise centrally in the vermis in children and more laterally in the hemispheres in young adults. There is a high risk of spread via CSF (one-third of cases) and it very rarely metastasizes outside the CNS, usually to bone. Recently, four molecular subgroups have been identified — wingless (WNT), sonic hedgehog (SHH), group 3 and group 4.

Presentation is with cerebellar symptoms and signs such as ataxia and obstructive hydrocephalus.

Patients require a posterior fossa craniotomy and tumorectomy. Often a ventriculoperitoneal shunt is required to relieve obstructive hydrocephalus and raised intracranial pressure. Medulloblastoma is one of the most radiation-sensitive CNS tumours. Radiotherapy is delayed if possible until after 3 years of age; prior to this high-dose chemotherapy may be pursued. Over 3 years radiotherapy to the posterior fossa and craniospinal axis is indicated followed in high-risk cases by further chemotherapy. Five-year survival is approximately 50%. Trials comparing

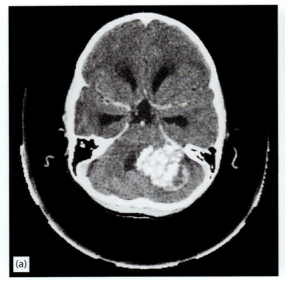 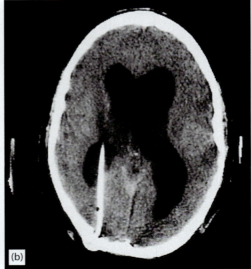

Figure 12.9 Ependymoma. (a) CT image showing a heavily calcified mass arising from the posterior fossa of a child. (b) CT image from the same child showing obstructive hydrocephalus leading to massive ventricular dilatation. A shunt has been inserted to relieve this.

chemotherapy (vincristine and CCNU) and radiotherapy with radiotherapy alone have not shown a substantial advantage for the combined modality treatment. A major issue is the impaired growth development and neuropsychiatric consequences of CNS irradiation in infants and young children.

CHORDOMA

This is a very rare tumour that presents in adult life, arising from notochord remnants in the axial skeleton anywhere from the sella turcica to the sacrum. In adults, these remnants persist in the nucleus pulposus of the intervertebral disc. Fifty percent are sacrococcygeal, 35% arise in the spheno-occipital region and 15% in the vertebral column. They are slow-growing, well-circumscribed, gelatinous, extradural tumours with areas of haemorrhage and necrosis, often reaching a large size and causing compressive symptoms. A characteristic histological finding is the so-called 'physaliferous' cells. They are locally invasive and can be confused with metastatic adenocarcinoma or chondrosarcoma, with less than 10% metastasizing to distant sites.

Radical excision should be attempted, although it is rarely possible, and post-operative radiotherapy is necessary in the majority, giving a 50% 5-year survival falling to 20% at 10 years. There are few published data regarding the use of chemotherapy, which is not particularly effective. A sarcoma-style protocol (e.g. doxorubicin and ifosfamide) can be used for palliation of symptoms refractory to radiotherapy or to control distant metastatic disease. In advanced disease, imatinib can dely progression although significant regression is unusual.

HAEMANGIOBLASTOMA

These are more common in children and form part of the von Hippel–Lindau syndrome. They are usually cerebellar in origin with the hemispheres affected more than the vermis. The tumour is slow growing, well circumscribed and associated with polycythaemia owing to ectopic secretion of erythropoietin.

LYMPHOMA

Primary cerebral lymphoma is rare but increasing in incidence (see also Chapters 16 and 20). It is associated with HIV infection but also occurs sporadically in older patients. It presents with symptoms of global cerebral dysfunction such as epilepsy, cognitive impairment and somnolence, or focal neurological signs. Chemotherapy schedules will include high dose (2–5 g/m^2) methotrexate to circumvent the BBB and achieve high CNS concentrations of drug. The role of WBRT remains under investigation. It results in considerable toxicity with significant effects on psychomotor function but may have an important role where there is an incomplete response to chemotherapy and where comorbidities preclude the use of high-dose methotrexate. Primary CNS lymphoma has a poor prognosis and is rarely cured however with radical chemotherapy and radiotherapy, the median survival is around 3 years.

METASTASES

These usually originate from cancers of the lung, breast, kidney, colon, pancreas and melanoma. Lung cancer is the most common primary (50%), particularly small cell and large cell variants, where one-quarter to one-half of patients will have cerebral metastases at autopsy. They are most frequent in the frontal and parietal lobes, usually rounded, well circumscribed and enhance on CT and MRI with intravenous contrast. They are often associated with cerebral oedema and can occasionally be confused with a cerebral abscess.

One-third will present as oligometastases defined when there are up to 3 metastases only (Figure 12.10 and 12.11); these patients should be considered for radical ablative treatment with surgical excision or stereotactic radiosurgery (SRS) provided their primary tumour is controlled and they have good performance status. Surgery in this setting should be followed by radiotherapy. SRS is now preferred as it is associated with less impact on cognitive function after treatment compared to whole brain radiotherapy. Median survival in this setting however remains poor at 8–12 months.

CNS tumours

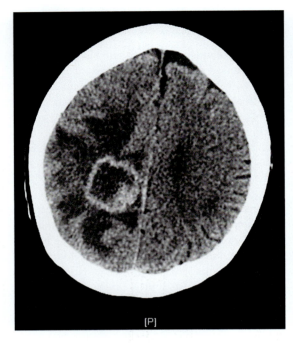

Figure 12.10 Solitary brain metastasis. Contrast-enhanced CT image of the brain showing a solitary metastasis arising in the right parietal region. This is typically well circumscribed and hypodense with ring enhancement, and associated with oedema of the surrounding brain.

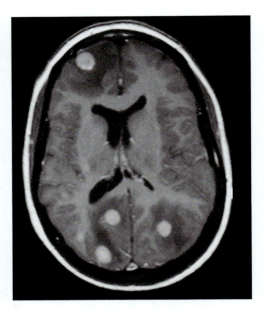

Figure 12.12 Multiple cerebral metastases. Transverse MRI of the brain.

Patients presenting with multiple brain metastases as shown in Figure 12.12 require careful evaluation as their prognosis is in general poor and the impact of treatment limited except in selected cases. This should include imaging of the brain stem and cervical cord where intramedullary metastases may

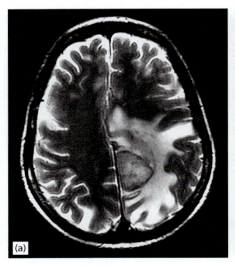
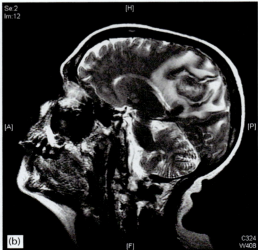

Figure 12.11 Solitary brain metastasis. There is much associated cerebral oedema. MRIs: (a) transverse view and (b) sagittal view.

Carcinomatous meningitis

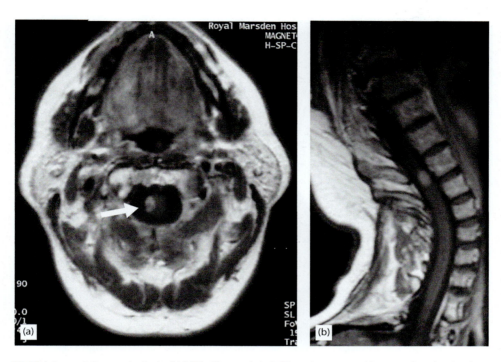

Figure 12.13 Intramedullary metastasis. (a) MRI of base of skull. There is an eccentric area of contrast enhancement within the cervical spinal cord corresponding to a metastasis. (b) Sagittal MRI showing a metastasis within the spinal cord.

occur as shown in Figure 12.13. Those with poor performance status, particularly those over 65 years with a lung primary should be considered for best supportive care rather than any oncological treatment having a median survival of around 2 months; those with good performance status, particularly when younger and with controlled primary tumours having a longer natural history such as breast cancer may benefit from whole brain radiotherapy (WBRT). Concern around the later cognitive deficits which can develop from WBRT has led to trials of hippocampal sparing techniques in an attempt to minimize this complication. The response rate for most symptoms such as headache, epilepsy and neurological disability is in the order of 80% and the net result is an improvement in functional independence for the majority of treated patients. Cranial nerve palsies are often less responsive.

Chemosensitive tumours such as germ cell tumours are managed aggressively with systemic chemotherapy, even if there are multiple sites of metastatic disease).

CARCINOMATOUS MENINGITIS

Tumour spread to the CNS can manifest as diffuse involvement of the meninges around the brain (Figure 12.14) and/or spinal cord. This is particularly seen in haematological malignancies (e.g. non-Hodgkin lymphoma), breast cancer, lung cancer and melanoma. It can present with non-specific symptoms such as headache, vomiting, meningism, lethargy, confusion or more focal neurological deficit, typically cranial nerve palsies. Such patients might have disease that extends along the optic nerves to involve the optic disc (Figure 12.15) or peripheral retina (Figure 12.16). Its onset and presentation is insidious, and it is easy to mistake some of the symptoms for other conditions, e.g. opiate toxicity. Diagnosis can be made from typical appearances on a contrast-enhanced MRI, although lumbar puncture is often necessary to obtain CSF for cytology and confirm the diagnosis. The diagnosis can sometimes remain elusive with negative imaging and CSF cytology, in which

CNS tumours

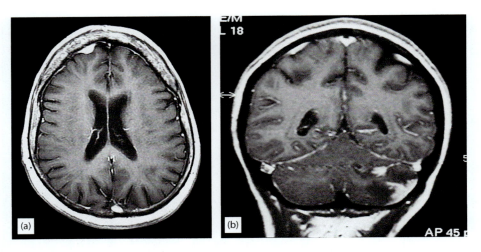

Figure 12.14 Meningeal carcinomatosis. MRI of the brain: (a) transverse view and (b) coronal view.

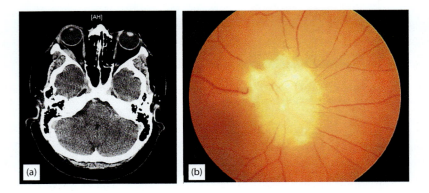

Figure 12.15 Optic nerve metastases. (a) Transverse CT image showing irregular thickening of the optic nerve. (b) Fundoscopy showing irregular, pale plaque of tumour at optic disc.

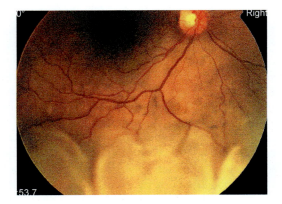

Figure 12.16 Choroidal metastasis. Fundoscopy showing a secondary retinal detachment and subretinal effusion.

case further cytological sampling of CSF is indicated. Treatment options include intrathecal instillation of chemotherapy agents, such as methotrexate, at twice weekly intervals via lumbar puncture or an Ommaya intraventricular catheter and/or cranial/craniospinal radiotherapy. The outlook for solid tumour carcinomatous meningitis is extremely poor, many patients dying within weeks of their diagnosis.

FURTHER READING

BMJ Best Practice: Brain Tumours. https://bestpractice.bmj.com/topics/en-us/262

Louis DN, Perry A, Reifenberger G et al. The 2016 World Health Organisation classification of tumors of the central nervous system: A summary. *Acta Neuropathol.* 2016;131(6):803–20.

Weller M, Wick W, Aldape K et al. Glioma. *Nat Rev Dis Primers.* 2015; 1, Article number: 15017.

SELF-ASSESSMENT QUESTIONS

1. Which three of the following are common features of CNS tumours?
   a. Hypothyroidism
   b. Cranial nerve palsy
   c. Raised intracranial pressure
   d. Epilepsy
   e. Taste disturbance
   f. Insomnia
   g. Mania

2. Which one of the following is true about pituitary tumours?
   a. Blindness is frequent
   b. Olfactory disturbance is frequent
   c. Binasal hemianopia is the commonest form of visual disturbance
   d. Epilepsy is rare
   e. Hemiparesis is sometimes seen

3. Which three of the following statements are true regarding the treatment of gliomas?
   a. Surgical excision is indicated for multifocal tumours
   b. Complete surgical excision is rarely achieved
   c. All types have a high mortality within 5 years of diagnosis
   d. They are very sensitive to radiotherapy
   e. Temozolomide crosses the blood–brain barrier
   f. Nitrosoureas are active drugs
   g. Chemotherapy leads to response rates of 30%–50%

4. Which one of the following is true about meningiomas?
   a. They are not well visualized by computed tomography
   b. They are readily identified by magnetic resonance imaging
   c. The majority are malignant in their behaviour
   d. Radiotherapy is used routinely after surgery
   e. Active treatment is always advisable

5. Which three of the following statements best describe brain metastases?
   a. Best seen by PET imaging
   b. Can be confused with cerebral abscesses
   c. Never treated surgically as they represent disseminated disease
   d. Usually multiple rather than solitary
   e. Produce symptoms distinct from those of a primary brain tumour
   f. Chemotherapy has no significant role in their management
   g. They usually lead to the death of the patient

6. Which one of the following is true about carcinomatous meningitis?
   a. Behaves more favourably than cerebral metastatic disease
   b. Associated with ocular spread of malignant disease
   c. Treated by systemic chemotherapy
   d. Usually seen with computed tomography images
   e. Intrathecal chemotherapy with cisplatin is a useful treatment

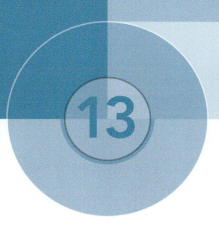

Head and neck cancer

Each year in the United Kingdom there are 12,000 cases of head and neck cancer with 4000 deaths accounting for 2% of all cancer deaths. Nearly 90% arise in the over 50s, the incidence is increasing with age and there is a strong male predominance with a male-to-female ratio of 2:1 for oral cancer and 5:1 for laryngeal cancer. Incidence rates vary greatly from region to region within each country, and the incidence and mortality rates are increasing. Worldwide, the highest incidence is in India and Sri Lanka where in some areas they account for up to 40% of the total. Other pockets of high incidence include South America and the Bas-Rhin region of France (oral cancer), and Newfoundland (lip). The head and neck regions are exposed to environmental carcinogens through the air we breathe and the food and drink we ingest. Each site will be dealt with individually, although cancer of the oral cavity will be described in detail as many of the basic principles are applicable to head and neck cancer in general. As a general rule, the prognosis worsens as the tumour site moves further down the aerodigestive tract from the lips.

CARCINOMA OF THE ORAL CAVITY

The oral cavity extends from the skin–vermilion junction of the lips to the junction of the hard and soft palates above and to the line of circumvallate papillae on the tongue below. This includes carcinoma of the lip, anterior two-thirds of tongue, floor of mouth, buccal mucosa, hard palate, retromolar trigone and lower alveolus.

AETIOLOGY

Tobacco accounts for 90% of oral cavity cancers today. Inhalation of tobacco smoke from cigarettes, pipes and cigars is the major cause of cancer of the floor of the mouth. As with lung cancer, the greater the amount smoked and the higher the tar content, the higher the risk. Chewing tobacco and betel nut, common in Asian cultures, carries a particularly high risk of carcinoma of the buccal mucosa and cancers arising in the retromolar trigone.

Heavy alcohol consumption is a major risk factor and high-alcohol mouthwashes have also been implicated. Alcoholics also tend to have poor nutrition, and their low intake of vitamins A and C might add to their risk of developing cancer. Human papilloma virus (HPV) infection, especially HPV 16, is associated with 12% oral cavity malignancies. In the past, chronic syphilitic glossitis was a major cause of carcinoma of the tongue.

Carcinoma of the lip is more common in those with outdoor occupations where ultraviolet exposure is greater, and this accounts for the predominance of this tumour on the lower lip.

Physical trauma from poor dentition can lead to malignant transformation at the site of trauma, usually the lateral border of the tongue. Historically, chronic heat trauma from clay-pipe smoking was associated with carcinoma of the lip.

PATHOLOGY

Macroscopically, the tumours can be frankly ulcerated, with raised, everted, nodular edges or papilliform.

Head and neck cancer

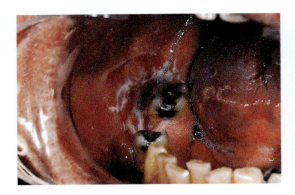

Figure 13.1 Leucoplakia. The retromolar region has a white, superficial, lace-like appearance. This may lead to the development of a squamous carcinoma.

They may also present as subtle areas of superficial denudation of the mucosa. Synchronous primaries sometimes occur either in the oral cavity or elsewhere in the aerodigestive tract. The tumour can be secondarily infected, and there may be surrounding white plaques—leucoplakia—which are premalignant (Figure 13.1).

Microscopically, 90% are squamous carcinomas, the remainder being adenocarcinomas, mucoepidermoid carcinomas, adenoid cystic carcinomas, lymphomas and melanomas. *In situ* carcinoma and/or dysplasia might be seen in the surrounding mucosa.

NATURAL HISTORY

Local infiltration into adjacent subsites of the oral cavity occurs with invasion of the deeper layers of the mucosa, reaching muscle in the case of the tongue and cheek, and even the underlying bone of the maxilla or mandible. Tumours of the lower alveolus tend to spread along the alveolus by insidious submucosal spread, so their microscopic extent can be much greater than appreciated macroscopically.

Lymph node spread is seen in a high proportion, e.g. 70% in carcinoma of the tongue, the incidence being greater with increasing tumour size and increasingly undifferentiated tumours. Tumours adjacent to the anatomical midline can spread to lymph nodes bilaterally. First station lymph nodes include those in the jugulodigastric, submandibular and submental groups. Second station lymph nodes are those of the jugular, and the upper and lower posterior cervical groups.

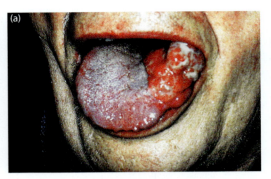

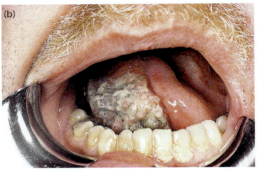

Figure 13.2 Carcinoma of the tongue. Such tumours will interfere with speech and swallowing.

Haematogenous spread is relatively uncommon at diagnosis and usually seen in the terminal phase of the disease, the lungs being the most common site, followed by bone.

SYMPTOMS

Many patients are asymptomatic, the tumour having been noticed at a routine dental examination, but some complain of soreness at the site of the tumour owing to chronic superficial ulceration. The initial presentation may be with a neck lump due to cervical lymph node enlargement. In locally advanced cases, pain might be more marked and radiate to the ear, while a fungating tumour will lead to halitosis. Bulky tumours of the tongue (Figure 13.2) will interfere with mastication and swallowing and lead to difficulty with speech.

SIGNS

Patients frequently have physical signs consistent with heavy smoking and alcohol intake. Oral hygiene is often poor with an increased incidence of dental decay and gum disease, and this should be noted as it is relevant to the planning of radiotherapy. A thorough ENT examination is mandatory, preferably by an ENT surgeon. The primary tumour should be described in detail with respect to its position (preferably supplemented by a drawing), size and depth of invasion. Areas of leucoplakia should be sought and care taken to exclude another primary tumour. The tumour should be palpated with a gloved finger to complement inspection, feeling for induration and mucosal irregularity. All patients should have fibreoptic endoscopy of the nasal fossa, nasopharynx, oropharynx, hypopharynx and larynx for full evaluation of the site of origin and local tumour spread. The neck should be palpated very carefully to detect enlarged lymph nodes, recording their distribution (preferably with a diagram), size, number, consistency, degree of tenderness and fixation to surrounding structures. Small tender lymph nodes are frequently due to associated infection in the region of the tumour rather than lymph node metastases.

DIFFERENTIAL DIAGNOSIS

Other benign causes of oral ulceration that should be considered include:

- Simple aphthous ulceration
- Lichen planus
- Herpes simplex
- Syphilis

INVESTIGATIONS

BIOPSY

A biopsy is essential in order to obtain tissue for histological analysis, and can be performed in an outpatient setting.

EXAMINATION UNDER GENERAL ANAESTHETIC

This allows detailed palpation of the tumour to define its precise size, position and extent of local invasion.

MAGNETIC RESONANCE IMAGING OF THE ORAL CAVITY AND NECK

This will give accurate assessment of the extent of the primary tumour and with contrast enhanced and diffusion weighted sequences identify abnormal lymph nodes. Extent of local infiltration and bone involvement are of particular importance when assessing the primary tumour.

ORAL PANTOMOGRAM (OPG)

This will evaluate invasion of the mandible or maxilla, and provides a detailed survey of the teeth, which will help plan any dental procedures that may be necessary prior to radiotherapy.

FINE-NEEDLE ASPIRATE OF ANY ENLARGED LYMPH NODES

This should be performed in the outpatient clinic and the specimen sent for immediate cytology. As the result may make a substantial difference to the proposed treatment, it is worth repeating the aspiration if a negative lymph node is still clinically suspicious.

WHOLE-BODY CT OR CT PET

This will assess the presence of distant metastases, in particular the lungs and liver as the most common sites. A synchronous second primary tumour in the lung or oesophagus should also be considered when interpreting these scans.

STAGING

The TNM staging is used:

- Tis: Carcinoma in situ
- T0: No evidence of primary
- TX: Primary cannot be assessed
- T1: 2 cm or less in greatest dimension
- T2: >2 but not >4 cm in greatest dimension
- T3: >4 cm in greatest dimension
- T4: Invasion of deep (extrinsic) muscle of tongue, skin, cortical bone or maxillary sinus
- N0: No regional lymphadenopathy

- N1: Single ipsilateral node 3 cm or less in greatest dimension
- N2: Single ipsilateral node >3 but not >6 cm in greatest dimension or multiple ipsilateral nodes not >6 cm or bilateral/contralateral nodes not >6 cm in greatest dimension
    - N2a: Single ipsilateral node >3 but not >6 cm in greatest dimension
    - N2b: Multiple ipsilateral nodes none >6 cm in greatest dimension
    - N2c: Bilateral/contralateral node(s) >6 cm in greatest dimension
- N3: Any node >6 cm in greatest dimension
- M0: No distant metastases
- M1: Distant metastases

TREATMENT

Patients should be discussed in a multidisciplinary team (MDT) meeting including a specialist, a head and neck surgeon and a clinical oncologist; oral surgeons, reconstructive surgeons, nutritionists and speech and language therapists also have an important role in assessing the patient.

Patients should be advised to stop smoking and drinking alcohol to lessen the risk of mucositis during radiotherapy or chest infections after an anaesthetic. Attention to nutrition is important as patients are frequently malnourished at presentation owing to neglect, oral soreness or dysphagia which will compromise their ability to tolerate major surgery or radical radiotherapy. The patient might require a softer consistency of diet or liquid supplements. A liquidizer can be very useful. All patients having radiotherapy should be referred to a dentist to have mild degrees of dental decay immediately dealt with by conservative measures while any teeth with serious decay should be extracted prior to radiotherapy to reduce the risk of complications such as radionecrosis following treatment.

RADICAL TREATMENT

Surgery

The aim of surgery is to remove the primary tumour with a margin adequate to encompass all microscopic spread with the reconstruction of any major tissue deficits. Surgery may also include excision of the regional lymph nodes. This may be the sole primary treatment, combined with radiotherapy or as salvage for local recurrence following radical radiotherapy. Surgery is sometimes the treatment of choice for locally advanced tumours, i.e. T3 and T4 tumours, as these are bulky tumours that may invade adjacent bone when they are particularly difficult to eradicate by radiotherapy alone. There is also an increased risk of osteonecrosis after radiotherapy when the bone is invaded and this is a particularly difficult management problem. However, radical surgery can involve a major resection of tissue, leading to severe functional morbidity. For example, resection of part of the tongue will result in some degree of dysarthria and possible difficulty in mastication of food and swallowing. Such symptoms can severely compromise the patient's quality of life. Therefore, T1, T2 and small bulk T3 tumours are usually best treated by radiotherapy with surgery reserved for local recurrence.

The surgeon can also perform a radical dissection of the cervical lymph nodes when these are involved. This is a major procedure involving removal of the ipsilateral nodes en bloc together with the internal jugular vein (IJV) and some other tissues such as the sternocleidomastoid and accessory nerve. The IJV cannot be sacrificed bilaterally, although a modified radical dissection can be performed on the contralateral side if necessary (IJV is preserved). Radiotherapy is indicated after neck dissection if three or more nodes are involved or if there is any evidence of extracapsular spread of tumour cells outside a lymph node.

Improvements in surgical techniques have resulted in more patients being able to benefit from reconstructive procedures after radical cancer surgery. This has lessened considerably the functional morbidity experienced after major resections of the tongue and other structures of the oral cavity.

Speech therapy is essential after major resections in the oral cavity, particularly of the tongue, floor of mouth and lips, which might result in speech and swallowing difficulties (Figure 13.3).

Radiotherapy

As with surgery, radiotherapy can be used as the sole primary treatment, combined with surgery or for salvage of local relapse after surgery. It has the

Carcinoma of the oral cavity

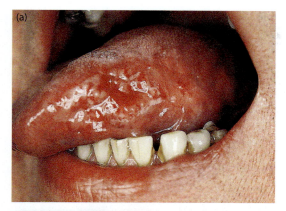

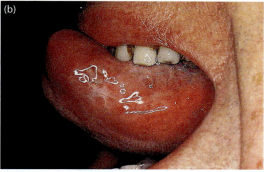

Figure 13.3 T1 squamous carcinoma arising from the lateral edge of the tongue: (a) before treatment and (b) 6 months after interstitial implant. Tongue function, speech and swallowing have been fully preserved.

advantage of having a greater chance of preserving the voice, speech and swallowing that surgery would compromise, and is therefore the treatment of choice for T1 and T2 tumours.

Usually, the treated volume will include the first station lymph nodes adjacent to the primary tumour as a prophylactic measure to eradicate subclinical tumour deposits, extended to include the whole cervical lymph node chain at risk if there are palpable lymph node metastases.

Radiotherapy gives poor local control when used alone for bulky T3 and T4 tumours, and therefore is usually given following surgery.

Modern techniques using intensity-modulated radiotherapy (IMRT) allows the high-dose radiation envelope to be matched in three dimensions to the shape of the tumour. It therefore spares the surrounding organs at risk such as the spinal cord and parotid salivary glands. This reduces morbidity and enables dose escalation. It also means re-treatment following failure of a previous course of radiotherapy can be considered and for achieving a varying dose across the treated volume, it can at the same time deliver lower doses to prophylactic sites and higher doses to macroscopic tumour.

Standard treatment will deliver a dose of 66–70 Gy to the primary tumour. Increasing the rate of delivery by giving the overall course in 5 weeks delivering six fractions instead of 5 per week has been shown to improve the outcome. HIV-associated head and neck malignancy is relatively more sensitive to radiation. Radiotherapy will often be given as chemoradiation (CRT) using cisplatin chemotherapy delivered weekly during radiotherapy to enhance its effect. Meta-analysis of over 60 trials suggests an 8% absolute survival advantage for the subgroup receiving CRT. Cetuximab, a monoclonal antibody targeting the epidermal growth factor receptor (EGFR) given during the course of treatment has also been shown to improve results over radiotherapy alone. Median overall survival was prolonged to 49 months compared with 29 months for radiotherapy alone, corresponding to 3-year survivals of 55% and 45% respectively. Mutations in the *K-ras* oncogene, which is involved in the growth of head and neck cancers, are associated with a decrease in response to cetuximab compared with tumours with 'wild-type' *K-ras*.

These modifications increase toxicity such as mucositis which is more severe with accelerated treatment and chemoradiation than with radiotherapy alone. Close nutritional support during treatment is essential and patients may require nasogastric feeding or a percutaneous endoscopic gastrostomy (PEG) to maintain nutrition during severe mucositis.

Chemotherapy

The most active agents are 5FU and cisplatin, which in combination will give an objective response rate of 60%–80%. Chemotherapy alone will not achieve cure. Adjuvant or neoadjuvant chemotherapy has no proven survival benefit except in the case of nasopharyngeal cancer when neoadjuvant chemotherapy improves the outcome for poorly differentiated tumours and adjuvant chemotherapy may also have a role.

Head and neck cancer

PALLIATIVE TREATMENT

Surgery

Major resection is not justified for the palliation of symptoms in incurable cases where there is a possibility of major post-operative morbidity with loss of function, but debulking might be necessary to avert respiratory obstruction or dysphagia. Tracheostomy is indicated if there is upper airway obstruction as this is a particularly distressing symptom.

Radiotherapy

Radiotherapy can be used in cases of locally advanced disease even when the prospect of cure is low, as it is of value in reducing tumour mass and relieving obstructive symptoms or preventing fungation.

Chemotherapy

Using 5FU and cisplatin, median survival is typically around 6 months. The addition of cetuximab to standard chemotherapy increases median survival by 2–3 months.

TUMOUR-RELATED COMPLICATIONS

Locally advanced tumours are often necrotic and infected, which can lead to halitosis, an unpleasant taste and local discomfort with associated anorexia. A course of an appropriate antibiotic such as metronidazole and chlorhexidine mouthwash can help. Obstruction of the aerodigestive tracts is very distressing and warrants urgent assessment for a tracheostomy. Trismus, dysphonia, dysphagia and salivary fistulae are all seen.

TREATMENT-RELATED COMPLICATIONS

SURGERY

Difficulty in mastication, swallowing, dysarthria and dysphonia result from surgical resection of structures involved in these processes. Poor healing is a particular problem following extensive surgery when the vascularity of the tissue has been compromised, especially if the tissues have been previously irradiated. Osteomyelitis can complicate surgery when there has been a resection of bone (e.g. mandibulectomy), which has become secondarily infected. Treatment is with high doses of the appropriate antibiotic and further surgery might be required to remove the sequestrum.

RADIOTHERAPY

The oral mucosa is very sensitive to radiation, the reaction beginning during the second week of radiotherapy as erythema and soreness, progresses to severe discomfort manifested as a fibrinous mucositis leading to dysphagia and difficulty in mastication. This can be lessened by advising patients to use a very soft toothbrush to avoid gingival trauma, regular mouthwashes to prevent secondary infection, avoid smoking, alcohol, spicy foods and food or drink that is very hot or very cold. Soluble aspirin 600 mg gargled and swallowed four times a day can relieve oral and oropharyngeal discomfort. Oral candidiasis should be treated promptly with a topical or systemic antifungal. Local anaesthetic lozenges are also useful. A dry mouth is very common during radiotherapy and might recover only partially or not at all. It results from radiation damage to the parotids and minor salivary gland(s) at the site of radiation beam entry and/or exit from the oral cavity, predisposing the patient to dental caries, making swallowing difficult and exacerbating any radiation mucositis. Loss of or altered taste will also occur. Artificial saliva sprays are the treatment of choice but oral hygiene is also important. Careful monitoring or nutrition is necessary and many patients will require nutritional support with some form of enteral nutrition and in some cases a prophylactic gastrostomy (PEG) may be placed to facilitate nutrition during treatment.

Trismus is a late complication of both surgery and radiotherapy and is due to fibrosis in and around the temporomandibular joint leading to restriction of jaw opening and closing. Osteonecrosis is a late complication of radiotherapy, usually affecting the mandible as the maxilla has a better blood supply. It can be precipitated by a dental infection or extraction many years after radiotherapy.

PROGNOSIS

The prognosis varies with site of origin, TNM stage and histological grade. In general, there is a high expectation of cure for all T1 and T2 tumours with a 5-year survival of 60%–90%, falling to less than 30% for T4 tumours.

SCREENING/PREVENTION

Dentists play a vital part in screening as they have the opportunity to inspect the oral cavity in many people on a regular basis, but unfortunately the people most at risk of cancer tend to be those who are least likely to attend a dentist. Long-term survivors should be kept under close surveillance in the clinic as many will develop second primaries, usually in the head and neck region and also in the lung and gastrointestinal tract.

Many cases of oral cavity cancer could be prevented by better patient education, i.e. by reducing tobacco smoking, chewing tobacco and betel nut and alcohol consumption. A diet rich in fruit and vegetables might also be protective.

RARE TUMOURS OF THE ORAL CAVITY

OTHER RARE CARCINOMAS

The palate and oral mucosa contain a number of minor salivary glands, which can develop mucoepidermoid carcinomas, adenocarcinomas and adenoid cystic carcinomas, treated by surgery with radiotherapy after incomplete excision or for inoperable tumours.

KAPOSI'S SARCOMA

The oral cavity, particularly the palate, is a relatively common site for this disease. This diagnosis should prompt serological testing to exclude HIV infection (see Chapter 20).

SOFT TISSUE AND BONE SARCOMAS

These are rare but include leiomyosarcoma, rhabdomyosarcoma, fibrosarcoma, malignant fibrous histiocytoma, osteosarcoma and Ewing's sarcoma.

METASTASES

Tumour cells can spread via the blood to the gingiva or lower alveolus, from which they can erode the overlying mucosa and mimic a primary carcinoma of the oral cavity. The lung is a common source of such metastases.

CARCINOMA OF THE OROPHARYNX

Each year in the United Kingdom there are almost 3000 cases of oropharyngeal cancer, with incidence roughly three times higher in men than women, reflecting a doubling in incidence over the last decade. The oropharynx comprises the tonsils, posterior third of the tongue, soft palate and posterior wall of the oropharynx down to the level of the hyoid bone. As the oropharynx is a direct extension of the oral cavity, tumours arising in this region are similar in their epidemiology, presentation and pathology. Of those developing oropharyngeal cancer, over 70% have evidence of prior infection with HPV, especially type 16, rising to one-half of those developing tonsil cancer. Such individuals are less likely to smoke or drink alcohol in excess, and much more likely to have had multiple oral sex partners. The relative risk for developing oropharyngeal cancer is around 3 for each of smoking and alcohol, but around 30 for HPV-infected individuals. HPV-associated cancers have a much better prognosis.

The structures comprising the oropharynx have a bilateral pattern of lymphatic drainage to the neck, which should be considered when planning treatment. Radiotherapy is the preferred treatment for all but the earliest tumours as radical resection of the tumour is likely to produce functional compromise greater than that from radiotherapy alone. It should be noted that the oropharynx is a site where lymphoid tissue is concentrated and where lymphoma is also seen.

CARCINOMA OF THE LARYNX

Each year in the United Kingdom there are 2200 cases of laryngeal cancer, 1800 cases in men and 400 cases in women, accounting for 0.8% of all cancer cases and leading to a total of 800 deaths per annum. These tumours are much more common in men with a male-to-female predominance of 10:1, predisposed to by smoking and 95% are squamous carcinomas. All patients complaining of a hoarse voice that has persisted longer than a month should undergo laryngoscopy to directly visualize the vocal cords. Glottic tumours arise on the vocal cords and present at an early stage with dysphonia. Tumours can arise above the cords (supraglottic) or below the cords (subglottic). These tumours present later in their natural history as they grow insidiously and have to reach a large size before the patient presents with dysphagia, stridor or symptoms from direct invasion of the glottis. A tumour in the supraglottic larynx can lead to referred pain in the ipsilateral ear.

The vocal cords have a poor lymphatic drainage and therefore lymph node metastases are less common at this site compared with a 70% incidence from supraglottic tumours, as the supraglottis has a rich lymphatic drainage. The TNM staging system is used for laryngeal tumours, the T stage is outlined as follows (N-staging is the generic head and neck version cited previously):

- Tis: Carcinoma *in situ*
- T0: No evidence of primary tumour
- TX: Primary tumour cannot be assessed

Supraglottis

- T1: Tumour limited to one subsite of supraglottis with normal vocal cord mobility
- T2: Tumour invades mucosa of more than one adjacent subsite of supraglottis or glottis or region outside the supraglottis (e.g. mucosa of base of tongue, vallecula, medial wall of pyriform sinus) without fixation of the larynx
- T3: Tumour limited to larynx with vocal cord fixation and/or invades any of the following: postcricoid area, pre-epiglottic tissues
- T4: Tumour invades through the thyroid cartilage and/or extends into soft tissues of the neck, thyroid and/or oesophagus

Glottis

- T1: Tumour limited to vocal cord(s) (might involve anterior or posterior commissure) with normal mobility
- T1a: Tumour limited to one vocal cord
- T1b: Tumour involves both vocal cords
- T2: Tumour extends to supraglottis and/or subglottis, and/or with impaired vocal cord mobility
- T3: Tumour limited to the larynx with vocal cord fixation
- T4: Tumour invades through the thyroid cartilage and/or to other tissues beyond the larynx (e.g. trachea, soft tissues of neck, including thyroid, pharynx)

Subglottis

- T1: Tumour limited to the subglottis
- T2: Tumour extends to vocal cord(s) with normal or impaired mobility
- T3: Tumour limited to larynx with vocal cord fixation
- T4: Tumour invades through cricoid or thyroid cartilage and/or extends to other tissues beyond the larynx (e.g. trachea, soft tissues of neck, including thyroid, oesophagus)

Laryngeal tumours can be treated by surgery or radiotherapy. A partial or total laryngectomy will have the disadvantage of changing the quality of the voice, and therefore radiotherapy is preferred for T1, T2 and small bulk T3 tumours. The prognosis from glottic tumours is excellent, reflecting their early presentation and low rate of lymphatic spread.

CARCINOMA OF THE HYPOPHARYNX

The hypopharynx extends from the level of the tip of the epiglottis to the lower border of the cricoid and comprises the pyriform fossae, posterior pharyngeal wall and postcricoid region. The tumours are squamous carcinomas that tend to present late with dysphagia. There is also an association with iron deficiency (Plummer–Vinson syndrome). Pharyngolaryngectomy has historically been the treatment of choice but with inevitably a significant degree of functional compromise. Combined modality treatment with chemotherapy and radiotherapy is now an established alternative, particularly for locally advanced disease.

CARCINOMA OF THE NASOPHARYNX

Each year in the United Kingdom there are 220 cases of nasopharyngeal cancer, 150 cases in men and 70 cases in women, leading to a total of 100 deaths per annum. This disease has a marked geographical variation, being more common in the Far East, particularly Southern China where it is endemic. In areas of high incidence, the disease is related to infection with the Epstein–Barr virus (EBV). In endemic areas, it has a peak incidence at a younger age (15–25 years vs. 40–60 years in developed countries) and a predominance of anaplastic tumours (squamous in developed countries). There is a lesser association with excess alcohol and tobacco consumption compared with other head and neck sites. Routes of spread include:

- *Nose*: Produces epistaxis, nasal discharge and blockage
- *Orbit*: Produces diplopia
- *Eustachian tube*: Blockage produces deafness
- *Cavernous sinus*: Causes palsies of cranial nerves 3, 4, 5 and 6
- *Cribriform plate*: Produces loss of smell
- *Pterygoid muscles and parapharyngeal space*: Produces inability to open jaw fully (trismus)

The TNM staging employed is as follows (generic N-staging):

- Tis: Carcinoma in situ
- T0: No evidence of primary tumour
- TX: Primary tumour cannot be assessed
- T1: Tumour confined to the nasopharynx
- T2: Tumour extends to soft tissues of oropharynx and/or nasal fossa
  - T2a: Without parapharyngeal extension
  - T2b: With parapharyngeal extension
- T3: Tumour invades bony structures and/or paranasal sinuses
- T4: Tumour with intracranial extension and/or involvement of cranial nerves, infratemporal fossa, hypopharynx or orbit

CT and MRI are the investigations of choice for delineating the locoregional extent of the tumour (Figure 13.4), CT being superior with respect to delineation of the skeletal anatomy, which is frequently involved by the tumour. Seventy percent will have overt or occult lymph node metastases with a tendency to bilateral involvement. The treatment of choice is chemoradiotherapy, typically using

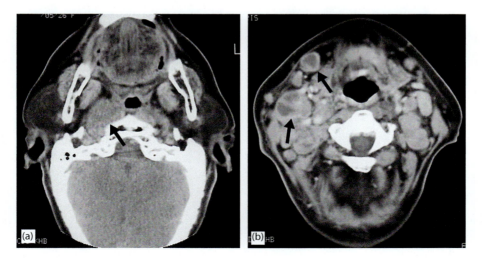

Figure 13.4 Nasopharyngeal carcinoma. (a) Transverse CT image of the base of skull. There is soft tissue within the nasopharynx, particularly on the right side. (b) CT image of the neck, of the same patient, showing multiple enlarged, necrotic lymph nodes consistent with nodal metastases.

cisplatin or cisplatin with 5FU. Additional chemotherapy prior to or after radiotherapy also improves outcome. The prognosis for squamous carcinoma is poor with a 5-year survival of less than 20% versus up to 50% for other histological types.

CARCINOMA OF THE PARANASAL SINUSES

These are rare tumours; sites of origin include the frontal, ethmoid, maxillary and sphenoid sinuses. The maxillary sinus is the most frequently affected. They are usually squamous carcinomas, frequently presenting late as the symptoms are mistaken for those of chronic sinusitis. By the time of diagnosis, they often spread beyond the bony walls of the sinus and have led to other symptoms from local invasion of adjacent structures, such as diplopia from orbital involvement (Figure 13.5), or epistaxis from nasal cavity involvement. They can also invade the cranial cavity. Radical surgery is hazardous owing to adjacent vital organs and therefore radiotherapy is the treatment of choice. Approximately 40% will survive 5 years after treatment. It should be noted that the sinuses are also a recognized site of extranodal lymphoma and plasmacytoma.

SALIVARY GLAND TUMOURS

The parotid gland forms the vast bulk of salivary gland tissue and therefore is the most common site for tumours (Figure 13.6), while tumours of the sublingual, submandibular and smaller glands distributed throughout the oral cavity are less common. There are several variants as described in the following.

PLEOMORPHIC ADENOMA

This is the most common salivary gland tumour constituting 75%, with a peak incidence at 30–50 years. It usually arises in the superficial lobe of the gland, is a benign tumour and therefore slow growing. Superficial parotidectomy is the initial treatment

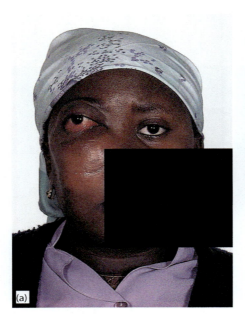
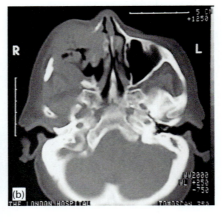

Figure 13.5 Carcinoma of the maxillary antrum. (a) Frontal view of face. Note the swelling of the right cheek owing to anterior spread from the antrum. Superior spread into the orbit has led to proptosis of the right eye. (b) CT image of the base of skull of the same patient showing destruction of the facial bones on the right side.

Salivary gland tumours

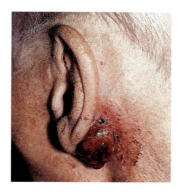

Figure 13.6 Adenoid cystic carcinoma of the parotid. Tumour fungation through the skin posterior to the left ear.

and post-operative radiotherapy is indicated if there is capsular rupture at the time of surgery or incomplete microscopic clearance. There is a small risk of transformation into a carcinoma.

ADENOLYMPHOMA

This is a benign, slow-growing tumour most commonly arising in the lower pole of the superficial lobe of the parotid. It is bilateral in 5%. The treatment of choice is surgery.

CARCINOMA

Each year in the United Kingdom there are 500–600 new cases per annum. This usually arises *de novo* but rarely can develop in a pleomorphic adenoma. Local infiltration may cause a facial nerve palsy, distinct from a benign tumour (Figure 13.7). Variants of carcinoma include:

- *Adenoid cystic carcinoma*: Slow-growing carcinoma and has a tendency for invasion along nerves and into the cranial cavity
- Acinic cell carcinoma arising from serous cells
- Mucoepidermoid carcinoma arising from mucin cells
- Adenocarcinoma
- *Squamous carcinoma*: Must be distinguished from a metastasis
- Undifferentiated carcinoma

The treatment of choice is resection of the lobe of origin followed by radiotherapy to the parotid.

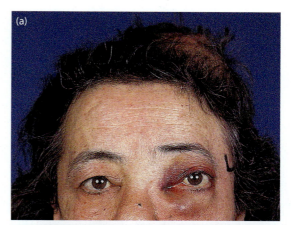

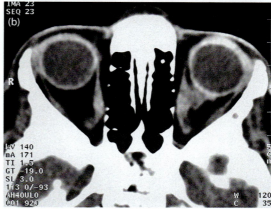

Figure 13.7 Orbital metastasis. This is most commonly seen in cancers of the breast, prostate and lung. (a) The left eye demonstrates non-axial proptosis. The patient has severe diplopia. (b) CT image through the orbits showing abnormal tissue in the lateral aspect of the left eye, pushing it forward.

Five-year survival varies between 20% and 80% depending on tumour type and histological grade.

LYMPHOMA

The parotid is a relatively common site of extranodal non-Hodgkin lymphoma. Typically, this will be a marginal zone (MALTOMA) or diffuse large B cell lymphoma. Localized disease (stage I or IIa) can be treated by low dose (24 Gy) radiotherapy alone if indolent and short-course chemotherapy followed by radiotherapy for more aggressive lymphomas. Full course chemotherapy will be needed if there is more widespread lymphoma.

Head and neck cancer

ORBITAL TUMOURS

These are all very rare, presenting because of a mass effect leading to proptosis and diplopia. Benign tumours include haemangioma, leiomyoma, rhabdomyoma, lipoma, fibroma, meningioma, neurofibroma, schwannoma, pseudotumour and 'malignant' granuloma, e.g. Wegener's granulomatosis. Malignant tumours include gliomas, rhabdomyosarcoma, leiomyosarcoma, malignant fibrous histiocytoma, fibrosarcoma, osteosarcoma, chondrosarcoma, Ewing's sarcoma, lymphoma, Langerhans' cell histiocytosis, melanoma, nephroblastoma, plasmacytoma and metastases, particularly from breast and lung cancers (Figure 13.7).

Tumours within the eye itself are also very rare, presenting with visual loss and strabismus. Benign tumours include naevi, leiomyoma, haemangioma and hamartoma. Malignant tumours include retinoblastoma, medulloepithelioma, melanoma and metastases.

With both sites, optimum management will aim to preserve vision in the affected eye as much as possible, and usually comprises radiotherapy alone, surgery alone or combined modality treatment.

FURTHER READING

Ahmed OA, Kelly C. Head and neck cancer: United Kingdom National Multidisciplinary Guidelines. *J Laryngol Otol*. 2016; 130(S2):S133–S141.

Colevas A, Yom SS, Pfister DG et al. NCCN guidelines insights: Head and neck cancers, version 1.2018. *J Natl Compr Canc Netw*. 2018; 16(5): 479–490.

SELF-ASSESSMENT QUESTIONS

1. Which three of the following statements are true for head and neck cancers?
   a. Account for 10,000 deaths per annum in the United Kingdom
   b. Overall, they are more frequent in men
   c. Laryngeal cancer is more frequent in women
   d. Associated with chronic gum disease
   e. Associated with human papilloma virus infection
   f. Associated with gonorrhoea
   g. High incidence in Asia

2. Which one of the following is not true about head and neck cancer?
   a. May be preceded by leucoplakia
   b. Lymph node involvement increases with size of primary tumours
   c. Adenocarcinoma is rare
   d. Three-quarters are squamous carcinomas
   e. The pattern of lymph node spread is predictable

3. Which three of the following statements are common presentations for head and neck cancers?
   a. Oral candidiasis
   b. Headache
   c. Enlarged cervical lymph node(s)
   d. No symptoms
   e. Diplopia
   f. Chronic mucosal ulcer
   g. Loss of taste

4. Which one of the following best describes the role of radiotherapy in head and neck cancer?
   a. Protons are the treatment of choice
   b. Only suitable for those where surgery is contraindicated
   c. Cannot be used to treat lymph gland areas
   d. Leads to permanent voice loss
   e. Has a high cure probability for small tumours

5. Which one of the following best describes the role of chemotherapy in head and neck cancer?
   a. Cisplatin is the mainstay of treatment
   b. Chemotherapy does not add to the toxicity of radiotherapy
   c. Adjuvant chemotherapy is given to most patients
   d. Cannot be given with cetuximab
   e. *K-ras* oncogene expression predicts for response to chemotherapy

6. Which three of the following are important prognostic factors for head and neck cancer?
   a. Lymph node involvement

b. Hepatitis seropositivity
c. Depth of invasion
d. Alcohol consumption
e. Size of tumour
f. Tobacco consumption
g. Trismus

7. Which one of the following best describes the role of radiotherapy in head and neck cancer?
   a. Best as single modality treatment
   b. The main toxicity is mucositis
   c. Has low probability of local control of tumour
   d. Unsuitable for treating involved lymph nodes
   e. Can only be used for tumours of oral cavity

8. Which three of the following are essential members of the head and neck cancer MDT?
   a. Specialist head and neck surgeon
   b. Gastroenterologist
   c. Dietician
   d. Chest physician
   e. Haemato-oncologist
   f. Dentist
   g. Clinical oncologist

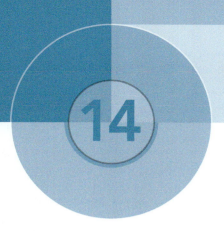

Endocrine tumours

THYROID CANCER

EPIDEMIOLOGY

Each year in the United Kingdom there are 1650 cases of thyroid cancer, 450 cases in men and 1200 cases in women, accounting for 2.9% of all cancer cases and leading to a total of 350 deaths per annum. Well-differentiated thyroid cancer has a high survival rate but accounts for 75% of thyroid cancer deaths. The overall incidence increases with age, papillary and medullary types typically arising in young adults, while follicular carcinomas and anaplastic cancers are usually seen in later adult life. There is a female predominance of 4:1 and a particularly high incidence in Iceland, Israel and Hawaii.

AETIOLOGY

Ionizing radiation is a recognized aetiological agent. Radiation-induced cancers have a latency of 5–40 years, with a peak at 15 years after exposure. Radiation induces papillary cancer, which has been described following childhood irradiation for thymic hyperplasia, ringworm and cervical lymphadenitis, and in atomic bomb survivors. A higher incidence of follicular cancer has been noted in endemic goitre areas where there is a dietary deficiency of iodine, while a higher incidence of papillary cancer is seen in areas where there is an excess of iodine in the diet. Multiple endocrine neoplasia (MEN – see end of this chapter) is a dominantly inherited condition, type 1 being occasionally associated with differentiated thyroid cancer while type 2 is associated with medullary cancer, which is more often multifocal and presents at a younger age than its sporadic counterpart.

Other rare associations include:

- Pendred syndrome (goitre and nerve deafness at birth)
- Gardener syndrome (polyposis of the bowel, osteomas and sebaceous cysts)
- Cowden disease (multiple hamartomas)

PATHOLOGY

The tumour usually appears as a firm, well-circumscribed lump, often with a pseudocapsule of compressed thyroid tissue at its periphery. The cut surface will have a characteristic glistening appearance of colloid if there is a significant follicular element. There can be haemorrhage and necrosis in anaplastic tumours, and it is sometimes multifocal. Follicular, papillary and medullary cancers tend to grow very slowly over many years, while anaplastic cancers are usually fast growing and locally invasive. Tumours may arise in ectopic thyroid tissue in the tongue, a thyroglossal cyst, sublingual, infrahyoid, pretracheal, mediastinal and pericardial regions.

Microscopically, thyroid cancer is characterized by invasion of the capsule and thyroid vasculature. There are four main types:

- Follicular carcinoma (50%)
- Papillary carcinoma (20%)
- Anaplastic carcinoma (25%)
- Medullary carcinoma (4%)

The presence of papillary structures is diagnostic of papillary carcinoma, although these tumours frequently contain a follicular component also. Follicular carcinoma must be distinguished from an adenoma. It is usually well differentiated with colloid held within follicles and there are no papillary elements. Anaplastic carcinoma is very poorly differentiated, usually with no identifiable follicular elements. Medullary carcinoma arises from the parafollicular ('C') cells, with the inherited form often multifocal in origin. Amyloid might be identified within the stroma and immunocytochemistry will be positive for the hormone calcitonin. *RET* gene testing can show a characteristic mutation in familial cases. Squamous carcinoma, clear cell carcinoma and Hurthle cell carcinoma are also recognized.

NATURAL HISTORY

The tumour initially spreads within the lobe of origin, contained by the capsule, but can then invade the contralateral lobe via the isthmus. Capsular invasion will lead to infiltration of surrounding structures such as the trachea, larynx, recurrent laryngeal nerves and skin. Papillary and medullary carcinomas have a propensity to metastasize to lymph nodes, the affected groups comprising the deep cervical, supraclavicular and paratracheal chains. All may give rise to distant metastases, the lung being the most common site, followed by the skeleton, liver, skin, brain and kidney. Lung metastases are often very numerous and small, sometimes giving a 'snowstorm' appearance. Follicular and anaplastic variants are the types most often associated with distant metastases.

SYMPTOMS

The most common presentation is with a painless, solitary lump in the neck. Some patients complain of a hoarse voice, which raises the suspicion of extracapsular extension leading to pressure on one or both of the recurrent laryngeal nerves innervating the vocal cords. Extrinsic compression of the pharynx or upper oesophagus will cause dysphagia, and could suggest retrosternal extension if the neck mass is small. Patients with medullary carcinoma sometimes complain of diarrhoea, which is thought to be due to secretion of prostaglandins by the tumour.

SIGNS

The patient will be euthyroid. The thyroid lump is usually confined to one side of the neck, moving with swallowing and protrusion of the tongue, non-tender, firm/hard in consistency and well circumscribed. There may be stridor as a result of recurrent laryngeal nerve palsy or extrinsic tracheal compression. Vocal cord palsy can be confirmed by flexible nasendoscopy (FNE). Extracapsular invasion can lead to loss of the normal laryngeal mobility. Lymphadenopathy can be palpable in the deep cervical and supraclavicular regions, while anaplastic tumours sometimes invade the overlying skin to produce induration, erythema and nodularity.

DIFFERENTIAL DIAGNOSIS

This includes:

- Benign tumours of thyroid, e.g. adenoma
- Other malignant tumours of thyroid, e.g. lymphoma and fibrosarcoma
- Metastases, e.g. carcinoma of the lung, hypernephroma and melanoma

INVESTIGATIONS

CHEST X-RAY

This should be performed in all patients to exclude obvious pulmonary metastases. These are usually small and numerous giving a 'snowstorm' appearance (Figure 14.1).

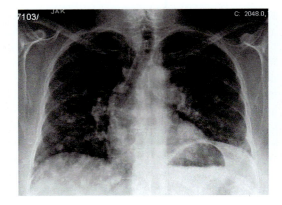

Figure 14.1 Multiple small lung metastases typical of thyroid cancer.

Thyroid cancer

THYROID ULTRASOUND AND FINE-NEEDLE ASPIRATION (FNA)

Carcinoma will give rise to a solid nodule rather than a cystic one and in either case FNA should be performed to obtain a cytological diagnosis.

FNA OF ENLARGED LYMPH NODES

This is essential to distinguish reactive lymph node enlargement from metastatic infiltration.

OPEN THYROID BIOPSY

This is required only in inoperable tumours when an FNA has proven negative or given an equivocal histological diagnosis.

ISOTOPE THYROID SCAN

In the case of thyroid cancer, administration of a tracer dose of technetium-99 or iodine-131 will give rise to a cold spot relative to the surrounding functioning thyroid tissue, giving useful information to the surgeon regarding its location and extent. Functioning adenomas will produce a hot spot.

CT SCAN OF THE NECK AND CHEST

This can be of value in assisting the surgeon to make a decision regarding operability of a large mass, particularly when retrosternal extension is suspected (Figure 14.2), or for radiotherapy planning at a later date. CT is also the most sensitive means of detecting small pulmonary metastases, which might be

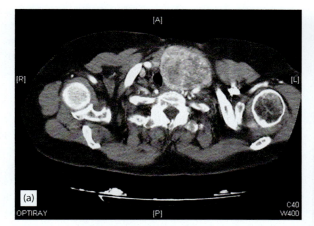

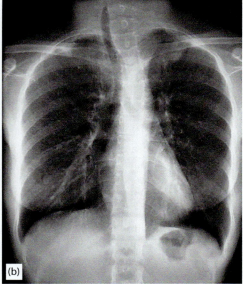

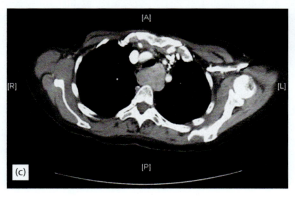

Figure 14.2 Medullary carcinoma of the thyroid. (a) CT scan of the neck showing a massive tumour arising from the left lobe of the thyroid, pushing the trachea to the right side of the neck. (b) Chest radiograph from the same patient. Note the soft-tissue mass in the neck and tracheal deviation. (c) CT scan of the thorax showing retrosternal extension of tumour that had not been appreciated from the chest radiograph.

below the spatial resolution of a radioiodine whole body scan.

SERUM MARKERS

Thyroglobulin can be used as a marker of differentiated thyroid cancer after ablation of normal thyroid tissue. Calcitonin will be raised in medullary carcinoma. These patients should also be screened for other MEN type 2 tumours, i.e. parathyroid adenomas (parathyroid hormone level) and phaeochromocytoma (blood catecholamine levels, urinary vanillylmandelic acid and bilateral adrenal MRI).

STAGING

- TX: Primary tumour cannot be assessed
- T0: No evidence of tumour
- T1: Tumour ≤2 cm limited to thyroid
- T2: Tumour >2 cm but not >4 cm in greatest dimension, limited to thyroid
- T3: Tumour >4 cm in greatest dimension, limited to thyroid or extrathyroid extension limited to the strap muscles
- T4: Tumour with gross extrathyroid extension into major neck structures
- NX: Lymph nodes cannot be assessed
- N0: No nodes involved
- N1: Regional nodes involved

TREATMENT

Small (<1 cm) well-differentiated tumours may be managed with local excision; other papillary or follicular cancers will require some form of thyroid ablation followed by hormone replacement therapy to prevent hypothyroidism and maintain thyroid stimulating hormone (TSH) at very low ('suppressed') levels to minimize the likelihood of recurrence of a TSH-dependent tumour.

RADICAL TREATMENT

SURGERY

This can be curative when used alone, the type of surgery being tailored to the stage of tumour. The smaller good prognosis cases may be managed by lobectomy whereas larger tumours or those with adverse features will require a total thyroidectomy with the aim of removing all thyroid tissue and any extracapsular extension. Care is taken to preserve the parathyroid glands and recurrent laryngeal nerves if possible. A cervical lymph node dissection should be undertaken when there is overt lymph node invasion.

RADIOIODINE (I-131)

Radioiodine is concentrated in the thyroid gland and can therefore be used for the diagnosis of locoregional and metastatic disease, for the ablation of a thyroid remnant and/or tumour persisting after surgery, and as a means of detecting early relapse. It is concentrated not only by normal thyroid tissue, but also by 70%–80% of well-differentiated thyroid carcinomas and their metastases (Figure 14.3). Radioiodine is given as an oral preparation using strict radiation protection procedures, with the large doses used for ablation of thyroid and tumour being given in an inpatient setting. Patient selection is important, as those with claustrophobia might not be suited to long periods left alone in a protected room. Urinary incontinence or dementia can pose a risk of contamination to staff, visitors or other patients in the ward. It emits β-particles (electrons) with a tissue range of only 2 mm, and it is these that ablate the thyroid/tumour. It also emits low-energy γ-photons, which are a radiation hazard to staff and visitors but allow external monitoring of the distribution, concentration and excretion of the isotope.

Radioiodine (1.1 GBq for better prognosis and 3.7 GBq for higher risk) is given after thyroid surgery to destroy any remaining normal thyroid tissue after total or near total thyroidectomy. There are several reasons to ablate the thyroid remnant:

- It can obscure occult disease in the neck or upper thorax on a whole body radioiodine scan.
- It may prevent a physiological rise in TSH on hormone therapy withdrawal and can therefore make follow-up thyroglobulin assays and whole body radioiodine scans less sensitive.
- It may be a source of new primary cancer or local recurrence.

Thyroid cancer

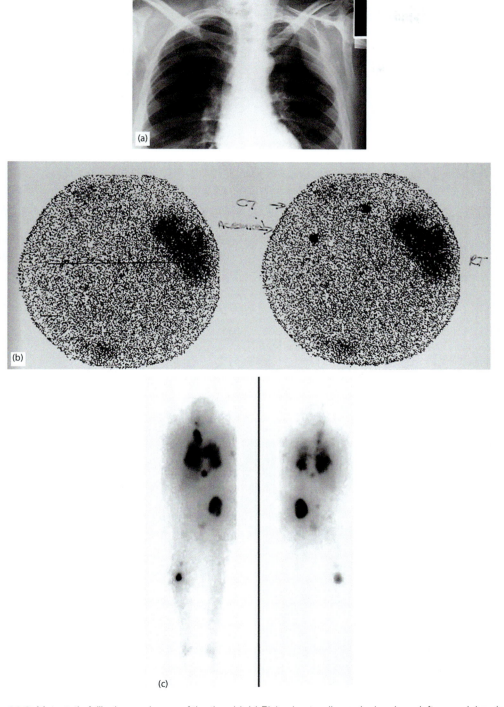

Figure 14.3 Metastatic follicular carcinoma of the thyroid. (a) Plain chest radiograph showing a left upper lobe pleural metastasis. (b) Iodine-131 uptake scan showing increased activity (dark) in the corresponding region. (c) Whole body iodine-131 uptake scan demonstrating widespread metastatic disease.

If whole body scans at any time demonstrate evidence of distant metastases, much higher therapeutic doses (e.g. 5.5 GBq activity) are given. Most patients will require one to three such treatments. The success of the treatment is determined by the avidity of the metastases for iodine.

EXTERNAL BEAM RADIOTHERAPY

External beam irradiation to the neck is used when there is residual papillary or follicular carcinoma in the neck that is not concentrating iodine-131, and is necessary in all cases of anaplastic carcinoma and incompletely excised medullary carcinomas.

PALLIATIVE TREATMENT

SURGERY

Tracheostomy may be necessary, particularly with anaplastic tumours causing tracheal compression (Figure 14.4) and when there are bilateral recurrent laryngeal nerve palsies leading to total vocal cord paralysis and upper respiratory airway obstruction.

RADIOTHERAPY

Death from asphyxiation owing to a rapidly growing anaplastic carcinoma is particularly unpleasant and distressing for all concerned and under such circumstances, even if the patient has distant metastases, radiotherapy to the neck is justified.

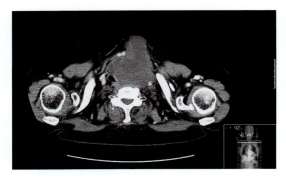

Figure 14.4 Anaplastic cancer of the thyroid. CT image of the lower neck showing a large mass on the left side pushing the trachea to the right.

CHEMOTHERAPY

This has no role in the curative treatment of thyroid cancer. Patients with anaplastic carcinoma and symptoms refractory to all other treatments can be considered for palliative chemotherapy. Responses are infrequent and short-lived. The tyrosine kinase inhibitors, sorafenib and sunitinib may be useful in patients with radioactive iodine refractory differentiated thyroid cancer.

HORMONE THERAPY

Elderly patients unfit for surgery with small, well-differentiated tumours can be treated by TSH suppression. Reducing the growth stimulation in this way using thyroxine in a dose sufficient to suppress TSH, may enable the patient to survive their natural life expectancy with an indolent tumour.

TUMOUR-RELATED COMPLICATIONS

Respiratory obstruction from extrinsic compression of the trachea or bilateral damage to the recurrent laryngeal nerves is seen with anaplastic carcinomas, while dysphagia can result from extrinsic compression of the cervical oesophagus and/or retrosternal extension. Superior vena cava obstruction is a rare complication associated with a large retrosternal tumour.

TREATMENT-RELATED COMPLICATIONS

SURGERY

Specific complications include risk of secondary haemorrhage during the postoperative period, laryngeal oedema, hypoparathyroidism causing hypocalcaemia and vocal cord palsy from damage to the recurrent laryngeal nerves leading to dysphonia and respiratory obstruction.

RADIOTHERAPY

External beam irradiation to the neck will result in an acute radiation laryngitis characterized by sore throat, dysphagia and dysphonia. Late complications include chronic laryngeal oedema, intense subcutaneous fibrosis leading to restricted neck movements and radiation chondritis of the tracheal cartilage rings.

RADIOIODINE

Severe adverse reactions to radioiodine are rare. Possible complications include nausea, acute parotitis, sore throat from radiation laryngitis and acute pneumonitis if there are miliary lung metastases. Rarely there may be myelosuppression, leukaemogenesis and induction of cancer elsewhere (there is some uptake in the salivary glands, stomach, colon and bladder). Acute thyroiditis is also recognized – this may cause temporary upper airway obstruction in severe cases. It settles quickly with corticosteroids. Radiation protection protocols should prevent radiation exposure to staff and relatives of those receiving high doses of radioiodine.

HORMONE REPLACEMENT THERAPY

Inappropriate dosage or poor patient compliance can lead to either hypothyroidism or hyperthyroidism. Hypothyroidism leads to a physiological rise in TSH, which may be detrimental if there is any occult residual disease.

PROGNOSIS

Differentiated thyroid cancer has a very good prognosis. Papillary carcinoma has the best prognosis of all with a long-term (40-year) survival of more than 90%, followed by follicular carcinoma (80%–90%) and medullary carcinoma (60%–70%). Of those with differentiated thyroid cancer, one-third will relapse after initial therapy. Two-thirds of such relapses will occur within the first decade of follow-up, and of those with distant metastases half will be cured by salvage therapy.

In contrast, most patients with anaplastic carcinoma will die within 6 months.

Children have an extremely good prognosis; young adults fare better than the elderly and women fare better than men, again reflecting the incidence of differentiated thyroid cancer in these groups. For differentiated thyroid cancer, age <15 or >45 years, male gender, tumour >4 cm, bilobar disease, extracapsular invasion, lymphatic invasion, non-iodine concentrating tumour and distant metastases at diagnosis are poor prognostic factors.

SCREENING/PREVENTION

Patients treated for differentiated thyroid cancer require life-long follow-up. This will involve regular thyroglobulin measurements. In the early post-treatment period whole body iodine uptake scans are performed. Thyroid hormone replacement therapy is usually withdrawn 2–6 weeks before such investigations. This precipitates a physiological rise in TSH, and therefore acts as a provocation test to facilitate detection of occult disease. In recent years, recombinant thyrotropin-α (Thyrogen®) given by intramuscular injection has been used for those individuals who do not have an adequate TSH response to hormone withdrawal, and for those where the transient myxoedema after hormone withdrawal is intolerable. A thyroglobulin level of >2 ng/mL 72 hours after TSH provocation usually warrants further investigation (neck ultrasound or MRI, CT scan of the thorax, whole body radioiodine scan) to exclude local relapse and distant metastatic disease.

Patients developing medullary carcinoma of the thyroid have a significant risk of having MEN type 2, particularly if aged 20–40 years with a multifocal carcinoma. A calcium provocation level of calcitonin (measured before, 2 and 5 minutes after intravenous calcium) might unmask an otherwise borderline level and is useful for screening members of MEN type 2 families who might have occult medullary carcinoma. Alternatively, risk-reducing thyroidectomy at an early age can be appropriate for those with familial medullary carcinoma even if calcitonin levels are normal.

RARE TUMOURS

LYMPHOMA

This constitutes less than 2% of extranodal lymphomas, with a median age at presentation of 65 years and a female predominance. It is invariably a non-Hodgkin lymphoma, usually marginal zone

(MALTOMA) or diffuse large B cell, and may be preceded by Hashimoto thyroiditis. It is staged and treated using the same principles as for lymphoma elsewhere and has a 5-year survival of about 40%.

TUMOURS OF THE PARATHYROID GLAND

These are rare and are sometimes part of MEN type 1 or 2. Adenomas are usually impalpable and solitary, and present with hyperparathyroidism (high serum calcium, low serum phosphate, hyperchloraemic metabolic acidosis, evidence of subperiosteal bone resorption on plain radiographs, e.g. of phalanges, nephrolithiasis). The glands can be imaged by radioisotope imaging using a technetium-99 scan (images the thyroid) followed by a thallium-201 scan (images both the thyroid and the parathyroids), subtraction of the two images giving an image of the parathyroids alone. Ultrasound or MRI of the neck is alternative, and venous sampling for parathyroid hormone is useful for tumours that cannot be visualized. Parathyroidectomy is the sole treatment. Carcinoma is extremely rare.

TUMOURS OF THE ADRENAL GLANDS

Tumours of the adrenal gland are rare, accounting for approximately 100 deaths per annum in the United Kingdom (Figure 14.5).

PHAEOCHROMOCYTOMA

This is a very rare tumour arising from the autonomic cells of the adrenal medulla, with a peak incidence at 35–55 years but can occur from infancy to old age. Recognized associations include:

- Multiple endocrine neoplasia type 2 (*RET* gene mutation)
- Neurofibromatosis I
- Von Hippel–Lindau syndrome
- Sturge–Weber syndrome
- Tuberose sclerosis

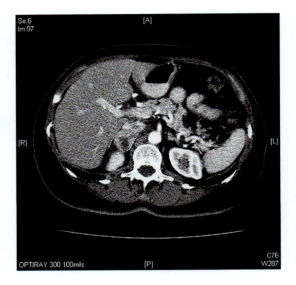

Figure 14.5 Phaeochromocytoma. CT image of the abdomen showing a heterogeneous mass arising above the upper pole of the right kidney.

Ninety-nine percent are found in the abdomen or pelvis, 90% of these in the adrenal medulla (Figure 14.5), the most common extra-adrenal site being adjacent to the aortic bifurcation. Other sites include the sympathetic chain, bladder, thorax (usually paravertebral) and carotid arch. The tumours can be very small or weigh several kilograms, are well circumscribed and slow growing, with 10% bilateral (70% of those arising in familial cases), 90% benign and 10% malignant (more likely for extra-adrenal tumours). They are rich in lipid and therefore yellow in cut section. Phaeochromocytomas arise from chromaffin cells of neural crest origin. The cells therefore stain with chrome salts and enzymes such as dopa decarboxylase and contain neurosecretory granules. As most tumours are benign, local invasion is unusual, although malignant tumours can infiltrate the underlying kidney and retroperitoneum. Lymphatic spread is unusual but malignant tumours can spread to lung, bone and liver. The classic presentation is with paroxysms of headache, postural dizziness, feelings of apprehension and fear, pallor, sweating, tremor, chest pain and palpitations. Attacks last minutes to hours and are followed by a feeling of exhaustion and muscle pain, and can be precipitated by emotion, exertion, posture, bending, pressure on tumour, foods or handling of tumour at operation. Thyrotoxicosis should be excluded as it might present in a similar manner. Half the patients have sustained hypertension, which may be difficult to control with conventional antihypertensive agents, while 70% have postural hypotension. Investigations include:

- Urinary vanillylmandelic acid (VMA)
- Meta-iodobenzyl guanidine (mIBG) imaging
- MRI scan of adrenals
- Selective venous sampling
- Selective angiography

VMA and catecholamines are measured using a 24-hour urine collection, and are useful screening tests during investigation of malignant hypertension. Urinary VMA is elevated in phaeochromocytoma, while high levels of adrenaline suggest an adrenal origin, high levels of noradrenaline suggest an extra-adrenal tumour and high levels of dopamine suggest a malignant phaeochromocytoma. CT is the best investigation for delineating site and size of primary and excluding gross tumour in the contralateral adrenal, but is limited by its resolution of 0.5–1 cm, which will miss some tumours.

Selective venous sampling is used to localize radiologically occult tumours, identifying their venous drainage using multiple venous samples that are tested for catecholamines. Selective arteriography is also of value when surgery is planned, as phaeochromocytomas have a rich vascular supply, but it may precipitate a hypertensive crisis.

Imaging with mIBG is useful for malignant tumours as part of staging or in the context of MEN type 2 when a multiplicity of tumours is possible. The compound is taken up by adrenergic tissue. It is of particular benefit in staging patients with malignant tumours, the iodine moiety being radioactive iodine-131 and therefore detectable by a gamma camera to give a whole body image. Uptake of mIBG opens up an additional therapeutic option for malignant tumours.

Laparoscopic unilateral adrenalectomy is the treatment of choice for those with a contralateral normal adrenal as it reduces the small but potentially fatal risk of acute adrenal insufficiency later in life associated with bilateral adrenalectomy. Adrenal cortex-sparing bilateral adrenalectomy is preferable to sacrificing both adrenals in their entirety for those with proven bilateral disease. Whatever surgery is planned, expert anaesthetic advice and preoperative alpha and beta blockades (e.g. phenoxybenzamine with propranolol or labetalol alone) are necessary as the tumour will be handled leading to a release of catecholamines. At laparotomy, it is important to inspect the contralateral adrenal for a second primary. In inoperable cases, phenoxybenzamine is a useful medical therapy, being an α-adrenergic receptor blocker. Alphamethyltyrosine inhibits hydroxylation of tyrosine to dopa, an intermediate compound in the synthesis of catecholamines and is a more toxic alternative. External beam radiotherapy and chemotherapy have no role in the curative treatment of these tumours, although the former is of value in palliating local symptoms from metastases. mIBG scan be used to treat metastatic disease if the tumour concentrates enough of it. Only one-third of patients will concentrate mIBG to an adequate degree within their tumours, and of these only one-third will show evidence of an objective response. With regards to prognosis, the vast majority will be cured by surgery alone. Even patients with malignant tumours can survive for many years, death often resulting from cardiovascular complications (e.g. myocardial infarction and cerebrovascular accident) rather than from metastatic disease. Annual biochemical screening, with MRI of the adrenals if it is abnormal, is recommended in asymptomatic MEN type 2 individuals or those who have previously undergone unilateral adrenalectomy.

ADRENAL CORTEX TUMOURS

Benign tumours are common at autopsy in the general population, but may be part of MEN type 1 disease. Most are non-functioning, the majority of functioning tumours arising in females. Of the functioning tumours, those arising in prepubertal patients are virilizing, while those in post-pubertal patients tend to produce Cushing syndrome, although Conn syndrome (primary hyperaldosteronism) may also result. A CT scan delineates the primary tumour if greater than 1 cm in diameter, although angiography is more sensitive, and treatment is by adrenalectomy.

Malignant tumours are rare, with a slight female predominance, arising at a younger age than most other carcinomas (median 35–55 years). Half are functioning and as with benign tumours are more frequent in females. Presentation is with vague abdominal symptoms, and up to one-third have signs of endocrine dysfunction, usually a combination of Cushing syndrome and virilism. Half have metastatic disease at presentation, haematogenous spread occurring to lung and liver. Investigation and treatment is as for benign tumours. In advanced disease metyrapone (250 mg–1 g qds) with physiological glucocorticoid replacement is useful for palliation of Cushing syndrome by inhibiting 2β-hydroxylase, but it might exacerbate virilism. Aminoglutethimide can be added if control is insufficient. An alternative is mitotane (o,p'-DDD), which causes necrosis and atrophy of normal adrenal tissue and differentiated carcinoma cells, reducing steroid output in 70% and giving objective tumour regression in one-third, although response is slow and glucocorticoid cover necessary.

CARCINOID TUMOURS

Carcinoid tumours form one of several types of gastroenteropancreatic (GEP) neuroendocrine tumours (see Chapter 9), but rarely can occur at sites outside the gastrointestinal tract.

EPIDEMIOLOGY

These are rare tumours arising at a younger age than carcinomas, with a peak incidence at about 50 years. There is no significant sex predominance or geographical pattern.

AETIOLOGY

It can be a feature of multiple endocrine neoplasia type 1.

PATHOLOGY

They usually arise submucosally and appear as a nodule, often red/brown in colour, yellow in cut section; they can be multifocal, and, unlike in carcinomas, ulceration is uncommon. Carcinoid is most common in the small bowel – 90% arise in the ileum, particularly the terminal segment, 7% in the jejunum, 2% in the duodenum and 2% in a Meckel diverticulum, but can arise elsewhere in the gastrointestinal tract, e.g. stomach, colon, rectum and other midline structures, such as thyroid, lung, bladder, testes, ovaries, common bile duct and pancreas. An encasement reaction characterized by a massive fibrous stroma can occur when the tumour reaches the mesentery and this predisposes to bowel obstruction. Carcinoids arise from APUD (amine precursor uptake and decarboxylation) cells, which are derived from the neural crest cells. Midgut-derived carcinoids characteristically stain with and reduce silver salts (argentaffin reaction), others stain with silver but cannot reduce it (argyrophilic reaction, e.g. gastric and bronchial carcinoids), while hindgut-derived carcinoids do not take up silver at all. Immunocytochemistry indicates staining for chromogranin, which is useful when the diagnosis is in doubt.

NATURAL HISTORY

The tumours are frequently slow growing and local infiltration of surrounding tissues is unusual. In contrast to a carcinoma, lymphatic spread is uncommon. Haematogenous spread is more common with larger primary tumours and is usually to the liver (Figure 14.6) as most tumours will arise in sites draining into the portal circulation. The primary tumour is often small compared with the bulk of liver metastases and symptoms of the carcinoid syndrome. Ileal tumours frequently metastasize, especially if more than 2 cm in diameter, while appendiceal, rectal and bronchial carcinoids rarely metastasize. The metastases are characteristically multiple and bulky compared with the primary, and can undergo spontaneous necrosis. The skeleton is sometimes a site of distant metastases and these may be osteoblastic.

SYMPTOMS

Symptoms depend on the site and size of the tumour. Asymptomatic carcinoids are often found incidentally at appendicectomy, when they are almost invariably benign. The patient might notice an abdominal mass if the tumour is large and superficial, or experience colicky abdominal pain if there is significant stenosis of the bowel lumen. Ultimately there could be symptoms of subacute small bowel obstruction. Bronchial carcinoids present with haemoptysis or

Carcinoid tumours

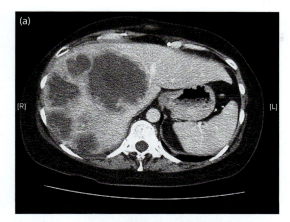

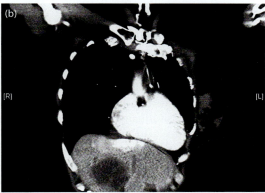

Figure 14.6 Carcinoid tumour with multiple liver metastases. (a) Transverse CT image. (b) Coronal CT image.

bronchial obstruction leading to recurrent chest infections. Carcinoid syndrome arises when there are liver metastases, so that the vasoactive tumour products, particularly 5-hydroxytryptamine (5-HT; serotonin), reach the systemic circulation. The syndrome can also arise from tumours originating outside the portal circulation (e.g. lung) or having spread outside it (e.g. a heavy burden of skeletal metastases). It comprises:

- Flushing – distribution may vary with site of primary
- Weals – from release of histamine
- Lacrimation
- Facial oedema
- Tachycardia and hypotension
- Wheezing
- Diarrhoea, borborygmi, abdominal colic and weight loss

A given patient will not necessarily have all these symptoms. There can also be hepatic pain from distension or if a large subcapsular metastasis infarcts. Attacks can be precipitated by alcohol, stress, emotion, ingestion of food and exogenous infusion of calcium, noradrenaline or pentagastrin.

SIGNS

The patient with advanced disease often looks remarkably well bearing in mind the bulk of liver metastases. They may appear malnourished if diarrhoea has been a particular problem, an abdominal mass might be palpable or in the case of a bronchial carcinoid there might be signs in the chest of pulmonary collapse or consolidation. Hepatomegaly is expected in patients with carcinoid syndrome from liver metastases. Auscultation of the heart can reveal tricuspid or pulmonary valve disease, although left-sided cardiac lesions have also been described with bronchial carcinoids, and there might also be signs of heart failure.

DIFFERENTIAL DIAGNOSIS

Other tumours arising at these sites should be considered, although none produces the carcinoid syndrome when there are liver metastases. It should be noted that rarely carcinomas at other sites can produce a carcinoid syndrome from 5-HT production, e.g. medullary carcinoma of the thyroid, small cell lung cancer.

INVESTIGATIONS

URINARY 5-HYDROXYINDOLEACETIC ACID (5-HIAA)

Twenty-four hour urinary 5-HIAA is elevated in those with carcinoid syndrome, reflecting metabolism of 5-HT. A false-positive result can be obtained if the diet at the time of urine collection is rich in bananas, pineapples, avocados or walnuts. Malabsorption syndromes (e.g. coeliac disease) can also cause modest elevations in 5-HIAA. Apart from 5-HT, carcinoids can produce histamine, kallikrein, motilin, enteroglucagon, neurotensin, substance P, prostaglandins, insulin, ACTH, glucagon, parathyroid hormone and calcitonin, most of which can be assayed if clinically relevant.

CHROMOGRANIN A

This is a characteristic serum marker.

COMPUTED TOMOGRAPHY/ MAGNETIC RESONANCE IMAGING

CT or MRI scan of the liver and site of primary tumour defines the locoregional extent of the primary tumour and will assess the liver for metastases.

HEPATIC ANGIOGRAPHY

This is of value if resection of liver metastases or embolization is planned.

STAGING

There is no formal staging system in routine clinical use.

TREATMENT

RADICAL TREATMENT

Surgery

The primary tumour should be completely excised as this offers the only chance of long-term cure, with 5-year survival of 90%. Radical lymph node resection is unnecessary, although obviously enlarged nodes should be cleared to ensure a complete resection of the tumour or at least significant cytoreduction.

PALLIATIVE TREATMENT

Dietary advice

Referral to a dietician for advice with regards to avoidance of substances may precipitate an attack of flushing and lessen diarrhoea and protein-losing enteropathy.

Surgery

In patients with symptoms from one large liver metastasis or multiple metastases confined to one lobe of the liver, resection should be considered reducing secretion of vasoactive peptides and therefore palliating symptoms. Careful supervision is essential during the perioperative period to avert a hypotensive crisis when the tumour is handled. Bypass of an intestinal obstruction might also be necessary.

Radiotherapy

Carcinoids are not sensitive to radiation, although low doses of radiation are useful for the palliation of painful skeletal metastases. Isotope therapy using mIBG (see the 'Phaeochromocytoma' section) should be considered if a preliminary scan shows uptake by the metastases.

Pharmacological measures

Both codeine phosphate (30–60 mg tds) and loperamide (up to 16 mg daily) are useful for the treatment of diarrhoea. The somatostatin analogue octreotide which is a potent inhibitor of the physiological effects of carcinoid tumours is the pharmacological treatment of choice. This can also have an antiproliferative effect on the tumour leading to disease stabilization. α-Interferon occasionally yields useful responses and can be combined with octreotide but has considerable toxicity.

Hepatic arterial embolization

This can benefit up to 80% of patients with symptomatic hepatic metastases, with palliation lasting up to 3 years. This procedure can be repeated as necessary.

Chemotherapy

Streptozotocin, cisplatin and etoposide and other combinations of drugs, have been used but with a partial response rate of 30% or less.

TUMOUR-RELATED COMPLICATIONS

As with any other gastrointestinal tumour, perforation, obstruction or intussusception can all occur. Ectopic hormone production is seen, the tumour producing growth hormone-releasing hormone leading to acromegaly or ACTH leading to Cushing syndrome. Pellagra is a rare syndrome characterized by glossitis, dermatitis in sun-exposed areas, diarrhoea and dementia, and is due to the tumour consuming tryptophan, which is a precursor for nicotinic acid. Heart failure might ensue in advanced cases from damage to the pulmonary and tricuspid valves.

TREATMENT-RELATED COMPLICATIONS

All cytoreductive treatments can release large amounts of vasoactive substances and therefore patients with bulky tumours should be pretreated with parachlorophenylalanine and cyproheptadine to avoid a serotonergic crisis.

PROGNOSIS

Carcinoid tumours are usually very slow-growing so that even patients with a heavy metastatic burden can survive for many years. Appendiceal carcinoids have an excellent prognosis as they are small, easily removed and rarely metastasize.

MULTIPLE ENDOCRINE NEOPLASIA (MEN)

MEN is rare and characterized as the name suggests by the occurrence of tumours involving more than one endocrine gland in a single patient. Various different genetic abnormalities have been linked to the MEN tumours.

TYPE 1

Dominant inheritance caused by a mutation of the *MEN 1* gene on chromosomal region 11q13. The involved glands include:

- Parathyroids (90%) – hyperplasia or adenoma; usually the presenting feature
- Pancreatic islets (80%) – adenoma, carcinoma or more rarely diffuse hyperplasia
- Anterior pituitary (65%) – adenoma
- Adrenal cortex (40%) – hyperplasia or adenoma
- Carcinoid tumours and lipomata – rare occurrences

TYPE 2

Dominant inheritance caused by a 10q11 chromosome region mutation affecting the *RET* gene. The involved glands include:

- Parafollicular cells of thyroid – medullary carcinoma (>95%); usually the presenting feature
- Adrenal medulla – phaeochromocytoma (50%)
- Parathyroids – hyperplasia or adenoma (<25%)

Subtype A (the commonest) has no mucocutaneous features while subtype B (5%) is characterized by multiple small subcutaneous or submucosal neuromas of the oral cavity and lips, autonomic ganglioneuromatosis and Marfanoid habitus. Familial medullary carcinoma of the thyroid forms a third subtype.

MIXED MEN

This demonstrates features of both types 1 and 2, usually pituitary adenomas and phaeochromocytoma.

FURTHER READING

Mallick U, Harmer C. *Practical Management of Thyroid Cancer*. Springer, New York, 2018.

Mitchell AL, Gandhi A, Scott-Coombes D, Perros P. Management of thyroid cancer: United Kingdom National Multidisciplinary Guidelines. *J Laryngol Otol*. 2016; 130(Suppl 2).

Raphael MJ, Chan DL, Law C, Singh S. Principles of diagnosis and management of neuroendocrine tumours. *Can Med Assoc J*. 2017; 189(10): E398–E404.

Yalsin S, Oberg K. *Neuroendocrine Tumours: Diagnosis and Management*. Springer, New York, 2015.

Endocrine tumours

SELF-ASSESSMENT QUESTIONS

1. Which three of the following statements are true for thyroid cancer?
   a. Commoner in men
   b. Accounts for more than 5000 cases per annum in the United Kingdom
   c. Medullary subtype is rare
   d. May be caused by exposure to ionizing radiation
   e. May be caused by thyroxine replacement therapy
   f. May be part of an inherited cancer syndrome
   g. Associated with prostate cancer

2. Which one of the following best describes follicular carcinoma of the thyroid?
   a. Associated with MEN type 2
   b. Rapidly growing
   c. Best treated with surgery and radioisotope therapy
   d. High risk of spread to liver
   e. Associated with a poor prognosis

3. Which three of the following statements are applicable to medullary carcinoma of the thyroid?
   a. Associated with MEN type 2
   b. May lead to a high serum calcium
   c. A high serum thyroglobulin is typical
   d. Associated with phaeochromocytoma
   e. It is a highly chemosensitive cancer
   f. It is a highly radiation-sensitive cancer
   g. Surgery is the mainstay of treatment

4. Which one of the following is not true about carcinoid?
   a. Often metastasizes to the liver
   b. May be slow growing
   c. 5-HIAA is a useful marker
   d. Is incurable
   e. Is not sensitive to radiation

15 Sarcomas

SOFT-TISSUE SARCOMAS

EPIDEMIOLOGY

There are over 3000 cases of soft-tissue sarcomas reported in the United Kingdom each year divided equally between men and women. In children, the predominant tumour is a juvenile rhabdomyosarcoma, which will be considered in the section on paediatric tumours. It has very different characteristics from the soft-tissue sarcomas of adults. In adults, these tumours can occur at any age, over 40% occurring in those >65 years.

AETIOLOGY

Usually there is no identifiable cause but the following factors may be of importance:

- *Chronic mechanical irritation*: Sarcomas can be induced in animal models but this does not appear important in humans.
- *Radiation*: A small number of sarcomas are undoubtedly related to previous therapeutic irradiation with tumours developing several years after exposure. Children are most at risk with a 16-fold increase in children receiving radiotherapy which is dose-related and also increased in those receiving additional chemotherapy.
- *Genetic*: Soft-tissue sarcomas are up to 200 times more common in individuals with a TP53 mutation, the most common manifestation being the Li–Fraumeni syndrome. In this syndrome they are associated with tumours of breast, brain, adrenal cortex and leukaemia in close relatives under the age of 45 years. They are also seen in patients with von Recklinghausen syndrome of familial neurofibromatosis when malignant change occurs within a pre-existing neurofibroma.
- *Chemical*: Angiosarcoma is associated with vinyl chloride exposure. Associations with pesticide use have not been confirmed.

PATHOLOGY

Sites for soft-tissue sarcomas include:

- Limbs (upper: 15%; lower: 45%)
- Retroperitoneum (16%)
- Viscera (bladder, bowel, uterus – 10%)
- Trunk (10%)
- Head and neck (4%)

Macroscopically, soft-tissue sarcomas are often large, fleshy tumour masses with associated haemorrhage and necrosis. They invade local soft tissues, nerves and blood vessels.

Microscopic classification of soft-tissue sarcomas is based on the finding of recognizable connective tissue elements within the tumour. There are some 50 different subtypes, with leiomyosarcoma, liposarcoma and pleomorphic sarcoma being the commonest. A classification of the soft-tissue sarcomas is shown in Table 15.1.

Histological grade is an important prognostic feature of sarcomas and a three-point scale is used to describe the degree of differentiation. This must,

Sarcomas

Table 15.1 Classification of soft-tissue sarcomas

Sarcoma subtype	Tissue type	Features
Fibrosarcoma	Fibrous tissue	Most common type, typically found in thigh
Liposarcoma	Fat	Lower extremity and retroperitoneum
Rhabdomyosarcoma	Skeletal muscle	Adult forms are alveolar or pleomorphic
Leiomyosarcoma	Smooth muscle	Uterus and gastrointestinal tract common, also limbs and retroperitoneum
Malignant fibrous histiocytoma (MFH)	Histiocytes	Especially legs, buttocks and retroperitoneum
Neurogenic sarcoma (neurofibrosarcoma)	Neural tissue	Arise within large nerves, e.g. sciatic, median, spinal roots
Synovial sarcoma	Uncertain	Arise around joints, especially thigh, foot, knee
Angiosarcoma	Blood vessels	Scalp, breast, liver
Lymphangiosarcoma	Lymph vessels	Sites of chronic lymphoedema, e.g. postmastectomy arm

however, be interpreted in light of the cell type. For example, angiosarcoma will usually appear well differentiated but is usually a highly malignant tumour. Similarly, virtually all synovial sarcomas can be regarded as high-grade tumours irrespective of their grading.

Molecular subtyping of sarcomas has become increasingly important with evidence emerging that differences will predict response to specific treatments.

NATURAL HISTORY

There is extensive local growth with infiltration of surrounding structures including blood vessels and nerves, and early blood-borne spread to lungs is the most common distant site.

Lymph node spread is relatively uncommon except for synovial and epithelioid sarcomas, alveolar rhabdomyosarcoma and angiosarcoma.

SYMPTOMS

Peripheral sarcomas present as a lump which may be present for some time before it becomes symptomatic. Retroperitoneal sarcomas can grow to a large size before manifestation of symptoms, the most common of which is backache. Rapid increase in the size of a pre-existing neurofibroma should alert the possibility of a malignant change to a neurofibrosarcoma.

SIGNS

At presentation, peripheral sarcomas are often large masses within soft tissue. Figure 15.1 shows a large soft-tissue sarcoma arising in the lower limb. Movement can become limited, particularly when close to joints. Retroperitoneal masses can be palpable through the abdomen.

DIFFERENTIAL DIAGNOSIS

Other benign soft-tissue masses should be considered, but it is recommended that any patient that is suspected of having a sarcoma be referred to a specialist sarcoma centre. Further investigations and biopsy to confirm and stage a sarcoma is best undertaken in a specialist sarcoma centre under the care of a multidisciplinary team.

INVESTIGATIONS

Routine investigations such as full blood count and blood biochemistry are usually unremarkable.

IMAGING

A CT scan of the chest should be performed in all patients diagnosed with a sarcoma to exclude metastases. A chest x-ray might also show pulmonary metastases (Figure 15.2).

Soft-tissue sarcomas

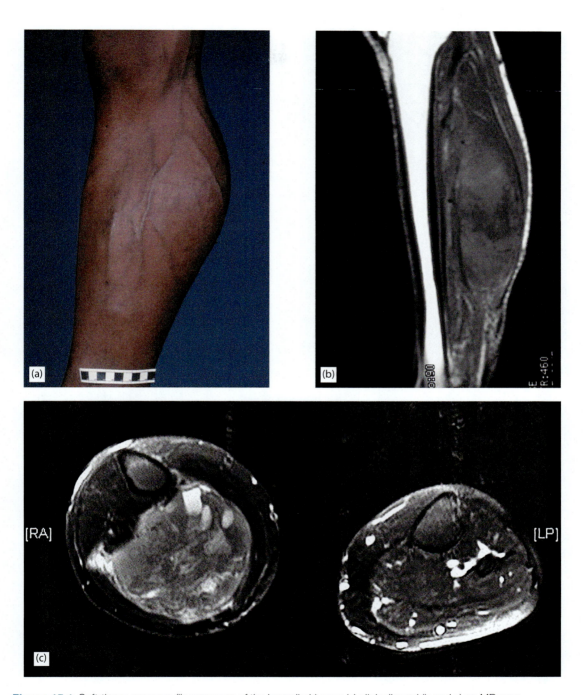

Figure 15.1 Soft-tissue sarcoma (liposarcoma of the lower limb) seen (a) clinically and (b and c) on MR scan, demonstrating the extensive involvement of the muscle compartment.

Sarcomas

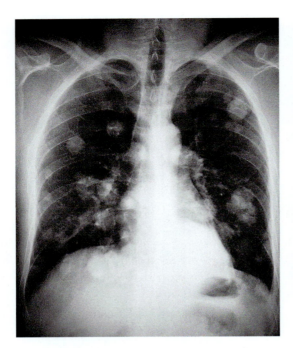

Figure 15.2 Chest x-ray demonstrating multiple pulmonary metastases from a soft-tissue sarcoma.

MRI of the primary site will give most precise definition of the soft-tissue extent and involvement of local structures as shown in Figure 15.3.

In some cases other imaging may be required, e.g. CT of the area involved or a PET scan.

BIOPSY

Biopsy of the primary lesion is essential to confirm the diagnosis and the type of sarcoma. Definition of a sarcoma can be difficult and, if a needle biopsy is not sufficient, an open biopsy is needed. It is important that this is performed in consultation with a specialist sarcoma surgeon who performs the definitive resection, as implantation at the biopsy site can occur; this should be included in the resection.

STAGING

Staging is based on the size of the primary tumour as follows:

- T1: Tumour <5 cm maximum diameter
- T2: Tumour >5 cm maximum diameter

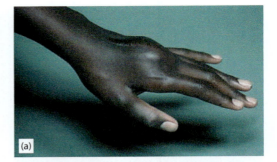
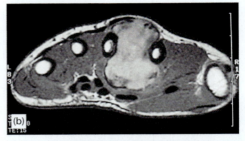
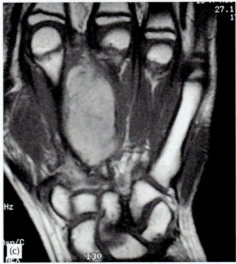

Figure 15.3 (a) Fibrosarcoma arising on dorsum of the hand and (b and c) MRIs showing details of precise anatomical location.

- N0: No nodes
- N1: Regional nodes

Grade is classified as follows:

- G1: Low grade
- G2: Intermediate grade
- G3: High grade

TREATMENT

Sarcoma management is complex and these tumours are relatively rare. They should be managed in specialist sarcoma centres by the specialized multidisciplinary teams.

LOCAL TREATMENT

Wide surgical resection including excision of any previous biopsy scar, combined with radiotherapy, which may be given pre- or post-operatively, enables conservation of the affected limb. Radiotherapy will include the tumour (or site of tumour if post-operative) and the surrounding soft-tissue compartment defined by site and natural barriers, e.g. fascial planes and bone. Amputation is avoided if at all possible but may be necessary for locally advanced tumours or those that progress despite radiotherapy.

Retroperitoneal tumours present a more difficult surgical problem and resection might not be possible. Preoperative radiotherapy may make surgery possible in some cases.

Radiation alone might control a soft-tissue sarcoma but a high dose is required and in general is inferior to the combination of surgery with irradiation.

The role of neoadjuvant or adjuvant chemotherapy remains limited to a few specific types of sarcomas. Soft-tissue sarcoma is not a particularly chemosensitive tumour. Meta-analyses suggest that there may be a small benefit for local and distant relapse-free survivals, but not for overall survival. Studies are ongoing finding the role of newer agents in tumours with a specific histological or molecular subtype.

Isolated limb perfusion with drugs such as melphalan might benefit locally advanced, unresectable limb tumours.

METASTATIC DISEASE

Chemotherapy has only limited activity. Doxorubicin remains the chemotherapy of choice for most sarcomas but in some subtypes or with certain molecular changes other agents may be indicated, e.g. ifosfamide in synovial sarcoma, paclitaxel in angiosarcoma and eribulin in liposarcoma. Trabectedin has been shown to have activity and other newer agents are showing promise in clinical trials.

Surgical resection (metastasectomy) or stereotactic ablative radiotherapy is the most successful treatment for limited lung metastases if feasible.

TUMOUR-RELATED COMPLICATIONS

Local effects owing to tumour size are the main problem associated with soft-tissue sarcomas. In general, paraneoplastic effects and systemic complications such as hypercalcaemia are not features of these tumours, although hypoglycaemia has been described as a rare association with massive retroperitoneal sarcomas.

TREATMENT-RELATED COMPLICATIONS

The emphasis of modern treatment is towards limb preservation. However, the effects of extensive resection and radiotherapy can lead to functional deficits in the limb with joint stiffness, loss of muscle power and limb oedema.

PROGNOSIS

The prognosis for peripheral limb tumours is better than that for sarcomas affecting the retroperitoneum, trunk or internal organs. With conservative limb-preserving treatment local control rates will be in the order of 80% with a 5-year survival around 60% depending on the tumour stage and grade. Patients with operable lung metastases have a 5-year survival of around 30% following metastasectomy.

FUTURE DEVELOPMENTS

The major change in the management of soft-tissue sarcomas has been in the development of limb-preserving treatment in the place of amputation. The main difficulty now lies in the prevention and treatment of systemic disease – currently treatments remain unsatisfactory but greater understanding of molecular pathways and drugs that can target these pathways are hoped to improve the situation.

RARE TUMOURS

EXTRAOSSEOUS EWING'S AND PRIMITIVE NEUROECTODERMAL TUMOURS (PNET)

These are rare soft-tissue tumours characterized by small round cells rich in glycogen morphologically identical to the classical Ewing tumour of bone (see the section 'Ewing sarcoma'). Extraosseous Ewing's is most common on the trunk and extremities, arising in soft tissue, distinct from bone, whilst PNET is most common in the chest, when it may be termed 'Askin tumour', and also the abdomen and pelvis. Management and prognosis follows that of classical Ewing tumour of bone (see the section 'Ewing sarcoma').

DESMOID TUMOURS

These classically arise in the abdominal wall in women postpartum but can occur at any site, presenting as a diffuse fibrous infiltrative tumour which, while pathologically benign, can cause serious effects by virtue of its relentless local growth. Surgical resection is the treatment of choice but when inoperable, slow regression is achieved following a radical dose of radiotherapy.

STEWART–TREVES TUMOUR

This is the name given to the rare development of a lymphangiosarcoma in the upper limbs of women with chronic lymphoedema secondary to the treatment of breast carcinoma. Treatment can be difficult owing to the pre-existing oedema and associated postoperative and postradiotherapy changes. Amputation might be necessary.

DERMATOFIBROMA

This is a benign tumour of the skin presenting as a fibrous nodule typically on the limbs, distinct from simple fibromas by the presence of histiocytes on microscopy. Its malignant counterpart is dermatofibrosarcoma protuberans, so-called because of its macroscopic appearance with an hour-glass shape pushing the epidermis outwards. It is usually found on the trunk and histologically it is essentially a fibrosarcoma.

OSTEOSARCOMA

EPIDEMIOLOGY

Osteosarcoma is the most common malignant tumour of the bone, although it is rare in relation to other malignancies. It occurs mainly in adolescents, particularly during the periods of active bone growth with a second peak of incidence in those over 60 years when it is related to Paget disease. It is almost twice as common in males as in females.

AETIOLOGY

No recognizable aetiological agent is present in the majority of cases. Paget's disease can be a pre-existing feature in adult osteosarcoma, as shown in Figure 15.4.

Osteosarcoma is a rare late effect following therapeutic irradiation. Historically, it is associated with radium dial painting and the use of thorium-based contrast agents, e.g. thorotrast, as contrast medium in diagnostic radiology.

It can occur as a component of the rare Li–Fraumeni syndrome in which bone or soft-tissue sarcomas are associated with a familial pattern of breast, brain and adrenal cortex tumours, and leukaemia. In these cases germ-line mutations of the $P53$ gene are found. An association with deletions in the retinoblastoma gene on the long arm of chromosome 13 is seen in 70% and other genetic changes including loss of heterozygosity on chromosomes 3q, 17q and 18p have also been described. Survivors of hereditary retinoblastoma have a relative risk of up to 500 for developing osteosarcoma with a latency of 10 years or more. It is seen in 15% of patients with bilateral retinoblastoma.

PATHOLOGY

The most common site for osteosarcoma is in a long bone, particularly around the knee, 30% arising from

Osteosarcoma

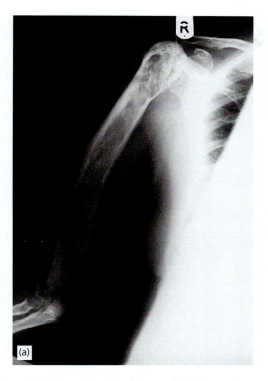 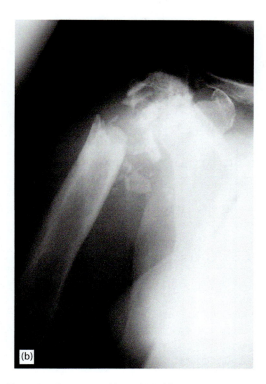

Figure 15.4 X-rays showing (a) pre-existing Paget disease of bone in a humerus within which (b) an osteosarcoma has subsequently developed.

the lower femur and 15% in the upper tibia; 10% arises in the humerus and the remainder can affect any bone, including the axial skeleton. Two principle groups are described, 'central (medullary)' and 'surface (peripheral)' tumours. The classical osteosarcoma is a central tumour and accounts for 95% of those seen.

Macroscopically, the tumour arises in the metaphysis and grows both eccentrically, expanding the cortex and raising the periosteum at its edges, and also along the medulla. Within the tumour are areas of haemorrhage and necrosis together with new bone formation in the subperiosteal regions to form the classic Codman triangles and sunray spicules seen on x-ray.

Pathological fracture through the tumour-bearing bone can occur.

Microscopically, there are two main populations of cells: a background stroma of spindle-shaped sarcomatous cells containing a matrix, which may be myxoid, cartilaginous or osteoid, together with multinucleate giant cells. Grading of osteosarcoma is not usual, all tumours being regarded as high grade.

NATURAL HISTORY

Local spread occurs within the bone of origin, typically the bone medullary cavity, and early blood-borne spread can occur, particularly to the lungs. Other bones may also be affected through blood-borne spread. Lymph node disease is not a prominent feature.

SYMPTOMS

There is usually pain in the bone and there may be a lump around the site of origin. There is sometimes a history of preceding trauma although no causal relationship exists. Symptoms from metastases include cough and haemoptysis but other features of malignant disease such as anorexia and weight loss are infrequent unless very advanced.

SIGNS

Swelling and deformity of the bone are seen. The area is often hot and red and an audible bruit might be heard. Thinning of the periosteum can result in a characteristic crackling on palpation and there may be crepitus if fracture has occurred. There is often an associated fever.

DIFFERENTIAL DIAGNOSIS

Other causes of bone swelling should be considered, including benign tumours such as osteochondromas and other malignant tumours.

INVESTIGATIONS

Routine investigations are often unremarkable, although there could be leucocytosis, and the alkaline phosphatase will be inappropriately raised. (However, in growing children and adolescents the normal range for alkaline phosphatase has increased during bone growth.)

RADIOGRAPHY

Plain x-ray of the affected bone will show local destruction of bone with the areas of new bone formation, which may form the classic Codman triangles and sunray spicules but more often are less well demarcated. There will be periosteal elevation and pathological fracture might be seen. In adults, coexisting Paget disease might be present, as illustrated in Figure 15.4.

CT OR MRI SCAN

Further details of the precise extent of bone destruction and spread within the medullary cavity will be found on CT or MRI scan, the latter being the investigation of choice.

CT scan of the lungs is important to identify pulmonary metastases.

ISOTOPE BONE SCAN

This will give further information on the extent of local bone involvement and also identify any bone metastases.

PET scanning might play a role in initial staging and response assessment, in particular distinguishing residual tumour from a postoperative change.

STAGING

The TNM staging for bone tumours is as follows:

- TX: Primary tumour cannot be assessed
- T0: Primary tumour not identified
- T1: Tumour ≤8 cm in maximum dimension
- T2: Tumour >8 cm in maximum dimension
- T3: Discontinuous tumours in the primary bone site

TREATMENT

The mainstay of modern treatment for osteosarcoma is a course of intensive chemotherapy together with local removal or irradiation of the site of origin.

Combination chemotherapy schedules are used. These typically include cisplatin, doxorubicin and high-dose methotrexate.

Following induction chemotherapy with a satisfactory response, conservative limb-preserving resection of the bone is undertaken. This might entail the use of an appropriate prosthesis or excision of the entire bone if expendable as in the case of a rib or the fibula. In children, a prosthesis that can be expanded to accommodate growth can be used as shown in Figure 15.5. In some cases the bone might be removed and sterilized with radiotherapy and then reimplanted to act as a scaffold for physiological new bone growth to remodel the bone.

For surgically unresectable disease, local radiotherapy will be given with the aim of delivering a dose of up to 60 Gy in 6 weeks. In certain sites, particularly in the spine close to the spinal cord, the dose can be limited by the tolerance of CNS tissue. Following local treatment chemotherapy will be continued for a total of around 20 weeks.

METASTASES

Following chemotherapy patients presenting with resectable lung metastases will be treated by metastasectomy alongside local surgery for the primary tumour.

Osteosarcoma

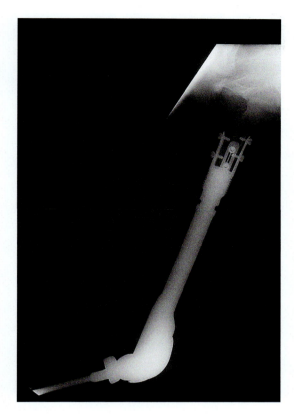

Figure 15.5 X-ray of extendable prosthesis used following resection of tumour from the lower femur.

RECURRENCE AND PALLIATION

Salvage treatment with further chemotherapy should be considered and may be successful but sometimes only palliative treatment will be indicated for relapsed disease. Local irradiation could be valuable for local pain and to arrest tumour growth through the skin. Amputation can be considered for recurrent disease but only when there is thought to be a realistic chance of long-term salvage.

Limited pulmonary metastases can be resected or ablated with radiofrequency ablation (RFA) or stereotactic radiotherapy.

TUMOUR-RELATED COMPLICATIONS

The principal complication is pathological fracture.

TREATMENT-RELATED COMPLICATIONS

The affected limb might have limitation of movement and muscle strength. Prostheses fitted to young patients who have not completed their growth will require revision from time to time. Following amputation, which might still be needed by a small number of patients, specific problems can include phantom limb pain, stump ulceration and chafing. Thoracotomy and metastasectomy can result in limited respiratory reserve depending on the extent of resection required, and postoperative pain in the thoracotomy scar is a well-recognized problem.

Chemotherapy will have considerable acute morbidity including nausea, vomiting, alopecia and mucositis. Longer term problems arise from nephrotoxicity related to the use of methotrexate or cisplatin, and neurotoxicity from cisplatin or vincristine. In children, growth retardation is sometimes seen with effects on subsequent maturation and fertility.

PROGNOSIS

Overall, with the use of modern chemotherapy-based schedules for treatment, the 5-year survival for non-metastatic osteosarcoma is between 40% and 50%. Prognosis is related to the size of primary tumour and response to neoadjuvant chemotherapy. In patients presenting with lung metastases, up to 20% could become long-term survivors and as many as 40% of those relapsing with pulmonary metastases can be salvaged. Elderly patients have a worse prognosis partly owing to the limitations of delivering intensive chemotherapy to this group. Those with tumours secondary to Paget disease have a 5-year survival of only 4%.

RARE TUMOURS

PAROSTEAL SARCOMA

This typically occurs in young adults, and is a peripheral tumour arising from the juxtacortical part of the bone metaphysis growing concentrically around the bone. The lower femur and upper tibia are the usual sites. Surgical excision is the treatment of choice. This is a low-grade malignancy with a low risk of metastases. Prognosis is better than that for an osteosarcoma, with a 5-year survival rate of 50%–70%. Occasionally, transformation into a high-grade osteosarcoma can be seen.

EWING SARCOMA

EPIDEMIOLOGY

Ewing sarcoma is the third most common sarcoma of bone affecting predominantly children and young adults, the maximum incidence being between the ages of 10 and 20 years. A rare extraosseous form of Ewing's is also recognized. The incidence of Ewing's in the United Kingdom is 0.3 in 100,000 and males are affected more than females; there are around 25 cases diagnosed each year in the United Kingdom and 200–250 in the United States. It is relatively rare in non-white populations.

AETIOLOGY

There is no recognized aetiological agent but a specific chromosomal translocation in Ewing's has been shown between chromosomes 11 and 22, and other similar translocations between chromosome 22 and chromosomes 21, 7 and 17 have also been described.

PATHOLOGY

Ewing's can affect any bone and is found in long bones, vertebrae and limb girdles, especially the pelvic bones where over 20% are found. Macroscopically, it arises in the diaphysis of the bone, growing subperiosteally. Periosteal reaction as it traverses the length of the bone can give rise to the characteristic onion peel appearance of the bone on an x-ray. To the naked eye the tumour contains areas of necrosis, and haemorrhage and cystic regions have also been seen.

Microscopically, Ewing's is composed of sheets of small round cells rich in glycogen. Ewing's is now considered to be one of the tumours in the group of PNET. The surface marker CD99 is characteristic for these tumours.

NATURAL HISTORY

There is local growth, the primary often reaching a considerable size, and blood-borne dissemination with metastases to lungs in particular. Lymph node metastases are not usually a major feature.

SYMPTOMS

Ewing's is typically painful and characteristically pain is intermittent in the early development of the tumour mass. There might be a preceding history of trauma but no causal relationship is recognized. Pathological fracture can occur. Lung metastases can cause cough or haemoptysis.

SIGNS

The tumour mass will be apparent as a palpable mass often tender to palpation. Associated fever, particularly in advanced cases, can be noted. Spinal Ewing's can result in neurological deficits.

DIFFERENTIAL DIAGNOSIS

Ewing's must be differentiated from other primary tumours of bone. Other round cell tumours that can affect bone should also be excluded, in particular lymphoma, neuroblastoma and anaplastic carcinomas.

INVESTIGATIONS

BLOOD CELL COUNT

A full blood count can demonstrate a raised white cell count and occasionally a mild anaemia might also be present.

BIOCHEMISTRY

Biochemical tests can be normal or show an inappropriately raised alkaline phosphatase.

RADIOGRAPHY

X-ray of the affected bone will show thinning of the diaphysis and in later stages extensive bone

Ewing sarcoma

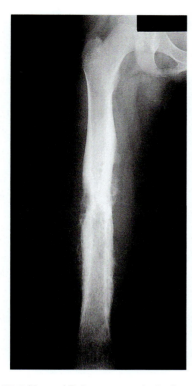

Figure 15.6 X-ray of Ewing sarcoma in the femur.

destruction (Figure 15.6). The characteristic onion peel appearance of successive layers of periosteal reaction can also be seen.

CT AND MRI

MRI shows greater details of the tumour mass, in particular soft-tissue invasion, and spread along the marrow cavity of the bone.

CT of the lungs is essential to exclude small volume lung metastases.

BIOPSY

Biopsy of the primary lesion is essential to confirm the diagnosis.

STAGING

There is no recognized staging system for Ewing sarcoma.

TREATMENT

CHEMOTHERAPY

The chemotherapy agents used initially typically include vincristine, ifosfamide, doxorubicin and etoposide (VIDE) followed by surgery and/or radiotherapy. Further chemotherapy with VIA (vincristine, ifosfamide and actinomycin D) and VAC (vincristine, actinomycin D and cyclophosphamide) may then be used to complete the therapy.

LOCAL TREATMENT

After 2–3 months of chemotherapy (VIDE), surgery and/or radiotherapy will be used to treat the primary tumour. For most patients, the aim will be to deliver a total dose of between 50 and 60 Gy in 5–6 weeks.

PALLIATIVE TREATMENT

Standard chemotherapy as described above is appropriate for widespread symptomatic metastases. Local symptoms of pain or bleeding can be better dealt with by local radiotherapy. In selected patients, high-dose chemotherapy with autologous marrow transplant could be an option.

TUMOUR-RELATED COMPLICATIONS

These include pathological fracture and spinal cord compression from rapid growth of spinal tumours.

TREATMENT-RELATED COMPLICATIONS

Chemotherapy can result in acute nausea, vomiting and alopecia. In the longer term, vincristine can be associated with a peripheral neuropathy and, in high doses, Adriamycin is cardiotoxic. For this reason actinomycin D is substituted once a tolerance dose has been reached.

High-dose radiotherapy to a limb can result in joint stiffness, skin changes and lymphoedema.

PROGNOSIS

The overall 5-year survival for patients without metastases treated with modern chemotherapy-based regimens is around 50%. This is determined particularly by the tumour size ranging from 70% in tumours <500 cm^3 to 35% in tumours >500 cm^3.

Local control rates can approach 90%, greater in long bones than in the pelvis.

OTHER BONE TUMOURS

CHONDROSARCOMA

This is the second most common bone tumour after osteosarcoma, typically affecting the pelvic bones, although it can also occur in the femur, humerus and scapula. It is a tumour of adults and usually slow growing. A primary might arise *de novo* from apparently normal bone, or a secondary when it arises within a pre-existing chondroma. Rarely (<5%) chondrosarcoma can be extraskeletal.

Initial treatment is radical surgical resection or, if it is inoperable, radiotherapy.

Well and moderately differentiated forms have a good prognosis and only metastasize late, if at all. There is, however, a high-grade variant, which has an aggressive course. These patients are treated with initial chemotherapy using drugs similar to the osteosarcoma schedules. The overall 5-year survival is around 35%.

OSTEOCLASTOMA (GIANT CELL TUMOUR)

This is a tumour arising in adults usually between the ages of 30 and 50 years, the most common sites being the long bones around the knee, radius and humerus. There is a characteristic 'soap bubble' appearance on x-ray with eccentric thinning of the cortex. Clinically this can be demonstrated, albeit rarely, by 'eggshell crackling' on palpation.

It is composed of two populations of cells, a background stroma of spindle cells, the differentiation of which defines the activity of the tumour, and scattered multinucleate giant cells. The majority are of low-grade malignancy and present a problem of local control rather than disseminated disease.

Wide surgical excision is the treatment of choice. Around one-third will recur locally and a further one-third will be high-grade tumours, which ultimately metastasize. Local irradiation can be of value for local recurrence; chemotherapy is not usually successful in a metastatic disease. The overall 5-year survival is around 65%–70%.

SPINDLE CELL SARCOMA

Tumours histologically identical to fibrosarcoma or malignant fibrous histiocytoma of soft tissue might be found as primary bone tumours. They are usually tumours of adults in the 30–60-year age group. Treatment is radical surgical excision. There has been some interest in giving adjuvant chemotherapy to this group of patients but to date there has been no evidence that this improves survival. The overall 5-year survival is in the range of 25%–40%.

Angiosarcomas also arise in bone and will be treated in the same way as the other spindle cell sarcomas of bone.

FURTHER READING

Casali PG, Abecassis N, Bauer S et al. Soft tissue and visceral sarcomas: ESMO-EURACAN clinical practice guidelines for diagnosis, treatment and follow-up. *Ann Oncol.* 2018 Oct 1; 29 (Supplement 4): iv51–iv67.

Casali PG, Bielack S, Abecassis N et al. Bone sarcomas: ESMO-PaedCan-EURACAN clinical practice guidelines for diagnosis, treatment and follow-up. *Ann Oncol.* 2018 Oct 1; 29 (Supplement 4): iv79–iv95.

Dangoor A, Seddon B, Gerrand C, Grimer R, Whelan J, Judson I. UK guidelines for the management of soft tissue sarcomas. *Clin Sarcoma Res.* 2016 Nov 15; 6: 20.

von Mehren M, Randall RL, Benjamin RS et al. Soft tissue sarcoma, version 2.2018, NCCN clinical practice guidelines in oncology. *J Natl Compr Canc Netw.* 2018 May; 16(5): 536–563.

SELF-ASSESSMENT QUESTIONS

1. Which of the following is true of soft-tissue sarcomas?
   a. They arise from epithelial cells
   b. They are common tumours arising equally in men and women
   c. They may be associated with the Li–Fraumeni syndrome
   d. In children the common form is an angiosarcoma
   e. The most common site is the upper limb

2. Which of the following is true of the pathology of soft-tissue sarcomas?
   a. Blood-borne spread is rare
   b. Synovial sarcomas are always high-grade tumours
   c. Angiosarcomas are usually well differentiated
   d. Radiation-induced sarcomas are usually well differentiated
   e. Synovial sarcomas arise from joint cartilage

3. Which three of the following apply to the presentation of soft-tissue sarcomas?
   a. Pain is a common feature of peripheral sarcomas
   b. Retroperitoneal sarcoma may present with chronic back pain
   c. Lung metastases may be the first manifestation
   d. Regional lymphadenopathy is common
   e. Rapid growth in a neuroma can be due to sarcomatous change
   f. Excision biopsy is the diagnostic procedure of choice
   g. May present with sudden pain due to intratumoral haemorrhage

4. In the treatment of soft-tissue sarcoma which of the following is true?
   a. Large tumours are best managed with initial chemotherapy
   b. Wide local excision should be followed by radiotherapy
   c. Angiosarcomas are best treated with radiation alone
   d. Metastatic disease will respond to cisplatin-based chemotherapy
   e. Radioisotope therapy has a role in selected cases

5. Which of the following is true of osteosarcoma?
   a. It is most common over 60 years of age
   b. The most common site for distant metastases is the liver
   c. In children it is usually associated with the Li–Fraumeni syndrome
   d. On x-ray it appears as a lucent defect in the cortex
   e. The most common site is in the long bones around the knee

6. In the treatment of osteosarcoma which of the following is true?
   a. Amputation is required for long-bone tumours
   b. Chemotherapy is only used in the palliation of metastatic disease
   c. Resection of lung metastases can be curative
   d. Chemoradiation is given for unresectable primary sites
   e. High-dose methotrexate is the chemotherapy of choice

7. Which three of the following are true of Ewing sarcoma?
   a. It arises from osteoclasts
   b. It is most common in the under 10 years age group
   c. Lymph node metastases are common
   d. Painless swelling is the common presentation
   e. It is composed of small round cells rich in glycogen
   f. X-ray shows a characteristic 'onion peel' appearance
   g. Prognosis is worse if the tumour volume is >500 cm^3

8. Which three of the following are true of bone tumours?
   a. Chondrosarcoma is most common in the spine
   b. Chondrosarcoma may arise within a pre-existing chondroma

257

Sarcomas

c. Lung metastases are frequent in osteoclastoma
d. Characteristic giant cells are found in the stroma of osteoclastoma
e. Liposarcoma may arise within bone
f. Malignant fibrous histiocytoma of bone is usually seen in childhood
g. Primary angiosarcoma of bone is well recognized

Lymphoma

Malignancies of the lymphoproliferative system are broadly classified into Hodgkin lymphoma and all other lymphomas, termed non-Hodgkin lymphomas. The classification of these is complex and many different systems have been described, of which the WHO classification has now gained international acceptance. A simplified clinical view is shown in Figure 16.1; a summary of the WHO classification is given in the 'Pathology' section of 'Non-Hodgkin lymphoma (NHL)'.

HODGKIN LYMPHOMA

EPIDEMIOLOGY

Each year in the United Kingdom there are 2100 cases of Hodgkin lymphoma, leading to a total of 300 deaths per annum. There is a bimodal age distribution, the two peaks of incidence occurring in young people aged 20–30 years and in later life over 70 years with over half of cases diagnosed over the age of 45 years. The UK incidence has increased by 20% in the past decade. Overall, it is almost twice as common in men as it is in women. In children, the sex difference is even more extreme, occurring almost exclusively in boys under the age of 10 years. It is rare in the Japanese and in the US black population, and particularly high in the Jewish populations of the United States and the United Kingdom.

AETIOLOGY

There is no proven aetiological agent responsible for the development of Hodgkin lymphoma.

Nodular sclerosing Hodgkin is more common in more affluent households and the reverse is seen for other subtypes, which are more common in less affluent households.

There is a strong association with infection with Epstein–Barr virus (EBV); EBV-associated Hodgkin seems particularly prevalent in those under 10 years and over 60 years, and in this group viral DNA can be identified in the cells in up to 50%.

Hodgkin lymphoma is observed to increase in patients with HIV infection, although it is less common than non-Hodgkin lymphoma in this group.

There is a three-fold risk in people who have a first-degree relative diagnosed with Hodgkin lymphoma.

PATHOLOGY

Macroscopically, Hodgkin lymphoma is usually found in lymph nodes, the spleen and the liver. More rarely, infiltration of the lungs, bone marrow, skin or central nervous system can occur. Typically, the nodes are relatively soft and uniformly enlarged. The spleen and liver appearances are of multiple nodules within their substance, the cut surface of which has been likened to that of a German sausage.

Microscopically, the diagnostic feature is the presence of binucleate cells called Reed–Sternberg cells. In addition, a wide variation of other cells including lymphocytes, neutrophils, plasma cells, eosinophils, histiocytes and fibroblasts is also found infiltrating the node or affected organ. There are four major histological subclassifications as shown in Table 16.1. Characteristically, the cells are of B-cell type and the

Lymphoma

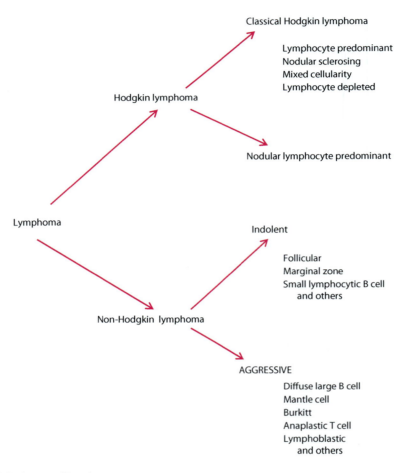

Figure 16.1 Clinical types of lymphoma.

Table 16.1 Histological subtypes of classical Hodgkin lymphoma

Subclass	Features	Prognosis
Lymphocyte predominant	Infiltrate of many small lymphocytes	Good
Nodular sclerosis	Node divided by fibrous bands. Cells may be rich in lymphocytes (type 1) or be of mixed type (type 2)	Type 1 – good Type 2 – moderate
Mixed cellularity	Mixed population of cells	Moderate
Lymphocyte-depleted	Fibrous node with Reed–Sternberg cells with few other cells	Poor

cell surface markers CD15 and CD30 can be identified on immunohistochemistry.

NATURAL HISTORY

Typically, stepwise involvement of adjacent node groups occurs. The most common nodes involved are those in the neck. In this situation spread is to adjacent nodes in the supraclavicular fossa, the axillae and the mediastinum before involving para-aortic nodes below the diaphragm. Extranodal involvement as a sole manifestation is rare and usually occurs in the context of extensive or bulky-node disease.

SYMPTOMS

Typically, the patient is aware of a painless enlarged node in the neck. This might have been present for many weeks or months but can develop more rapidly.

'B' symptoms are characteristic of lymphomas and are as follows:

- Fever >38°C often with typical remittent pattern (Pel–Ebstein fever)
- Weight loss of >10% body weight
- Night sweats

Other uncommon but characteristic symptoms include generalized and often intractable itching and alcohol-induced pain in the enlarged nodes. Although the lymph nodes themselves are usually painless, there might be some backache from para-aortic nodes and left-sided abdominal pain from splenic enlargement.

SIGNS

Enlarged lymph nodes can be present in any site, but most commonly in the neck. Typically, the nodes of Hodgkin lymphoma are described as firm and rubbery as opposed to the hard craggy nodes of carcinoma. Palpable hepatosplenomegaly or an abdominal mass owing to para-aortic or mesenteric nodes might also be present. Inguinal and pelvic lymphadenopathy can be associated with oedema of the lower limbs, although arm oedema is an unusual complication of axillary lymphadenopathy from lymphoma. Mediastinal lymphadenopathy might present with the signs of superior vena cava obstruction.

DIFFERENTIAL DIAGNOSIS

The main differential diagnosis is between Hodgkin lymphoma and non-Hodgkin lymphoma. Other causes of lymphadenopathy will also be considered including infection, which can be pyogenic, tuberculous or viral, e.g. EBV or CMV (cytomegalovirus), toxoplasmosis and other neoplastic conditions such as leukaemia or carcinoma.

INVESTIGATIONS

BLOOD COUNT

A full blood count may show mild anaemia and leucocytosis with a raised lymphocyte count but is frequently normal.

ERYTHROCYTE SEDIMENTATION RATE

ESR can be raised, particularly in more aggressive forms of the disease.

BIOCHEMISTRY

Serum lactate dehydrogenase is a sensitive index of disease activity and of prognostic importance. Serum albumen is important in the prognostic index.

Routine biochemical blood tests can show evidence of hepatic infiltration with raised alkaline phosphatase and γ-glutamyltransferase. More profound hepatic disturbance is rare. Obstruction of the renal tracts by enlarged nodes can cause renal failure. Hypercalcaemia is a recognized but rare finding in Hodgkin disease.

BONE MARROW EXAMINATION

Unlike non-Hodgkin lymphoma, bone marrow involvement is unusual in the absence of other soft-tissue involvement, i.e. stage 4 disease. Bone marrow examination is no longer routine for those patients presenting with stage 1–3 nodal disease in the absence of B symptoms.

RADIOGRAPHY

Chest x-ray can show widened mediastinal shadow owing to enlarged nodes or, more rarely, lung parenchymal infiltration. Pleural effusion is also a recognized finding.

CT AND MRI

CT scan of chest, abdomen and pelvis gives the most accurate assessment of internal lymphadenopathy and is the imaging of choice for staging in lymphoma. There is less experience of MRI in Hodgkin lymphoma but wider availability and the use of new contrast agents could broaden its role in the future.

PET CT SCAN

Additional staging information can be seen on fluorodeoxyglucose (FDG) PET scans with normal size nodes demonstrating increased uptake indicative of lymphoma. This can also show bone marrow involvement with Hodgkin lymphoma, avoiding the need for a formal bone marrow examination. PET can also have an important role in response assessment and follow-up.

BIOPSY

A tissue diagnosis is mandatory to confirm the diagnosis and define the histological subtype of Hodgkin lymphoma. This will usually take the form of an open lymph node biopsy where there is an accessible node in the neck, axilla, supraclavicular fossa or groin. Mediastinoscopy or laparoscopy could be required where there are no other sites accessible for biopsy.

STAGING

The staging of Hodgkin lymphoma follows the Ann Arbor classification:

- *Stage 1*: Involved lymph nodes limited to one node area only
- *Stage 2*: Involved lymph nodes involving two or more adjacent areas on one side of the diaphragm only
- *Stage 3*: Involved lymph nodes on both sides of the diaphragm
- *Stage 4*: Involvement of extranodal organs denoted by the following suffixes:
  - M – Bone marrow
  - D – Skin
  - H – Liver
  - S – Spleen

Each stage is further subclassified 'A' or 'B' according to the absence or presence, respectively, of B symptoms (see the section 'Symptoms' of Hodgkin lymphoma).

TREATMENT

Hodgkin lymphoma is both radiosensitive and chemosensitive and most patients can expect to be cured of their disease. Since this disease frequently affects young people who will live for many years after successful treatment, there is now considerable emphasis laid not only on the efficacy of the treatment, but also on achieving cure with minimal long-term morbidity.

LOCALIZED DISEASE (STAGES 1A AND 2A)

The standard approach to early localized disease involves treatment comprising:

- Short course chemotherapy, typically three or four cycles of ABVD (Adriamycin, bleomycin, vinblastine and dacarbazine) followed by
- Radiotherapy treating a volume including only those areas initially affected

A favourable group can be identified which only require two cycles of chemotherapy and radiotherapy. The need for radiotherapy in patients who achieve a complete response to chemotherapy has been investigated, and particularly in those with a negative FDG PET scan, the improvement in relapse-free survival (around 5%) should be balanced against potential late toxicities, especially second tumours and cardiac effects.

Hodgkin lymphoma is much more sensitive to radiation than the common epithelial cancers and requires only 30 Gy given over 3 weeks, or 20 Gy in 2 weeks for the 'favourable' subgroup (compared with 60–70 Gy for a squamous carcinoma).

Relapse in these patients can in most cases be salvaged using chemotherapy.

ADVANCED DISEASE (STAGES 1B, 2B, 3 AND 4)

Although there may be only limited nodal disease apparent, the presence of B symptoms is a poor prognostic feature and implies more widespread disease. For this reason stages 1B and 2B disease are included in this category together with those patients who have widespread node disease or involvement of

Hodgkin lymphoma

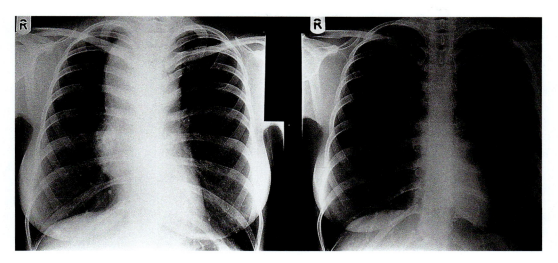

Figure 16.2 Chest x-ray before and after four cycles of chemotherapy for bulky mediastinal Hodgkin lymphoma.

systemic organs. Chemotherapy is given to these patients.

Prior to starting chemotherapy male patients should have the opportunity to consider sperm banking as subsequent fertility cannot be guaranteed after chemotherapy.

All patients undergoing chemotherapy should be well hydrated and started on allopurinol to prevent tumour lysis syndrome (see Chapter 21). Response can be rapid; an example of a chemotherapy response on treating bulky mediastinal nodes from Hodgkin lymphoma is shown in Figure 16.2.

CASE HISTORY

HODGKIN LYMPHOMA

A 23-year-old man presented to his GP with a 1-month history of an enlarging lump in the left side of his neck. On examination, he was found to have a 3 cm enlarged gland in the left deep cervical region with a further 2 cm node in the left supraclavicular fossa. These were non-tender and there were no associated foci of infection to find. On further questioning, however, he admitted to episodes of fever and several nights when he awoke drenched with sweat. A biopsy of the lymph node was undertaken and this showed nodular sclerosing Hodgkin lymphoma. Further investigations showed a normal full blood count but an ESR of 53 mm/hr, normal biochemistry but, on CT scan, other areas of enlarged lymph nodes in the anterior mediastinum and para-aortic region with marked splenomegaly. A bone marrow examination was clear. A CT PET scan showed increased FDG uptake in lymph nodes in the neck, mediastinum, para-aortic region and in the spleen. A diagnosis of stage 3B Hodgkin lymphoma was made. He was recommended to receive combination chemotherapy. Prior to starting chemotherapy he was counselled with regards to future fertility and, an initial sperm count being normal, semen was taken for cryopreservation.

He underwent combination chemotherapy using Adriamycin, bleomycin, vinblastine and dacarbazine (ABVD) for which he attended the hospital outpatient chemotherapy unit on a fortnightly basis. After each visit he had 24 hours of nausea, which was controlled by taking ondansetron 4 mg twice daily for the first 2 days after chemotherapy. By the fourth week of chemotherapy his hair was thinning and he needed to shave only once every other day.

One week after the third chemotherapy injection he developed a high fever and felt generally unwell. As instructed by the chemotherapy unit he attended for a blood count, which showed that he had haemoglobin of 10.3, a total white blood cell count of 0.9 with a neutrophil count of 0.2 and a platelet count of 73. Admission to the oncology ward was arranged on the same day and he was treated with intravenous gentamicin and tazocin. Within 24 hours

Lymphoma

his temperature had settled. He was treated with 5 days of high-dose intravenous antibiotics by which time his neutrophil count had risen to 1.3 and he could be safely discharged from hospital. He proceeded with his next course of chemotherapy uneventfully but with each subsequent course he received 5 days of GCSF injection mid-cycle.

After his second course of ABVD chemotherapy, a further PET CT scan was undertaken. This showed that the enlarged lymph nodes in the neck had disappeared but there was a residual abnormality of 2 cm in size in the mediastinum and a 1.5 cm node remaining in the para-aortic region which was negative on PET with no increase in FDG over the background mediastinal blood level. He continued with four more courses of ABVD chemotherapy. This was followed by further CT PET scan, which showed that the residual abnormalities in the mediastinum and para-aortic region had resolved and there was no FDG uptake at those sites or elsewhere. He was therefore considered to be in complete remission and no further treatment was given. On completion of chemotherapy he noted that his nails had developed marked changes with loosening of the nail bed and a brownish discoloration. He was reassured that these were normal reactions to the administration of bleomycin chemotherapy, and over the next few months these changes grew out as new nail advanced. His hair regrew normally but it was some months before his energy levels returned and he was able to resume a normal lifestyle.

He continued to attend the oncology clinic initially at 3-month intervals but later at less frequent intervals. Five years later he remains fit and well with no signs of active disease and has been discharged from regular review. He has recently gotten married and his wife is pregnant with their first child, his fertility having been preserved despite his chemotherapy.

SPECIFIC CHEMOTHERAPY

Early schedules used were based upon MOPP (mustine, vincristine, procarbazine and prednisolone). While effective at giving complete remission rates of up to 80%, there is significant toxicity and modifications have been developed to minimize this morbidity.

LOPP or ChlVPP replaced mustine with chlorambucil and in the case of ChlVPP, vincristine is replaced by vinblastine.

Anthracycline-based (i.e. Adriamycin or its analogues) schedules such as ABVD (Adriamycin, bleomycin, vinblastine and dacarbazine) are highly active and are now recognized as the chemotherapy of choice for Hodgkin lymphoma. These schedules are associated with less long-term toxicity and randomized trials have shown cure rates to be at least equivalent to earlier schedules. Most patients will receive six to eight courses of standard chemotherapy. In patients having a complete response on CT PET scan after two cycles the chemotherapy may be reduced by omission of bleomycin to reduce the risk of pneumonitis.

For patients who have a number of adverse risk factors more intensive schedules can be advantageous; an example is the BEACOPP schedule.

Radiotherapy is only indicated in this group of patients where complete remission is not achieved at the end of chemotherapy; in this setting the involved field radiotherapy delivering 30 Gy in 3 weeks will improve the prognosis of partial responders similar to those who achieve a complete response with chemotherapy.

TREATMENT FOR RELAPSE

Of those patients given initial chemotherapy for advanced disease, around 40% will either relapse or fail to achieve a sustained complete remission. Retreatment with the same or alternative chemotherapy regimens can result in further regression of disease for around 50%, but of these only 15%–20% will achieve long-term remission. It is therefore in this group of patients that more intensive treatment using high-dose chemotherapy and peripheral blood stem cell autograft is indicated. With such techniques, long-term survival can be achieved in over 30% of patients relapsing after conventional chemotherapy for Hodgkin lymphoma.

A new agent, brentuximab, an antibody directed against the CD30 surface antigen has high activity in Hodgkin lymphoma and can achieve second remissions in many patients failing first-line therapy; current trials are assessing its efficacy in first-line combination schedules.

TUMOUR-RELATED COMPLICATIONS

Massive lymphadenopathy can have consequences as a result of local pressure, although in general lymphoma tends to grow around structures rather than directly invade them. In the mediastinum dysphagia and superior vena cava obstruction can occur. In the abdomen, renal failure from ureteric obstruction and lower limb oedema from pelvic node enlargement are seen.

TREATMENT-RELATED COMPLICATIONS

RADIOTHERAPY

For many patients, there are few, if any, sequelae; however, long-term effects are now seen as patients cured in their 20s and 30s are followed-up for several decades. Potential problems are shown in Table 16.2.

CHEMOTHERAPY

Acute toxicity includes nausea and vomiting, alopecia and bone marrow depression. Neutropenic sepsis is a potential hazard of any such treatment, the risk of which can be minimized by the use of colony-stimulating factor (GCSF). Peripheral neuropathy can develop from the use of vincristine or, less commonly, vinblastine.

Table 16.2 Late effects of radiotherapy for Hodgkin disease

Site	Late radiation effects
Neck	Hypothyroidism, laryngeal oedema or fibrosis
	Treatment in puberty may induce thyroid cancer, loss of muscle and soft-tissue bulk causing asymmetry
Mediastinum	Pneumonitis and lung fibrosis
	Pericarditis
Spinal cord	Myelitis
Abdomen	Increased incidence of peptic ulceration
Pelvis	Amenorrhoea in women and sterility if gonads included in radiation field

Adriamycin has specific dose-related cardiotoxic effects and bleomycin can cause lung damage at high doses. Neither of these effects will be expected in standard treatment schedules but might become a potential hazard in patients requiring retreatment. Bleomycin also results in characteristic changes to the nails and skin.

The anthracycline-containing schedules such as ABVD have the advantage of preserving fertility.

SECOND MALIGNANCIES

There is increasing concern regarding the incidence of second malignancies in patients who are cured of their Hodgkin lymphoma. There is an ongoing risk with time from treatment, which appears to be rising to over 15% in patients who have survived for 20 years or more. In the early years, occasional leukaemias or non-Hodgkin lymphomas are diagnosed but the major problem is an increasing risk of solid tumours, which develop towards the end of the first decade after treatment with an ongoing incidence thereafter. More intensive regimes, in particular escalated BEACOPP, give high doses of etoposide which can result in a specific form of AML.

The greatest concern is the incidence of breast cancer in young women where a relative risk (RR) between 2 and 4 for breast cancer in women between the ages of 25 and 35 years when irradiated has been reported and an RR of over 20 for those under the age of 20. In smokers, there is also a dramatic increase in lung cancer related to both radiation and chemotherapy exposure where the relative risk of developing lung cancer is again over 20.

CARDIAC DISEASE

Whilst it has been recognized for some time that anthracyclines cause dose-related cardiomyopathy, more recently it has become clear that there is an increase in deaths from cardiac disease related to both chemotherapy and radiotherapy in long-term follow-up. Features which seem to predict for this include supradiaphragmatic radiotherapy and the use of anthracycline and vincristine chemotherapy. Survivors of treatment for Hodgkin lymphoma should minimize their cardiac risk factors and increasingly are being offered regular cardiological assessment with early intervention.

PROGNOSIS

Overall, the prognosis for patients diagnosed with Hodgkin lymphoma is good. Virtually all patients presenting with early localized disease will be cured and with intensive chemotherapy over 80% of those with advanced disease (stages 3B or 4) can also be expected to be cured.

Seven important prognostic factors have been identified, which now comprise the international prognostic index. These are:

- Age >45 years
- Male
- Stage IV disease
- Haemoglobin <10.5 g/dL
- Total white blood cell count >16 × 10^9/L
- Lymphocyte count <0.6 × 10^9/L
- Serum albumin <40 g/L

FUTURE PROSPECTS

Increasingly, the emphasis in Hodgkin lymphoma now is to maintain the very high cure rates obtained while reducing morbidity. This can be achieved by individualizing treatment according to stage and risk factors. New, less toxic chemotherapy schedules could be appropriate for low-risk patients whilst the more intensive weekly drug schedules combined with involved field radiotherapy might be needed for those with high-risk disease. The use of PET scans early in chemotherapy could be valuable in identifying patients in whom treatment can be minimized and conversely intensified where early response is unsatisfactory. Modern radiotherapy techniques enable smaller volumes to be treated and lower doses will reduce the probability of late effects.

NON-HODGKIN LYMPHOMA (NHL)

EPIDEMIOLOGY

Each year in the United Kingdom there are around 13,500 cases of NHL. It is slightly more common in men (7700 cases) than in women (6300 cases) and is the sixth commonest form of cancer, accounting for a total of 5000 deaths per annum.

The incidence increases with age, being relatively unusual under the age of 50 years with 70% of cases diagnosed over the age of 60 years. NHL is as common in white, black and Asian populations, although different subtypes may predominate.

AETIOLOGY

No single aetiological agent has been identified to account for the common forms of lymphoma found in the United Kingdom.

INFECTIVE AGENTS

- EBV is associated with Burkitt lymphoma found predominantly in Africa.
- Human T-cell lymphotropic virus type 1 (HTLV1) is associated with T-cell lymphoma found in the Caribbean and Japan.
- HIV infection is also associated with an excess of lymphomas, which is probably a feature of the immunosuppressed status rather than a direct causation by virus. The RR for a high-grade lymphoma in HIV infection is 400.
- *Helicobacter* is closely associated with gastric mucosal-associated lymphoid tissue-type lymphomas (MALTomas) and eradication of *Helicobacter* has been accompanied by regression of gastric lymphoma in a high proportion of cases.
- *Chlamydophila psittaci* has been associated with orbital lymphoma responding to treatment with doxycycline.

ALTERED IMMUNE STATUS

In addition to HIV, NHL is also increased in other disease states associated with a depressed immune system including rheumatoid arthritis, coeliac disease and hypogammaglobulinaemia, and following iatrogenic immune suppression after renal transplantation. There are also associations with autoimmune disease such as Hashimoto thyroiditis with thyroid lymphoma and Sjögren disease with salivary gland lymphoma.

IRRADIATION

This could also be a factor in the development of NHL and increased incidences have been seen following exposure in Hiroshima and Nagasaki, and after low-dose therapeutic irradiation to the spine for ankylosing spondylitis.

PATHOLOGY

NHL describes a spectrum of neoplastic conditions as a result of which many complex and confusing classifications have arisen. The majority of NHL arise from the B lymphocyte but there is a well-recognized group which are T-cell-derived neoplasms. Rare forms of histiocytic neoplasm also occur.

Macroscopically, NHL will occur as a mass of neoplastic lymphoid tissue, which can reach a considerable size. Ulceration, necrosis and haemorrhage are unusual. It can arise in recognized lymph node chains but, unlike Hodgkin lymphoma, extranodal lymphoma is relatively common with up to 50% involving sites such as Waldeyer's ring, the gastrointestinal tract, skin and bone.

Microscopically, the appearances are complex and interpretation can be difficult. In broad terms, lymphomas can be low grade or high grade. Features of low-grade lymphoma are the preservation of follicular architecture and cellular composition of well-differentiated small lymphocytes. In contrast, high-grade lymphomas are characterized by diffuse infiltration of the node or extranodal site with large undifferentiated lymphoid cells. The current international classification for NHL is the WHO classification shown next, which attempts to define disease entities rather than a pure morphological categorization. Increasingly, there is a move towards subclassifying lymphoma according to molecular subtypes.

A simplified listing omitting some rarer subvariants is as follows:

- Mature B-cell neoplasms
  - Chronic lymphocytic leukaemia/small lymphocytic lymphoma
  - B-cell prolymphocytic leukaemia
  - Splenic marginal zone lymphoma
  - Hairy cell leukaemia
  - Lymphoplasmacytic lymphoma
  - Waldenstrom macroglobulinaemia
  - Monoclonal gammopathy of undetermined significance (MGUS)
  - Plasma cell myeloma
  - Solitary plasmacytoma of bone
  - Extraosseous plasmacytoma
  - Extranodal marginal zone lymphoma of mucosa-associated lymphoid tissue
  - MALT lymphoma
  - Nodal marginal zone lymphoma
    - Paediatric nodal marginal zone lymphoma
  - Follicular lymphoma
  - Mantle cell lymphoma
  - Diffuse large B-cell lymphoma (DLBCL), NOS
    - Germinal centre B-cell type
    - Activated B-cell type
    - T-cell/histiocyte-rich large B-cell lymphoma
    - Primary DLBCL of the central nervous system (CNS)
    - Primary cutaneous DLBCL, leg type
    - EBV1 DLBCL, NOS
    - EBV1 mucocutaneous ulcer
    - DLBCL associated with chronic inflammation
    - Lymphomatoid granulomatosis
    - Primary mediastinal (thymic) large B-cell lymphoma
    - Intravascular large B-cell lymphoma
    - ALK1 large B-cell lymphoma
  - Plasmablastic lymphoma
  - Primary effusion lymphoma
  - Burkitt lymphoma
  - Burkitt-like lymphoma with 11q aberration
  - B-cell lymphoma, unclassifiable, with features intermediate between DLBCL and classical Hodgkin lymphoma
- Mature T and NK neoplasms
  - T-cell prolymphocytic leukaemia
  - T-cell large granular lymphocytic leukaemia
  - Chronic lymphoproliferative disorder of NK cells
  - Aggressive NK-cell leukaemia
  - Adult T-cell leukaemia/lymphoma
  - Extranodal NK-/T-cell lymphoma, nasal type
  - Mycosis fungoides

- Sézary syndrome
- Primary cutaneous anaplastic large cell lymphoma
- Peripheral T-cell lymphoma, NOS
- Angioimmunoblastic T-cell lymphoma
- Anaplastic large-cell lymphoma, ALK1
- Anaplastic large-cell lymphoma, ALK2

The histological diagnosis of lymphoma is now supported by a range of specific monoclonal antibody stains. Distinction from a poorly differentiated small cell carcinoma is made using the leucocyte common antigen (LCA). Distinction of one subtype of lymphocyte from another has become a complex science. Monoclonal antibody stains to identify surface markers can differentiate B cells from T cells from histiocytes, and a large library of stains has now been built up to enable subtyping of a suspected lymphoma. Increasingly specific genetic signatures are used to subtype lymphoma.

Despite this relatively complex classification, in practice most lymphomas can be divided into low-grade indolent lymphomas or more aggressive intermediate/high-grade types, which will define their natural history, management and prognosis as shown in the box.

Indolent (low-grade): 40% having a long natural history but rarely if ever cured

- Follicular lymphoma with any of the following cell types:
  - Small cleaved cells
  - Mixed small and large cleaved cells
- Well-differentiated diffuse small cell lymphocytic lymphoma

Aggressive (intermediate/high-grade): 50% having a shorter natural history with a fatal course unless treated with combination chemotherapy with which long-term cure is possible

- Follicular lymphoma containing predominantly large cells (grade 3)
- Diffuse lymphoma containing any of the following cell types:
  - Small cleaved cells
  - Mixed small and large cells
  - Predominantly large cells
- Immunoblastic
- Peripheral T-cell lymphoma

Rarer types: Requires different management

- Lymphoblastic: aggressive requiring leukaemia-type treatment
- Small non-cleaved cells as in Burkitt lymphoma: poorly responsive to standard chemotherapy requiring more intensive schedules
- Mycosis fungoides: skin lymphoma having long natural history
- MALTomas, arising in mucosal surfaces, usually low: in stomach respond to anti-*Helicobacter* therapy

NATURAL HISTORY

Indolent low-grade lymphoma can remain asymptomatic for many years and, in the elderly, have little impact upon their life expectancy.

A high-grade immunoblastic or lymphoblastic lymphoma is an aggressive often rapidly fatal condition.

Extranodal lymphoma can have a relatively benign course as in a low-grade skin lymphoma, existing as purplish nodules requiring little other than gentle local treatment from time to time. In contrast, it can follow an aggressive course as in a high-grade lymphoma of the bowel or central nervous system.

In general, NHL, unlike Hodgkin lymphoma, does not have a clear pattern of contiguous spread from one area to the next. Dissemination is often wide and unpredictable following a pattern closer to that of a carcinoma with relatively frequent involvement of organs such as the lung and CNS.

SYMPTOMS

NHL usually presents with a painless lump in a lymph node area, most commonly the neck but also the axilla or groin. There can be backache owing to enlarged para-aortic nodes or upper abdominal pain from hepatosplenomegaly.

'B' symptoms as described for Hodgkin lymphoma are also an important feature, namely weight loss, fever and night sweats.

Other symptoms relate to the site of origin of an extranodal lymphoma. NHL arising in Waldeyer's ring therefore will cause local symptoms similar to those of a carcinoma in these regions, with local pain or discomfort, and epistaxis or nasal discharge where the nasopharynx is involved. Gastrointestinal lymphoma usually presents with an acute abdominal event owing to haemorrhage, perforation or obstruction. CNS lymphoma can cause symptoms of raised intracranial pressure with headache, vomiting and fits. Focal neurological features can cause bulbar palsy, diplopia, limb weakness and altered sensation. Skin lymphoma usually presents as asymptomatic lumps but mycosis fungoides has a characteristic pretumour phase often lasting many years with chronic skin change, which can be itchy and resemble dermatitis in its clinical symptoms.

SIGNS

Enlarged lymph nodes will be palpable, typically painless, firm, 'rubbery' nodes clinically indistinguishable from those of Hodgkin lymphoma but different from the hard craggy nodes of carcinoma. At extranodal sites lymphoma often has a characteristic purplish appearance, stretching overlying surfaces and ulcerating only rarely. Hepatosplenomegaly is a common finding in both nodal and extranodal lymphoma.

INVESTIGATIONS

BLOOD COUNT

A full blood count can show signs of mild anaemia or pancytopenia if there is bone marrow involvement. A high white blood cell count composed predominantly of lymphocytes can also be found and is a relatively poor prognostic sign.

ERYTHROCYTE SEDIMENTATION RATE

The ESR will be raised; an ESR >40 mm/hr is a further poor prognostic feature.

BIOCHEMISTRY

The serum lactate dehydrogenase (LDH) is a marker of disease activity and prognostic.

Routine biochemistry can show signs of hepatic infiltration. Renal failure is an occasional complication of massive para-aortic node enlargement causing ureteric obstruction. Immunoparesis can be present and paraproteinaemia can occur. Hypercalcaemia is associated with HTLV-associated lymphomas.

RADIOGRAPHY

The chest x-ray might show mediastinal or hilar lymphadenopathy; more rarely infiltration of the lung parenchyma, pleural nodules or a pleural effusion will be found.

CT SCAN

Contrast enhanced CT will demonstrate enlarged lymph nodes and abnormalities in extranodal sites and is currently the investigation of choice for staging. Figure 16.3 demonstrates extensive lymphadenopathy in the neck and para-aortic region on CT scan.

POSITRON EMISSION TOMOGRAPHY COMPUTED TOMOGRAPHY (PET CT)

FDG PET CT can give additional information showing evidence of active disease in normal-sized lymph nodes resulting in upstaging in relation to the CT stage, an example of which is shown in Figure 16.4. It can also be useful in assessing a response, a negative PET scan at completion of treatment having a high predictive power for long relapse-free survival.

BONE MARROW EXAMINATION

Bone marrow examination will be required in all cases to assess the possibility of marrow infiltration.

OTHER IMAGING

Other imaging might be indicated depending on the site of origin. For bowel lymphoma a full barium series is performed since multiple foci of disease are well recognized. An MR scan of the brain will be performed for CNS lymphoma, which can be further extended to image potential spinal disease.

Lymphoma

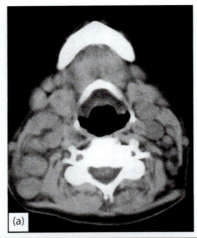

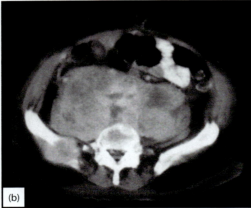

Figure 16.3 CT scans showing (a) extensive cervical lymphadenopathy and (b) para-aortic lymphadenopathy in non-Hodgkin lymphoma.

CEREBROSPINAL FLUID (CSF) EXAMINATION

CSF examination for lymphoma cells will be required for central nervous system (CNS) lymphoma and can also be considered for other types of lymphomas that have a high risk of CNS involvement, in particular diffuse large cell and lymphoblastic lymphomas and those affecting the testis, tonsil or nasal sinuses.

DIFFERENTIAL DIAGNOSIS

The main differential diagnosis rests between NHL and Hodgkin lymphoma. Epithelial tumours should

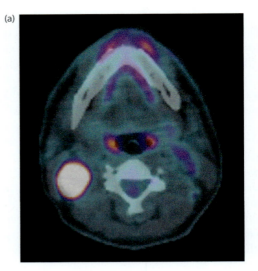

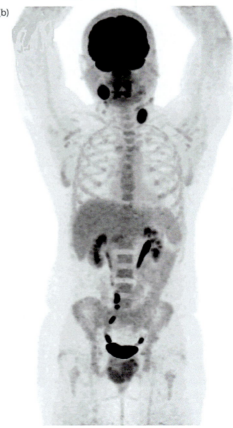

Figure 16.4 PET CT scan demonstrating localized non-Hodgkin lymphoma in the neck on fused CT PET axial scan (a) and whole body uptake scan (b).

be considered where NHL arises in extranodal sites. It might be difficult to distinguish clinically an indolent diffuse small lymphocytic lymphoma with extensive bone marrow involvement from chronic lymphocytic leukaemia, and lymphoblastic lymphoma from acute lymphoblastic leukaemia.

STAGING

The Ann Arbor staging system is used for NHL as for Hodgkin lymphoma (see the section 'Staging' of 'Hodgkin lymphoma') with the further addition of a suffix 'E' where the lymphoma has arisen in an extranodal site. For example, an NHL arising in the tonsil with involved nodes in the neck would be stage 2 by virtue of the presence of two or more sites all on the same side of the diaphragm and be designated stage 2E, having arisen in an extranodal site.

TREATMENT

Treatment is based on histological grade and stage.

INDOLENT LOW-GRADE NHL

(Common types are follicular and diffuse small cell lymphoma in WHO-REAL classification.)

This is a condition that is rarely curable unless early stage but usually has a long clinical course.

Localized low-grade NHL (stage 1A) is treated using local radiotherapy. The involved area only is treated, using low doses of 24 Gy in 2.5 weeks.

In the management of more advanced stage disease there is no proven advantage of immediate treatment in the asymptomatic patient who does not have bulky disease or potential organ failure. Such patients will often be kept under surveillance until symptoms arise or they develop bulk disease or compromised bone marrow function, or other major organs are perceived under threat, e.g. early hydronephrosis from enlarging nodes. The administration of a short course of rituximab, four weekly infusions, will delay the need for further treatment and has been shown to be an alternative cost-effective approach.

The first-line chemotherapy of choice for this group of lymphomas is R-Bendamustine comprising rituximab and bendamustine which has now replaced RCHOP (rituximab, cyclophosphamide, Adriamycin, vincristine and prednisolone) in this setting. In elderly patients, an alternative is to use RCVP (rituximab, cyclophosphamide, vincristine and prednisolone) or single-agent oral chemotherapy, of which the most popular is chlorambucil or cyclophosphamide: 70%–80% of patients will enter remission with such treatment.

The subsequent relapse-free period can be prolonged with maintenance rituximab given every 2 months for 2 years.

Relapse

Low-grade lymphoma that is not localized is never cured, although survival for many years is to be expected. When relapse does occur further chemotherapy will be given; second-line treatment can include RCHOP or fludarabine often in combination with Adriamycin or mitoxantrone and dexamethasone (FAD or FMD), which appear more active than the single drugs alone. Local sites causing symptoms can be irradiated. Rituximab (see the section 'Indolent low-grade NHL') will also achieve responses in chemotherapy-resistant disease.

Patients who achieve a second remission after relapse can benefit from proceeding to more intensive chemotherapy using either high-dose schedules such as BEAM (BCNU, etoposide, cytosine arabinoside and melphalan) with a stem-cell autograft or a low-dose allograft.

Transformation

Richter syndrome refers to the transformation from a low-grade to a high-grade lymphoma, which can occur in up to 15% of patients presenting initially with low-grade lymphoma. For this reason re-biopsy of recurrent disease, particularly where there has been a period free from detectable disease or a change in growth rate is observed, should be considered before treatment.

Palliation

Steroids alone in moderate doses (40–60 mg of prednisolone) can have a valuable antitumour effect as well as conferring general effects such as improvement in appetite and general well-being.

Single-agent etoposide or vincristine can be used for progressive advanced disease at relapse. Hemi-body irradiation, a valuable palliative treatment for widespread NHL, is no longer responsive to chemotherapy.

AGGRESSIVE HIGH-GRADE LYMPHOMA

(Common type is a diffuse large cell lymphoma according to the WHO-REAL classification.)

This is a much more dangerous condition than low-grade lymphoma and in general requires more intensive therapy.

Nodal lymphoma

Localized high-grade B-cell NHL (stages 1A and 2A) is best treated with a short course of chemotherapy (typically three courses of RCHOP [rituximab, cyclophosphamide, Adriamycin, vincristine and prednisolone] followed by local irradiation to the involved sites delivering a dose of 30 Gy in 3 weeks or six cycles of RCHOP chemotherapy alone).

Advanced disease (stages 1B, 2, 3 or 4) is treated with chemotherapy. As for Hodgkin lymphoma, consideration should be given to sperm banking for young males and all patients should be well hydrated and started on allopurinol to prevent tumour lysis syndrome (see Chapter 21).

Specific chemotherapy

Usually, combination chemotherapy is given, of which the most widely used for B-cell lymphoma is RCHOP, rituximab, cyclophosphamide, Adriamycin, vincristine and prednisolone and for T-cell non-cutaneous lymphoma CHOP alone as there is no CD20 receptor on T cells. The first four drugs are given intravenously on day 1 of a 21-day cycle with oral steroids on the first 5 days. Allergic reactions to the monoclonal antibody rituximab can be seen on initial exposure and so the infusion is given slowly for the first cycle, speeding up on subsequent cycles if no reaction is seen. A total of six to eight courses is usually given, the standard dictum being to deliver two courses of chemotherapy beyond complete clinical remission. Rapid responses can be seen after only one cycle of treatment, as illustrated in Figure 16.5.

Combined modality treatment

Sites of original bulky disease are often irradiated on the basis that these are frequently the sites of initial relapse and recent studies have shown an improved outcome for patients receiving radiotherapy in this setting.

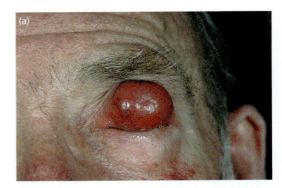

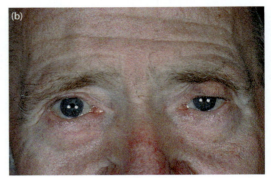

Figure 16.5 Conjunctival lymphoma (a) before and (b) after one cycle of CHOP chemotherapy.

High-dose chemotherapy and autograft

The procedure of peripheral blood stem cell (PBSC) collection from the blood subsequently using the stem cells to reseed the marrow after treatment has become a routine procedure enabling high-dose marrow ablative chemotherapy schedules to be given safely in patients up to the age of 65–70 years; beyond this there is an increasing morbidity and mortality, which must be carefully considered.

PBSCs are obtained by using bone marrow stimulation with chemotherapy followed by colony-stimulating factors such as GCSF. This increases the number of PBSCs in the peripheral circulation, which are then 'harvested' during plasmapheresis. These cells are stored in liquid nitrogen until needed for reinfusion after an ablative dose of chemotherapy (or radiotherapy).

Ablative high-dose chemotherapy such as BEAM (carmustine, etoposide, cytosine arabinoside and melphalan), which result in ablation of the bone marrow as well as residual lymphoma, can then be given followed by PBSC infusion to reseed the marrow. The role of high-dose chemotherapy in advanced high-grade NHL is principally in relapse or disease refractory to initial chemotherapy. In recurrent disease, challenge with conventional dose chemotherapy is essential to select those with chemosensitive disease. In this group further treatment with high-dose chemotherapy will result in prolonged remission in over 60%. There is, however, no value in proceeding to such treatment in those patients having relapsed disease who are unresponsive to initial chemotherapy, and who unfortunately have a poor prognosis.

Mantle cell lymphoma

This often occurs in the elderly and whilst indolent forms can be seen, as it usually follows an aggressive course and is relatively unresponsive to standard RCHOP chemotherapy. More intensive schedules including CNS prophylaxis and cytosine arabinoside are more successful as is ibrutinib, a tyrosine kinase inhibitor.

Lymphoblastic lymphoma

This form of high-grade lymphoma has a particularly aggressive course and resembles acute lymphoblastic leukaemia in many of its features, for example a propensity to spread to the CNS. Results from standard lymphoma chemotherapy are poor and most of these patients will be treated in protocols similar to those for acute lymphoblastic leukaemia (ALL), including CNS prophylaxis.

Burkitt lymphoma

This is a distinct high-grade lymphoma defined histologically as a diffuse small non-cleaved cell lymphoma. It is common in certain parts of Africa where an association with EBV infection is apparent, but is a rare lymphoma in Europe and the United States. Results from standard lymphoma treatment are poor and current schedules use more intensive chemotherapy including CNS prophylaxis.

Extranodal lymphoma

In general, these lymphomas are high grade and will be treated in the same way as lymphomas arising in nodes. There are, however, certain features of management particular to specific sites.

Waldeyer's ring lymphomas

These usually arise in the tonsils or nasopharynx and will be treated in the same way as nodal lymphomas, localized disease receiving three cycles of RCHOP followed by involved field radiotherapy, and more advanced disease receiving six to eight cycles of RCHOP.

Gastrointestinal tract lymphomas

These often present as a surgical emergency with obstruction or perforation when patients proceed to laparotomy at which bowel resection is performed. The diagnosis of NHL having been made, these patients will be treated with chemotherapy. A well-recognized hazard of initial chemotherapy in these patients is that of intestinal perforation as the lymphoma in the bowel wall regresses, and careful observation as an inpatient is usually recommended for the first course of treatment. Irradiation is difficult in these patients as it is a problem to demarcate clearly the affected area using standard localization techniques, and the bowel tolerates irradiation poorly.

A distinct pathological entity is the MALToma found particularly in the stomach and small bowel. Initial management of MALTomas in the stomach should be a course of anti-*Helicobacter* therapy using omeprazole and antibiotics such as ampicillin or tetracycline with metronidazole. Responses are seen in over 90% of patients but close gastroscopic surveillance is required to detect those patients who relapse and then require standard lymphoma chemotherapy.

Skin lymphomas

These are often low grade (lymphoma cutis) and require only gentle local treatment from time to time, but more extensive high-grade lymphoma can develop, as shown in Figure 16.6. Mycosis fungoides is a characteristic T-cell skin lymphoma, which has a long pretumour phase before developing into the characteristic skin infiltration, which can be widespread. It responds poorly to chemotherapy. Less severe forms can respond to PUVA (psoralens and ultraviolet A exposure) and for others local irradiation is required. In widespread disease, the entire body can be affected when irradiation of the whole body with electrons will be required.

Lymphoma

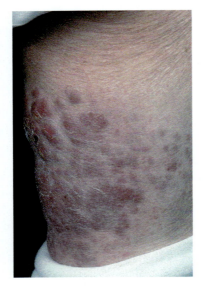

Figure 16.6 Infiltration of the skin with characteristic features of primary skin lymphoma.

CNS lymphoma

This has a poor prognosis. It has a propensity to seed throughout the CNS via CSF circulation. Management will include high-dose methotrexate chemotherapy and radiotherapy despite which most patients will still relapse after only a relatively short time. Two distinct populations have now emerged: those with sporadic primary CNS lymphoma and those where it is associated with HIV infection. The prognosis for the latter is particularly poor. In patients who do survive after radiotherapy there are concerns with regards to long-term psychometric function.

TUMOUR-RELATED COMPLICATIONS

Given the great heterogeneity of NHL, a vast range of clinical complications can arise, most of which have been covered in this chapter.

CASE HISTORY

NON-HODGKIN LYMPHOMA

A 53-year-old man presents to his GP having had a sore throat for the past few weeks with discomfort on swallowing. On examination he is found to have enlargement of the left tonsil and a 2 cm lymph node palpable in the left side of the neck. He is referred urgently to an ENT surgeon who performs an excision biopsy of the tonsil. Histology of the tonsil shows diffuse large cell non-Hodgkin lymphoma. He is referred to the oncologist who undertakes various staging investigations. MR and PET CT scans show no evidence of further lymphadenopathy other than that detectable clinically in the neck. His bone marrow is normal and other blood tests including a full blood count, ESR, biochemical profile, immunoglobulins and serum lactate dehydrogenase are all normal. He is recommended to receive a short course of chemotherapy to be followed by radiotherapy.

Chemotherapy is started with a cycle of combination treatment using rituximab, cyclophosphamide, Adriamycin, vincristine and prednisolone (RCHOP). He is warned about the possibility of infertility but has decided that he does not wish to store sperm having completed his family many years ago. An echocardiogram is also performed to check cardiac function before he receives anthracyclines, and this is also normal with a left ventricular ejection fraction of 65%. Following his first cycle of RCHOP chemotherapy he has some transient nausea but otherwise no significant side effects. Three weeks later he receives a second cycle of RCHOP chemotherapy. By this time he has noted marked thinning of his hair but otherwise remains well and reports that the lump previously palpable in his neck has already disappeared. A third course of RCHOP chemotherapy is repeated after 3 more weeks.

Two weeks later he attends the radiotherapy planning clinic where a cast for a head shell is made. His head is placed in the correct position for the treatment and a close-fitting plastic shell is made. A CT scan for radiotherapy planning is then taken with him in position wearing the shell. These are used by the oncologist to define the areas to be treated and from this a plan of the radiation beams is defined by the radiation physicists. A week later he attends for the beam positions to be checked, x-ray images of the beams to be taken to check their accuracy, and marks made on the shell for them to be lined up against during his subsequent treatment. A week later he attends for his first of 15 daily radiotherapy treatments. He feels perfectly well during the procedure other than some minor discomfort on being kept still in the shell. By the end of the first week he notices some slight discomfort on swallowing again and as he continues treatment in the second week he becomes increasingly uncomfortable with pain on swallowing particularly hot foods. He also notices that the skin where the x-ray beams enters his face and neck has become red and starts to feel tight and uncomfortable, as if he had been exposed to excess sun. He is given dietary advice and later aspirin mucilage to take before food. He continues treatment on a daily basis through the third week. At completion of treatment he has marked skin reddening and some early peeling of the skin over the neck. Swallowing is very uncomfortable and he is warned to expect this to continue for a few days before a slow improvement develops. Two weeks later the skin is feeling itchy and peeling but he is otherwise comfortable. His throat has improved considerably and he is starting to return to a normal diet without the need for regular medication.

Three months after treatment his symptoms have resolved completely and the follow-up PET CT scan shows no evidence of detectable lymph node enlargement or other abnormalities. Examination of his oropharynx shows no abnormalities either. He is told that he is in complete remission.

He is seen regularly in the outpatient clinic. Five years later he remains well with no signs of recurrence of his lymphoma and is discharged from routine follow-up.

Mass effects can be caused by malignant nodes or lymphomatous tissue compromising normal function so that, for example, mediastinal disease could cause SVC obstruction or dysphagia, abdominal disease could cause renal failure owing to ureteric obstruction, and pelvic disease could cause oedema of the lower limbs.

Gastrointestinal lymphoma can cause bowel haemorrhage, obstruction or perforation.

CNS lymphoma can cause focal neurological damage or obstructive hydrocephalus.

TREATMENT-RELATED COMPLICATIONS

RADIOTHERAPY

This can cause late toxicity related to site, e.g. irradiation of Waldeyer's ring can cause dry mouth, taste loss and dental problems. Abdominal and pelvic irradiation can result in postradiation bowel and bladder changes.

CHEMOTHERAPY

During treatment bone marrow depression, with the risks of neutropenic sepsis, occurs together with nausea, vomiting, alopecia and mucositis.

Rapid tumour regression can result in complications, in particular perforation at the site of gastrointestinal lymphoma, estimated to occur in around 5% of patients with lymphoma in this site, and tumour lysis syndrome (see Chapter 21).

In the longer term, Adriamycin can cause dose-related cardiotoxicity, and bleomycin is associated with dose-related pneumonitis and lung fibrosis together with peripheral skin changes.

Infertility can result, particularly in males, after combination chemotherapy, although pregnancy is seen in women even after high-dose chemotherapy.

Second malignancy in patients with NHL is becoming more apparent as the results of treatment improve and more patients survive to develop a new malignancy. It is estimated that the risk of developing acute myeloblastic leukaemia in the first 5 years following treatment is between 6% and 8% and as with Hodgkin lymphoma appears most marked in patients treated with both chemotherapy and radiotherapy. There is a less clear association with the development of solid tumours (i.e. cancers or sarcomas) as yet, but since it is known that this risk increases with time over 20 or 30 years it is likely to emerge as cohorts of cured patients are followed for this length of time.

PROGNOSIS

There are four major independent prognostic features in non-Hodgkin lymphoma:

- Age
- Performance status
- Stage (3 or 4 worse than 1 or 2)
- Serum lactate dehydrogenase

These have been validated and are referred to as the International Prognostic Index (IPI).

The overall prognosis for indolent low-grade lymphoma is better than that for intermediate or high-grade lymphomas, with median survivals of 8–10 years reported from most centres.

Early localized disease will be associated with high cure rates, over 90% for indolent lymphoma and 85% for aggressive forms following radiotherapy preceded in the latter by short-course chemotherapy.

Extranodal lymphoma, even when localized, tends to have a worse prognosis than nodal lymphoma; Waldeyer's ring and skin do better than the gastrointestinal tract, which does better than the CNS.

More advanced aggressive high-grade NHL will respond to chemotherapy in most patients with complete regression of disease in 70%–80%; however, long-term survival rates tend to fall below 50% at 5 years from treatment.

FUTURE PROSPECTS

The main areas of development in the management of NHL are concerned with individualizing treatment according to risk factors and lymphoma subtype with more sophisticated definition of subtypes using molecular profiling.

RARE TUMOURS

NODULAR LYMPHOCYTE-PREDOMINANT HODGKIN LYMPHOMA (NLPHL)

NLPHL accounts for around 5% of Hodgkin lymphomas and is a distinct entity characterized histologically by cells that are negative for the cell markers CD15 and CD30 but positive for CD20.

Clinically, it typically presents with localized lymphadenopathy and has an indolent course. Optimal management varies between nothing more than observation after excision biopsy to involved site radiotherapy. In more advanced disease, management is analogous to that of Hodgkin lymphoma but includes rituximab in combination schedules such as R-ABVD or RCHOP as for non-Hodgkin lymphoma.

MALIGNANT HISTIOCYTOSIS

This is a rare form of lymphoma characterized by systemic symptoms of fever, weight loss, generalized lymphadenopathy, hepatosplenomegaly and pancytopenia. Histiocytic lymphoma is typically associated with coeliac disease, when it presents as a multicentric bowel lymphoma. It may respond to lymphoma-type chemotherapy but the prognosis is generally much worse than that for other forms of lymphoma.

CASTLEMAN DISEASE

This is probably not a neoplasm but a hamartomatous condition of lymphoid tissue. It can present in a similar manner to lymphoma and histological differentiation can be difficult. It is uncertain whether active treatment other than simple excision of affected nodes is of value, although there are reports of successful regression after irradiation.

WALDENSTRÖM MACROGLOBULINAEMIA

This is lymphoplasmacytic lymphoma typically producing an IgM paraprotein and as such needs to be distinguished from myeloma. This is usually clear from the clinical findings, which are those of a lymphoma with lymph node and splenic involvement. Bone marrow examination shows infiltration with lymphoma rather than plasma cells. Haemolytic anaemia owing to cold agglutinins is a further rare feature. Management and prognosis are similar to those of other low-grade non-Hodgkin lymphomas.

FURTHER READING

Chaganti S, Illidge T, Barrington S et al. Guidelines for the management of diffuse large B-cell lymphoma. *Br J Haematol*. 2016 Jul; 174(1): 43–56.

Dreyling M, Ghielmini M, Rule S et al. Newly diagnosed and relapsed follicular lymphoma: ESMO Clinical Practice Guidelines for diagnosis, treatment and follow-up. *Ann Oncol*. 2016 Sep; 27(Suppl 5): v83–v90.

Follows GA, Ardeshna KM, Barrington SF et al. Guidelines for the first line management of classical Hodgkin lymphoma. *Br J Haematol*. 2014 Jul; 166(1): 34–49.

Herst J, Crump M, Baldassarre FG et al. Management of early-stage Hodgkin lymphoma: A practice guideline. *Clin Oncol (R Coll Radiol).* 2017 Jan; 29(1): e5–e12.

Non-Hodgkin lymphoma: Diagnosis and management NICE guideline [NG52] Published date: 2016 Jul https://www.nice.org.uk/guidance/ng52

Swerdlow SH, Campo E, Pileri SA et al. The 2016 revision of the World Health Organization classification of lymphoid neoplasms. *Blood.* 2016; 127: 2375–2392.

Tilly H, Gomes da Silva M, Vitolo U et al. Diffuse large B-cell lymphoma (DLBCL): ESMO Clinical Practice Guidelines for diagnosis, treatment and follow-up. *Ann Oncol.* 2015 Sep; 26(Suppl 5): v116–v125.

SELF-ASSESSMENT QUESTIONS

1. Which of the following is true of Hodgkin lymphoma?
   a. It arises from immunoblasts
   b. It is most common in middle age
   c. It is associated with previous infection with EB virus
   d. It is common in Japan and the Caribbean
   e. There is an increased risk in identical and non-identical twins

2. Which of the following is true of the pathology of Hodgkin lymphoma?
   a. The cells stain with T-cell surface markers
   b. The presence of large binucleate cells is characteristic
   c. Extranodal sites are frequently involved
   d. Splenic involvement is rare
   e. The lymphocyte-depleted subgroup has the best prognosis

3. Which three of the following are typical in Hodgkin lymphoma?
   a. Alcohol-related pain
   b. Hypercalcaemia
   c. Eosinophilia
   d. Raised levels of α-fetoprotein (AFP)
   e. Anaemia
   f. Lymphocytosis
   g. Hypercalcaemia

4. Which of the following is *not* a routine staging investigation in Hodgkin lymphoma?
   a. CT scan of chest, abdomen and pelvis
   b. ESR
   c. Full blood count
   d. Bone marrow examination
   e. Liver function tests

5. In the treatment of Hodgkin lymphoma which of the following is true?
   a. The common chemotherapy includes high-dose steroids
   b. Radiotherapy alone is preferred for stage I and II disease
   c. Rituximab is added to combination chemotherapy
   d. Tumour lysis is common
   e. Late complications include secondary breast cancer

6. Which three of the following are important adverse prognostic factors in Hodgkin lymphoma?
   a. Age <45 years
   b. Male sex
   c. Haemoglobin <10.5 g/dL
   d. Serum albumin <40 g/dL
   e. B symptoms
   f. Lymphocytosis
   g. Mediastinal mass

7. Which of the following is true of non-Hodgkin lymphoma?
   a. It is less common than Hodgkin lymphoma
   b. It is most common in childhood
   c. In the stomach, may be associated with *Helicobacter* infection
   d. Is related to HTLV-I infection in China
   e. Is characterized by a translocation from chromosome 9 to 22

8. Which of the following is regarded as an indolent (low-grade) lymphoma?
   a. Burkitt lymphoma
   b. Follicular lymphoma
   c. Mantle cell lymphoma
   d. Peripheral T-cell lymphoma
   e. HTLV-associated T-cell lymphoma

Lymphoma

9. Which three facts about the treatment of non-Hodgkin lymphoma are true?
   a. The standard chemotherapy for aggressive disease is ABVD
   b. Rituximab improves results with chemotherapy for T-cell lymphomas
   c. Localized indolent lymphoma may be cured by radiotherapy alone
   d. MALToma of the stomach is best treated by surgical resection
   e. Stage IV follicular lymphoma may need no active treatment
   f. Mycosis fungoides is treated initially with amphotericin
   g. Lymphoblastic lymphoma is treated with acute leukaemia therapy

10. Which three of the following are adverse prognostic factors in aggressive types of non-Hodgkin lymphoma?
    a. Age
    b. Performance status
    c. Weight loss
    d. Haemoglobin
    e. Lymphocyte count
    f. Serum albumin
    g. Serum lactate dehydrogenase

Haematological malignancy

LEUKAEMIA

Neoplastic conditions of the haemtopoietic and lymphoid systems are closely related. Subclassifications of leukaemias and lymphomas tend to be complex but clinical management is usually based on a more simple and pragmatic division of leukaemias into acute or chronic, lymphoid or myeloid. There are around 9000 cases of leukaemia registered per year in the United Kingdom and these account for over 4000 deaths each year.

Acute leukaemia is subclassified by its cell of origin into two broad groups: lymphoblastic and myeloblastic. Chronic leukaemias are malignancies of cells that have differentiated beyond the blast stage. They are subdivided into chronic granulocytic leukaemia and chronic lymphocytic leukaemia. Despite their names, they do not necessarily have a more protracted natural history, and the prognosis for chronic leukaemia is overall no better than for acute leukaemia.

ACUTE LYMPHOBLASTIC LEUKAEMIA

EPIDEMIOLOGY

Each year in the United Kingdom there are almost 800 cases of acute lymphoblastic leukaemia (ALL) leading to 250 deaths per annum. ALL is less common than acute myeloid leukaemia, affecting males and females in equal proportions. It is predominantly a malignancy affecting children with over 40% occurring in the 2–5-year-old age group when it predominates in boys.

AETIOLOGY

Down's syndrome is associated with a higher incidence as are other less common genetic syndromes including neurofibromatosis, Bloom syndrome, Fanconi anaemia and ataxia telangiectasia.

Environmental agents, e.g. viruses, might be implicated. Clustering of cases in certain areas of the United Kingdom has been described. There is an increased incidence in affluent and industrialized areas but no specific environmental agent has been identified.

Chromosomal translocations have been identified: around 25% of B-cell ALL cases have a t(12;21)(p13;q22) translocation and more than 50% of T-cell ALL cases have mutations involving the *NOTCH1* gene involved in the regulation of normal T-cell development and which can potentiate the overexpression of the oncogene *c-myc*. The most frequent translocation in adults is t(9;22), the Philadelphia chromosome, which is also found in chronic myeloid leukaemia.

Radiation exposure might be implicated, although postradiation leukaemia is more commonly myeloblastic.

PATHOLOGY

Lymphoblastic leukaemia is characterized by the presence of large immature lymphoblasts throughout the reticuloendothelial system. These cells are distinguished from other cells such as

Table 17.1 Staining characteristics of acute lymphoblastic leukaemia compared with acute myeloid leukaemia

Type	PAS	TdT	Sudan black
ALL	+	+	−
AML	−	−	+

Abbreviation: PAS, periodic acid Schiff; TdT, terminal deoxyribonucleotidyl transferase.

myeloblasts by their staining, as presented in Table 17.1, although classification of leukaemias now has become much more sophisticated based on molecular profiling.

In addition to de novo ALL, up to 15% of cases represent transformation into an acute phase from chronic granulocytic leukaemia (CML). These are characterized by possessing the Philadelphia chromosome. Other chromosomal changes that may be identified and relate to a worse outcome are translocations affecting chromosome 4, t(4;11), deletions of chromosome 7 and trisomy 8.

Based on the molecular signature, the 2016 WHO classification lists nine subtypes of ALL with two other 'provisional' entities as follows:

- B-lymphoblastic leukaemia/lymphoma, not otherwise specified (NOS)
- B-lymphoblastic leukaemia/lymphoma with recurrent genetic abnormalities
- B-lymphoblastic leukaemia/lymphoma with t(9;22)(q34.1;q11.2); BCR-ABL1
- B-lymphoblastic leukaemia/lymphoma with t(v;11q23.3); KMT2A rearranged
- B-lymphoblastic leukaemia/lymphoma with t(12;21)(p13.2;q22.1); ETV6-RUNX1
- B-lymphoblastic leukaemia/lymphoma with hyperdiploidy
- B-lymphoblastic leukaemia/lymphoma with hypodiploidy
- B-lymphoblastic leukaemia/lymphoma with t(5;14)(q31.1;q32.3); IL3-IGH
- B-lymphoblastic leukaemia/lymphoma with t(1;19)(q23;p13.3); TCF3-PBX1
- Provisional entity: B-lymphoblastic leukaemia/lymphoma, BCR-ABL1–like
- Provisional entity: B-lymphoblastic leukaemia/lymphoma with iAMP21

NATURAL HISTORY

Progressive infiltration of the bone marrow and subsequent bone marrow failure ensue. It may also affect other sites, in particular the CNS, where diffuse meningeal infiltration can be seen, and the testes in males.

SYMPTOMS

Patients present with bone marrow failure, which results in:

- Malaise, lethargy, effort dyspnoea or angina owing to progressive anaemia
- Infection owing to leukopenia
- Bleeding in the form of epistaxis, haematuria or haemoptysis owing to thrombocytopenia

Bone pains can also be present. There are also general symptoms of malignancy including fever, sweats and weight loss.

SIGNS

These may include:

- Peripheral lymphadenopathy
- Splenomegaly
- Palpable liver
- Purpura, particularly on the lower limbs, and also other signs of recent haemorrhage from the nose or oral cavity
- Signs of infection, with fever and oropharyngeal or chest signs

DIFFERENTIAL DIAGNOSIS

Other types of acute leukaemia or high-grade non-Hodgkin lymphoma should be considered, as should other causes of pancytopenia, including aplastic anaemia. Infection with Epstein–Barr virus can give a similar picture, with abnormal blast cells seen in the peripheral blood.

INVESTIGATIONS

Blood count

A full blood count will show pancytopenia. The blood film will reveal the presence of lymphoblasts.

Erythrocyte sedimentation rate

The ESR will be raised.

Liver function

Liver function tests might be abnormal.

Radiography

Chest x-ray or CT scan can show evidence of leukaemic infiltration or more commonly infection. A mediastinal mass of lymph nodes might be seen.

Bone marrow examination

A bone marrow aspirate and trephine is required to confirm the diagnosis with an excess (>5%) of abnormal lymphoblasts. Specific stains will then be applied to subtype the cells into common, T, B or null ALL together with molecular profiling to complete full classification.

STAGING

There is no formal staging system for the leukaemias. However, the important features that determine prognosis are:

- Subtype, common ALL having a good prognosis
- Total white blood cell count, a total count of more than 20,000 being associated with a poor prognosis

Other favourable features are female sex, young age and the absence of a mediastinal mass.

TREATMENT

Treatment intensity is now based on risk stratification. The most important parameters in this are age above or below 10 years and total white cell count above or below 50,000. High WBC and older age groups represent higher risk and may demand more intensive treatment. CNS or testicular involvement at presentation is also a high-risk feature.

The treatment of acute leukaemias can be considered in three phases: induction, consolidation and maintenance. Alongside this, intensive supportive treatment might be necessary with blood products and antibiotics. In the United Kingdom, most centres will treat patients within the national UKALL protocols through which modifications to treatment schedules have been tested in prospective randomized studies.

Induction

Induction consists of vincristine and prednisolone and L-asparaginase and sometimes the addition of an anthracycline such as Adriamycin or daunorubicin and in high-risk cases an alkylating agent such as cyclophosphamide. Imatinib mesylate will be indicated in those patients with the t(9;22) translocation. Remission rates of >95% in children and 80%–90% in adults are achieved. Induction therapy will usually continue over a period of 8 weeks.

Consolidation (intensification)

This will be necessary once remission is achieved, i.e. when abnormal leukaemic cells are no longer detectable in the peripheral blood and bone marrow, to ensure eradication of any relatively resistant cells surviving the induction phase. Various drug schedules are in use including further exposure to the initial induction agents and high-dose methotrexate. Prophylactic treatment to the CNS will be included since this site accounts for 30%–40% of all relapses including intrathecal injections of methotrexate. The use of low-dose cranial irradiation (18 Gy) is also included in some protocols but omitted in others because of concerns over late toxicity to brain function.

Maintenance

Chemotherapy will continue beyond the intensification phase for a total of 2–3 years using methotrexate and mercaptopurine with the dose adjusted to bone marrow tolerance through regular blood count monitoring.

Bone marrow transplantation

High-dose chemotherapy with allogeneic (donor) stem cell or bone marrow transplantation is considered for poor-risk patients who achieve initial remission. This is particularly the case for adults who have a much worse prognosis from ALL than children, especially those with Philadelphia chromosome present on the leukaemic cells. Bone marrow transplantation is also indicated for children who relapse with bone marrow disease after initial chemotherapy.

Bone marrow transplantation is an intensive treatment which involves exposure of the patient to very high doses of chemotherapy, usually cyclophosphamide or melphalan, and whole body irradiation. This has the effect of completely ablating the bone marrow, which then has to be replaced. This may be from a matched donor (allograft) or from the patient's marrow previously collected and stored while in remission (autograft). The patient's marrow can be treated with monoclonal antibody techniques in an attempt to purge it further of residual leukaemic cells.

Intensive support is required for the period from marrow ablation to the re-establishment of the grafted marrow, which might be 3–4 weeks. During this time blood and platelet transfusions are required. Antibiotic prophylaxis is given with aggressive treatment of any febrile episode using high-dose broad-spectrum antibiotics for bacterial, viral and fungal infections. Despite this, even in experienced units, a mortality rate of around 5% is expected from the procedure, usually owing to neutropenic infection or pneumonitis. Mortality is in general related to age, and bone marrow transplantation is a hazardous undertaking in patients over the age of 50.

A further complication of allograft bone marrow transplantation is that of graft-versus-host disease in which the graft marrow reacts against the host tissues. This may manifest itself in a number of ways, most commonly through hepatic dysfunction, gastrointestinal disturbance and skin rashes. Various attempts have been made to reduce this event by treating the donor marrow to remove T lymphocytes, which are the principal cell type involved, and by the use of immunosuppressive agents such as methotrexate or azathioprine.

Relapse treatment

When ALL has failed to respond to first-line chemotherapy or has relapsed following initial treatment, the usual pattern of relapse is as with bone marrow disease. CNS relapse occurs in up to 10% of cases despite CNS prophylaxis and will require treatment with local irradiation and intrathecal therapy. Testicular relapse is also well recognized representing a further site where chemotherapy has poor penetration. It is treated with local irradiation.

Salvage chemotherapy takes the form of using standard induction chemotherapy as previously described with alternative drugs added such as cytosine arabinoside. For those with a matched donor available, bone marrow transplantation is indicated.

TUMOUR-RELATED COMPLICATIONS

Pancytopenia with consequent anaemia, leukopenia predisposing to infection and thrombocytopenia-related haemorrhage can occur.

TREATMENT-RELATED COMPLICATIONS

- Tumour lysis syndrome is a rare complication arising as a result of the breakdown of large numbers of lymphoid cells when chemotherapy is initiated, which is discussed in full in Chapter 21.
- Bone marrow suppression with a particular risk of neutropenic sepsis is also seen.
  - Adolescents in particular are at risk of osteonecrosis and pancreatitis.
- Bone marrow transplantation carries the added risks of graft-versus-host disease and prolonged immunosuppression.
- Total body irradiation during marrow transplantation can cause pneumonitis.
- CNS prophylaxis in young children could have effects on later intellectual development. Attempts are constantly being made to minimize this effect by reducing the dose and overall use of CNS irradiation.
- Testicular irradiation will result in sterility but not impotence.

PROGNOSIS

The prognosis for childhood ALL is age-related. In babies <12 months the cure rate is 44%, increasing in children aged 1–9 years to 88%; in adolescents aged 10–15 years it is 73% and for adults it falls to 69%. Philadelphia-positive ALL has a worse outcome than other types of ALL.

ACUTE MYELOID/MYELOBLASTIC LEUKAEMIA

EPIDEMIOLOGY

Each year in the United Kingdom there are 3000 cases of AML leading to a total of 2500 deaths per annum. AML has an incidence of 1 in 200 males and 1 in 250 females in the United Kingdom, affecting more males. In children, it is most common under the age of 4 years but is less common in children than ALL, accounting for 20% of childhood leukaemias. In adults, it is typically seen in the over 40 age group; 55% of cases are found in the over 70 age group and the highest incidence is in the over 85 age group.

AETIOLOGY

- *Radiation exposure*: Increased incidence of AML appeared in populations exposed to radiation after the nuclear explosions in Hiroshima and Nagasaki. After therapeutic or diagnostic use of radiation it is a rare but recognized event.
- *Chemotherapy agents*: These include, in particular, alkylating agents such as chlorambucil and procarbazine when AML is usually preceded by a period of myelodysplasia. Topoisomerase II inhibitors, of which etoposide is the most common example, are also associated with an increased incidence of secondary AML, typically not preceded by myelodysplasia and associated with a specific gene rearrangement affecting 11q23.
- *Environmental agents*: Benzene exposure has been associated with the development of AML.
- *Genetic predisposition*: An increase in Down syndrome, trisomy 8 and syndromes associated with defects in DNA repair including Bloom syndrome, ataxia telangiectasia and Fanconi anaemia is seen.

The vast majority of cases of AML (over 90%) have no clear association with environmental agents and appear to arise de novo.

PATHOLOGY

AML encompasses a much broader pathological spectrum of disease than ALL. The characteristics

Table 17.2 Subtypes of acute myeloid leukaemia

AML subtype	Cell type
M0	Undifferentiated myeloblastic
M1	Undifferentiated myeloblastic without maturation
M2	Differentiated myeloblastic
M3	Promyelocytic
M4	Myelomonocytic
M5	Monoblastic
M6	Erythroleukaemia
M7	Megakaryoblastic

of the myeloblast are positive staining with Sudan black and peroxidase stains. Eight subtypes based on morphological and cytochemical differences are now recognized; their features are outlined in Table 17.2. The common forms are M1 and M2.

Clinically, all these forms of AML behave in a similar manner. Around half of all patients with AML will have chromosomal abnormalities. Recognized changes include trisomy of chromosome 8, deletions affecting chromosome 5 or 7, abnormalities of chromosome 11 and FLT3 mutations, all of which are poor prognostic features. A more complex classification based on molecular profiling by the WHO defines the following subgroups:

- AML with recurrent genetic abnormalities
- AML with myelodysplasia-related features
- Therapy-related myeloid neoplasms
- AML, not otherwise specified
- Myeloid sarcoma
- Myeloid proliferations related to Down syndrome
- Blastic plasmacytoid dendritic cell neoplasm

An important difference in the definition of AML between the two classifications is that the WHO defines the disease with only 20% of blasts in the marrow compared to the previous requirement for 30%.

NATURAL HISTORY

There is progressive infiltration of the bone marrow with subsequent bone marrow failure. Testicular and CNS involvement is relatively rare. CNS involvement is most common in monoblastic AML. Extramedullary involvement is more common than with ALL, with infiltration of liver and spleen in over 50% and characteristic skin and gum infiltration in myelomonocytic and monoblastic leukaemias.

SYMPTOMS

Symptoms include bone marrow failure causing fatigue, recurrent infections and haemorrhage. There is also associated fever, sweats and weight loss. Scattered bone pains may also occur.

SIGNS

These may include:

- Signs of anaemia, bruising, purpura and recurrent infection
- Hepatosplenomegaly
- Lymphadenopathy (less common than in ALL)
- Gum hypertrophy with associated gum bleeding, particularly in myelomonocytic and monoblastic forms of AML

DIFFERENTIAL DIAGNOSIS

Other forms of acute leukaemia and non-Hodgkin lymphoma together with aplastic anaemia and myelofibrosis should be considered.

INVESTIGATIONS

Blood count

A full blood count will show pancytopenia with the presence of primitive blast cells on examination of the blood film.

Biochemistry

Routine biochemistry may show abnormalities in liver function owing to infiltration.

Radiography

Chest x-ray could show signs of infection or, more rarely, leukaemic infiltration.

Coagulation studies

There can be coagulation abnormalities, particularly with promyelocytic leukaemia associated with disseminated intravascular coagulation.

Bone marrow examination

The diagnosis will be confirmed on examination of the bone marrow and the subtype of AML determined by specific stains.

TREATMENT

Induction

This consists of chemotherapy in the form of daunorubicin and cytosine arabinoside. Some schedules have included a third drug such as thioguanine (DAT) or etoposide but the added value is uncertain. Complete regression can be achieved in up to 85% of patients on first exposure to these agents. It is highly dependent on age, the complete response rate in patients over 55 years of age falling to only 45% compared to 60%–70% in children.

Consolidation

Consolidation therapy in AML may be in the form of further chemotherapy for patients with good risk disease, and autograft transplant or allogeneic transplant for those with unfavourable features.

Chemotherapy will comprise high-dose cytosine arabinoside. Patients with CNS disease will also require cranial irradiation and intrathecal methotrexate but prophylactic CNS treatment is not generally recommended in contrast to that in ALL.

Allogeneic transplant is often used in high-risk cases with better outcomes from matched donor transplants than from sibling donors due to the positive effect of graft-versus-host disease. In other groups, it will be reserved for relapse.

In older adults, the toxicity and treatment-related mortality of such intensive treatment is often not feasible. Low-dose cytosine arabinoside or azacytidine is of value in this group with complete remission rates approaching 20%.

Maintenance therapy has not been shown to have great value in AML.

Relapse treatment

Relapse carries a poor prognosis; re-induction chemotherapy using cytosine arabinoside-based schedules or combination schedules with mitoxantrone, etoposide or cyclophosphamide followed by allogeneic transplantation for those under 55 years with an HLA-matched donor gives the best chance of salvage. Autologous transplant can be considered for older patients up to 65 years but is less effective.

TUMOUR-RELATED COMPLICATIONS

These include in particular the effects of pancytopenia including anaemia, susceptibility to infection and haemorrhage.

TREATMENT-RELATED COMPLICATIONS

Tumour lysis can occur with induction chemotherapy, and prophylaxis with fluids, allopurinol or rasburicase should be given. Chemotherapy is also associated with further bone marrow depression and, in particular, the risk of neutropenic sepsis. High-dose cytosine arabinoside may be associated with treatment-related deaths in 10%, especially in older patients. Bone marrow transplant has its own specific risks of infection, graft-versus-host disease, radiation-induced pneumonitis and treatment-related mortality ranging from 5% to 40% increasing with age.

PROGNOSIS

The prognosis for AML is not as good as for ALL but has improved considerably in recent years with the use of bone marrow transplantation. Overall, around 40% of all patients are cured of AML. Cure rates of around 50% are to be expected in those undergoing transplantation in first remission and 25% for those undergoing transplantation in the second remission. Prognosis is however closely related to age with only 25% of adult AML being cured overall compared to 50%–60% of cases in infants. The outlook is worse for older patients (>40 years) who have a lower rate of initial remission and are less able to tolerate intensive chemotherapy regimens or bone marrow transplantation.

Poor prognostic features at presentation include a high white cell count $>100 \times 10^9/L$ and disseminated intravascular coagulation associated with M3. Other features associated with a poor prognosis are AML secondary to previous treatment, previous myelodysplasia and CNS disease. The M0 and M7 subtypes have a worse prognosis as do those expressing CD34, bcl-2, monosomy 7, monosomy 5/del(5q), 3q abnormalities, and FLT3-ITD with a high-allelic ratio.

RARE TUMOURS

Promyelocytic leukaemia (M3) is characterized by the t(15;17) translocation. It is particularly sensitive to anthracyclines and to all-trans-retinoic acid (ATRA), which can alone induce remissions. Standard induction therapy will therefore include ATRA with cytosine arabinoside and daunorubicin. ATRA is also included in maintenance treatment with mercaptopurine for 2 years after induction. Cure rates of over 80% with these schedules are achieved.

Chloroma or isolated granulocytic sarcoma is a localized tumour of myeloblasts. Around two-thirds will progress to widespread AML; localized treatment with surgery or radiotherapy is not appropriate and these tumours should be treated as for AML.

SCREENING AND FUTURE PROSPECTS

Patients at risk of treatment-related AML, typically survivors from intensive chemotherapy treatment for germ cell tumours or lymphoma, are screened with regular examination of the peripheral blood.

CHRONIC MYELOCYTIC (GRANULOCYTIC) LEUKAEMIA

Each year in the United Kingdom there are 750 cases of CML leading to a total of over 200 deaths per annum.

CML increases in incidence with age; it is rarely diagnosed below the age of 30 and the median age is 60 years with the highest incidence in the over 85 age group. Its annual incidence in the United Kingdom is around 1 in 840 men and 1 in 1180 women.

AETIOLOGY

There are no recognized environmental agents, although an increased risk in those populations exposed to excess radiation has been documented.

PATHOLOGY

CML represents neoplastic proliferation of granulocyte precursors and is characterized by an excess of metamyelocytes and myelocytes in the peripheral blood. Promyelocytes and myeloblasts can also be present and often there is an excess of basophils and eosinophils.

Philadelphia chromosome is present in around 80% of patients, formed by a translocation from chromosome 9 to chromosome 22 or less frequently another chromosome. Additional chromosomal abnormalities frequently develop in the acute phase of CML (the blast crisis).

The translocated fragment from chromosome 9 is a proto-oncogene, *ABL*, which translocates to the breakpoint cluster region (BCR) of chromosome 22. This results in a chimeric fusion gene *BCR-ABL* which encodes for a protein having tyrosine kinase activity. This is outside the tight control mechanisms that govern the normal expression of *ABL*. The downstream events from this are related to both proliferation and apoptosis of haemtopoietic progenitor cells leading to a massive accumulation of myeloid cells.

NATURAL HISTORY

There are three phases to the disease: chronic, accelerated and blast phase. An initial indolent period typically lasting 3–5 years gives way to rapid progression leading to a fulminating blast crisis indistinguishable from an acute leukaemia but in general is less responsive to treatment.

Blast crisis is usually myeloblastic in type although lymphoblastic crises may occur. Occasionally, the blast crisis might be the first clinical manifestation of the disease when it can be distinguished from a de novo acute leukaemia by the presence of Philadelphia chromosome.

SYMPTOMS

Around 85% are diagnosed in the chronic phase and two-thirds of these will be asymptomatic detected on a blood test. In the remainder CML can present with:

- Symptoms of anaemia or thrombocytopenia owing to bone marrow failure
- Abdominal distension and discomfort from splenic enlargement which may be massive
- Bone pain
- General features of an active leukaemic process such as fever and weight loss and also itching
- Very high white count resulting in hyperviscosity of the blood causing confusion and headache
- Priapism

SIGNS

These may include:

- Clinical signs of anaemia and purpura
- Massive splenomegaly
- Hepatomegaly
- Lymphadenopathy – usually not prominent

DIFFERENTIAL DIAGNOSIS

Myelofibrosis can also present with a large spleen and pancytopenia. In the acute phase, differentiation between de novo acute leukaemia and blast crisis of CML can be difficult unless the preceding history is known, but can be resolved by the finding of Philadelphia chromosome.

INVESTIGATIONS

Blood count

The peripheral blood usually has a characteristic picture with a very high white blood cell count between 100 and 1000×10^9/L of which the majority will be metamyelocytes with other granulocyte precursors. This is usually associated with a mild thrombocytopenia and anaemia. Basophilia is also a characteristic finding.

Bone marrow examination

This will show a hypercellular picture with an excess of granulocyte precursors. Areas of myelosclerosis can also be seen. Philadelphia chromosome can be demonstrated in myeloid, erythroid and megakaryocytic cell lines.

Imaging

Abdominal ultrasound or CT scan will confirm the extent of hepatomegaly and splenomegaly.

Other investigations

Other characteristic abnormalities are a low leukocyte alkaline phosphatase and raised serum B12 and

B12 binding proteins. Blast crisis is characterized by the appearance of more primitive blast cells and on bone marrow these will comprise over 50% of the myeloid population.

TREATMENT

Chronic phase

Initial treatment is aimed at reducing the peripheral blood white cell count to $<15 \times 10^9$/L and to alleviate symptoms of splenomegaly.

Chemotherapy using imatinib mesylate, a specific inhibitor of the *BCR-ABL* tyrosine kinase, is now the treatment of choice. It is given orally as a single daily dose and with this after 12 months over 80% of newly diagnosed patients will be in cytogenetic remission. Treatment is continued indefinitely whilst in remission.

In patients failing to achieve remission with imatinib, defined by the detection of BCR-ABL1 transcripts >10% at 3 months, second-line treatment with an alternative TKI such as dasatinib or nilotinib will be considered.

In patients who have BCR-ABL1 transcript levels >10% after 6 months of second-line therapy, an HLA-matched donor allogeneic transplantation is recommended.

Older patients and those with no donor can be considered for autologous transplant procedures.

The traditional treatments for CML – busulphan, hydroxyurea and α-interferon – are now only used in those with advanced disease refractory to imatinib and unfit for intensive chemotherapy.

Splenic irradiation is useful in the palliation of local symptoms from a large spleen and the effects of hypersplenism in disease refractory to chemotherapy.

Leukapheresis will achieve rapid reduction of very high white cell counts. The patient's blood is passed through a cell separator, being returned through a continuous flow into a second intravenous cannula. This results on average in a 35% reduction in white cell count with each procedure, and also has the advantage of providing large numbers of redundant granulocytes, which can be used for therapeutic transfusion in other patients. However, no effect on the natural history of the CML process is achieved by regular leukapheresis and it is therefore generally used only when hyperviscosity is a predominant feature.

Acute phase

The treatment of the blast crisis is essentially that of the acute leukaemia into which the CML transforms. In around 70% this will be an AML, around 5% may have a mixed picture and the remaining 25% will manifest ALL. As with de novo acute leukaemia, an ALL blast crisis has a better prognosis with around 40% of patients reverting to a chronic phase with simple induction therapy such as vincristine and prednisolone. Bone marrow transplantation could be of value in those patients achieving remission from their acute phase.

TUMOUR-RELATED COMPLICATIONS

There might be bone marrow failure resulting in anaemia, reduced resistance to infection and a bleeding tendency from thrombocytopenia. This can be exacerbated by the effects of gross splenomegaly, causing the phenomenon of hypersplenism with pooling of blood within the large spleen. Massive splenomegaly can also cause local pain and might impair gastric emptying. Local areas of infarction can occur within the spleen, causing acute pain.

Large numbers of white cells in the circulation can cause hyperviscosity with headache, confusion, visual disturbance and priapism.

TREATMENT-RELATED COMPLICATIONS

Imatinib results in bone marrow depression and close monitoring of the peripheral blood count is required; titrating the dose is necessary in the first few weeks of administration. Tumour lysis is seen on rare occasions and prophylactic cover with fluids and allopurinol is important. Other side effects from imatinib include nausea, muscle cramps, and fluid retention causing periorbital and peripheral oedema.

Splenic irradiation or surgical splenectomy can be hazardous because of thrombocytopenia and a subsequent predisposition to infection, particularly pneumococcal pneumonia.

PROGNOSIS

The use of imatinib and second-line TKI drugs has made a dramatic change to the survival chances in patients with CML. The 5-year survival in patients in the chronic phase under 70 years of age is now similar to that of the age-matched population. The principal cause of death is acute blast crisis, particularly in older patients for whom intensive treatment is not appropriate. Prognostic indices use age, platelet count, splenomegaly and peripheral blast counts to define good, intermediate and poor-risk groups and molecular response to first-line TKI exposure.

FUTURE PROSPECTS

Further developments are related to new more active TKI agents currently in clinical trials.

CHRONIC LYMPHOCYTIC LEUKAEMIA

Each year in the United Kingdom there are 3700 cases of CLL leading to a total of 1000 deaths per annum. CLL represents the end of the leukaemic spectrum where the classification merges with that of non-Hodgkin lymphoma. CLL is a neoplastic proliferation of the same cell type as lymphocytic lymphoma, the differentiating feature being the extent of bone marrow infiltration.

EPIDEMIOLOGY

CLL affects a somewhat older age group than CML, with 60% diagnosed in the over 70 age group. The incidence in men is 1 in 155 and in women 1 in 250.

AETIOLOGY

The only specific aetiological agent relates to the use of herbicides in agricultural workers and an association with exposure to Agent Orange as used in the Vietnam War has been confirmed. No other environmental factors for the common form of CLL seen in Europe and North and South America have been recognized.

First-degree relatives are three times more likely than the general population to also develop CLL or another lymphoid malignancy.

Around half of all patients with CLL have demonstrable chromosomal abnormalities. The most common of these is a deletion on chromosome 13q seen in 55%, trisomy of chromosome 12 in 18% and a deletion on chromosome 11q in 16%.

The rarer T-cell variant can be associated with HTLV-I infection, as found in Japan and the Caribbean.

PATHOLOGY

The cell of origin for CLL is in most cases a B lymphocyte, although in 5% there might be markers of T-cell origin. The B-cell type will demonstrate surface immunoglobulin, which may be either kappa or lambda, and the surface antigens CD5, CD19, CD20 and CD23. The characteristic finding in the peripheral blood is a large number of mature lymphocytes with a total lymphocyte count of $>5 \times 10^9/L$ being required to confirm the diagnosis. This is associated with bone marrow infiltration by immature lymphocytes, which should account for more than 30% of the total marrow. Three patterns of marrow involvement have been described: interstitial, nodular or diffuse. As with non-Hodgkin lymphomas, diffuse appearance is associated with a worse prognosis than the more focal forms.

NATURAL HISTORY

The natural history spans many years. Ultimately, death occurs usually owing to bone marrow failure or to transformation into a high-grade lymphoma.

SYMPTOMS

CLL can be asymptomatic for many years sometimes. When symptoms do appear they include:

- Painless lymphadenopathy
- Anaemia
- Recurrent infections
- Fever, sweats and weight loss

SIGNS

These include:

- Peripheral lymphadenopathy
- Splenomegaly
- Hepatomegaly – usually only mild

INVESTIGATIONS

Blood count

A full blood count will reveal anaemia, thrombocytopenia and a high total white cell count, which on examination of the blood film consists of predominantly small, round lymphocytes.

Bone marrow examination

This will confirm the diagnosis with the finding of excess lymphoid cells, at least 30% of which will be immature forms.

Biopsy

Lymph node biopsy can be performed and will show the infiltration of involved nodes with well-differentiated lymphocytes, usually in a diffuse pattern.

Other tests

Hypogammaglobulinaemia is a common association. Haemolytic anaemia might be associated with CLL with elevated conjugated bilirubin and a positive Coombs test. In HTLV-associated CLL, hypercalcaemia and hyponatraemia are characteristic features.

DIFFERENTIAL DIAGNOSIS

Other small-cell non-Hodgkin lymphoma should be considered, particularly mantle cell and lymphoplasmacytic subtypes.

STAGING

There are two staging systems in use: the Rai and the Binet system; both are similar and classify patients into good, intermediate and poor risk (Table 17.3).

Table 17.3 Rai classification for chronic lymphocytic leukaemia

Stage	Features	Risk
0	Lymphocytosis in blood and marrow	Good
I	Lymphocytosis and enlarged nodes	Good
II	Lymphocytosis and large spleen/liver	Intermediate
III	Lymphocytosis and anaemia	Poor
IV	Lymphocytosis and thrombocytopenia	Poor

TREATMENT

Because CLL has a long indolent course and most patients present with no clinical signs or symptoms but simply an abnormal blood count, treatment is considered only when patients are symptomatic or when there are signs of bone marrow failure in the presence of very high peripheral white cell counts. No benefit to earlier treatment in the asymptomatic patient has been demonstrated.

When treatment is required, the standard chemotherapy schedules are based on fludarabine and alkylating agents; a common schedule is FCR (fludarabine, cyclophosphamide and rituximab). Ibrutinib is a new agent with TKI activity which may replace these older drugs as first-line CLL treatment. Steroids can also be used and are of value when the disease becomes refractory to alkylating agents, but there is no evidence that adding them to chemotherapy in the early management of the disease is of value. In refractory disease cladribine, ofatumumab, an anti CD20 antibody, or alemtuzumab, an anti CD52 monoclonal antibody with profound antilymphocyte activity may be used.

Low-dose irradiation will result in rapid shrinkage of enlarged node masses or splenomegaly. Doses as low as 20 or 30 Gy over 2–3 weeks are usually sufficient and associated with little or no morbidity.

Currently, stem-cell autograft and bone marrow transplantation has no established role in CLL.

TUMOUR-RELATED COMPLICATIONS

The associated hypogammaglobulinaemia results in a high incidence of infections.

There can be chronic anaemia, which can have a haemolytic component requiring regular transfusions. Thrombocytopenia may also persist.

The rare HTLV-related CLL is sometimes associated with hypercalcaemia.

TREATMENT-RELATED COMPLICATIONS

Oral alkylating agents are usually relatively trouble free, provided careful attention is paid to the blood count and treatment stopped when there are signs of significant bone marrow depression. Fludarabine may exacerbate haemolytic anaemia.

With a large tumour burden there is always the possibility of provoking hyperuricaemia owing to cell lysis on initiation of chemotherapy. This should be prevented by the administration of allopurinol and ensuring adequate fluid intake.

PROGNOSIS

While remissions are usually readily achieved in CLL, cures are rare. Many patients will live with their disease for several years, the median survival being around 8–12 years, with many patients having had the disease for some years before diagnosis.

The HTLV-associated T-cell form of CLL is a far more aggressive disease, however, and some patients succumb within a few months, although a more chronic form similar to sporadic CLL is also seen.

Other poor prognostic features are CD38 positivity, ZAP 70 positivity and chromosomes 12, 11q- and 17p-.

RARER FORMS OF LEUKAEMIA

PROLYMPHOCYTIC LEUKAEMIA

This is related to CLL, presenting in elderly men with splenomegaly and very high white cell counts. The cells are larger than the mature lymphocytes seen in CLL and the disease has a more aggressive course.

HAIRY CELL LEUKAEMIA

This is a chronic leukaemia occurring in the middle aged and is more frequent in men than women, sometimes classified as a variant of CLL, distinguished immunohistochemically by cells that are positive for CD19 and 25 but negative for CD5. It is rare, accounting for around 2% of all cases of adult leukaemia. Typically, it presents with massive splenomegaly and pancytopenia. The characteristic finding is of 'hairy cells' in the peripheral blood and bone marrow. These are B lymphocytes with cytoplasmic projections giving them a 'hairy' appearance under the microscope.

Hairy cell leukaemia usually has a long indolent course. It responds to treatment with interferon with which it may remain in remission for many years before it becomes resistant and bone marrow failure develops. The new purine analogue drugs pentostatin and cladribine are also highly active in this disease and can be used instead of interferon.

MULTIPLE MYELOMA

EPIDEMIOLOGY

Each year in the United Kingdom there are 5500 cases of multiple myeloma leading to a total of around 3000 deaths per annum. The incidence has increased by almost 15% in the last decade.

Almost half of the cases are diagnosed in the over 75 age group; the incidence in men is 1 in 115 and in women 1 in 155. It is more common in black than in white or Asian people.

AETIOLOGY

There are no recognized aetiological agents for multiple myeloma. An increased risk in those exposed to excess radiation after the atomic bombing and in radiologists prior to formal radiation protection has been seen. It has been suggested that the origin of the paraprotein production could be as a host antibody response to a foreign protein but no consistent antigen has been identified.

PATHOLOGY

Multiple myeloma is one of a spectrum of plasma cell neoplasms ranging from benign monoclonal gammopathy through solitary plasmacytoma to multiple myeloma. All these conditions are characterized by a neoplastic proliferation of B cells producing a characteristic paraprotein. Transformation within this group of conditions is well recognized, with around 20% of benign monoclonal gammopathies and 60% of apparent solitary plasmacytomas eventually developing multiple myeloma.

Cytogenetic abnormalities are found in around 50% but no single characteristic change is recognized. The most common is found in the *14q32* gene locus but many others have also been reported.

Deletion of 13q-14 and deletion of 17p13 are poor prognostic features.

NATURAL HISTORY

Three phases in the evolution of multiple myeloma have been described, but not all will be seen in an individual patient:

- Monoclonal gammopathy
- Smouldering myeloma, which is usually asymptomatic with low levels of paraprotein and 10%–20% plasma cells in bone marrow
- Typical myeloma, with symptoms, rising paraprotein levels and >20% plasma cells in bone marrow

Once established, myeloma affects the bone marrow, bones and kidneys. Bone invasion is facilitated by the release of chemicals, which act as osteoclast-activating factors, including interleukins (in particular IL-1 and IL-6), tumour necrosis factor (TNF) and macrophage colony-stimulating factor (MCSF). Renal damage occurs from the deposition of paraprotein and amyloid formation, hypercalcaemia and hyperuricaemia.

SYMPTOMS

Symptoms of multiple myeloma typically present in three ways:

- Bone marrow infiltration causes anaemia; thrombocytopenia is usually not prominent but more commonly there may be a bleeding disorder owing to the effects of macroglobulinaemia
- Bone destruction results in local pain, pathological fracture or neurological complications such as nerve root or spinal cord compression – bone pain is present in two-thirds of patients presenting with myeloma
- Metabolic and biochemical disturbance occurs, including:
  - High levels of paraprotein causing hyperviscosity, resulting in confusion and headache
  - Renal failure, which is present in around one-third of patients as defined by a raised blood urea and creatinine causing nausea, vomiting, malaise, fluid retention or itching
  - Hypercalcaemia, which is present in around one-third of patients who present with myeloma resulting in thirst, polyuria, dyspepsia, nausea, vomiting, constipation or confusion

SIGNS

Clinical signs of myeloma can be few. Patients might be clinically anaemic and bone lesions present as locally tender or even swollen areas. There can be rib or spinal tenderness.

Patients presenting with pathological fracture will have obvious signs of swelling, tenderness and deformity.

Cord compression can present with weakness of the lower limbs, sphincter disturbance and neurological signs of an upper motor neuron lesion. In contrast, cauda equina compression from disease in the lumbosacral spine will result in lower motor neuron weakness.

Hyperviscosity causes confusion. Papilloedema and retinal haemorrhage are also described.

DIFFERENTIAL DIAGNOSIS

There are few conditions outside the spectrum of plasma cell neoplasms that will mimic myeloma; however, there are rare forms of non-Hodgkin lymphoma that may produce high levels of paraprotein and cause initial confusion.

Waldenström macroglobulinaemia (lymphoplasmacytic lymphoma) will also present with a paraprotein but none of the other features of myeloma and must be distinguished from benign monoclonal gammopathy (see Chapter 16).

Other causes of bone metastases including primary tumours of the breast, lung, thyroid and prostate should be considered.

Patients who present with a solitary plasma cell lesion might have a true solitary plasmacytoma as shown in Figure 17.1, but 60%–70% will eventually manifest the characteristic features of widespread multiple myeloma, particularly when it is found in a bone site.

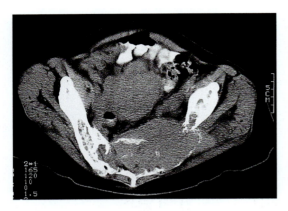

Figure 17.1 Solitary plasmacytoma arising in the ilium showing large soft-tissue mass and bone destruction. This patient has an associated plasma paraprotein but no evidence of other sites of bone involvement and a normal bone marrow.

INVESTIGATIONS

BLOOD COUNT

A full blood count can show anaemia and the ESR will be raised. The blood film might have rouleaux formation.

BIOCHEMISTRY

Biochemical tests will show a raised total protein and there might be hypercalcaemia, renal failure with raised urea and creatinine and hyperuricaemia.

PROTEIN ELECTROPHORESIS

This will demonstrate the characteristic M band containing the paraprotein, which can also be quantitatively measured. These will be an IgG in around 50% of patients, IgA in 20%, IgM in 10% and light chain in only 10%. Other rare types of paraprotein include IgD (2%) and heavy chain fragments (1%). In 1% of patients there might be two different M proteins and in 1% the paraprotein may be absent.

SERUM β_2-MICROGLOBULIN

Serum β_2-microglobulin is also raised in many patients and is an important marker of disease both for prognosis and for monitoring treatment.

URINE TESTS

Proteinuria could be present and, on electrophoresis of the urine, Bence–Jones protein might be detected.

BONE MARROW EXAMINATION

This will show infiltration with plasma cells; infiltration with more than 20% plasma cells is diagnostic.

RADIOGRAPHY AND SCANS

An x-ray skeletal survey might show lytic bone lesions, many of which are asymptomatic. Typical appearances of lesions on the x-ray of the skull are shown in Figure 17.2. Because the bone metastases of myeloma are usually predominantly lytic with little osteoblastic reaction, they often do not show on isotope bone scan or might be seen as cold areas rather than hot spots. MRI will also demonstrate bone lesions well, and whole skeleton MRI is an alternative staging investigation where available (Figure 17.3). FDG PET is also increasingly used as a staging investigation to provide a more sensitive evaluation of the whole skeleton.

OTHER TESTS

Other investigations can be considered where indicated, including plasma viscosity, plasma volume and rectal biopsy for amyloid.

STAGING

A number of criteria for the diagnosis of myeloma have been defined:

- 1: Presence of a monoclonal 'M' protein in serum or urine
- 2: Bone lesions owing to a plasma cell infiltrate
- 3: Marrow plasma cells accounting for >10% of marrow infiltrate
- 4: Associated features: anaemia, hypercalcaemia or renal failure

Diagnosis is confirmed on demonstration of any two of criteria 1–3.

Staging of myeloma is based on recognized prognostic factors, which include haemoglobin,

Multiple myeloma

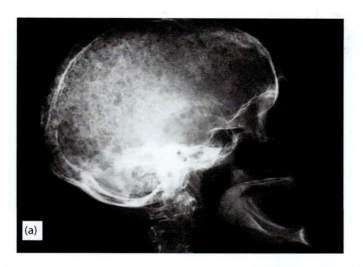

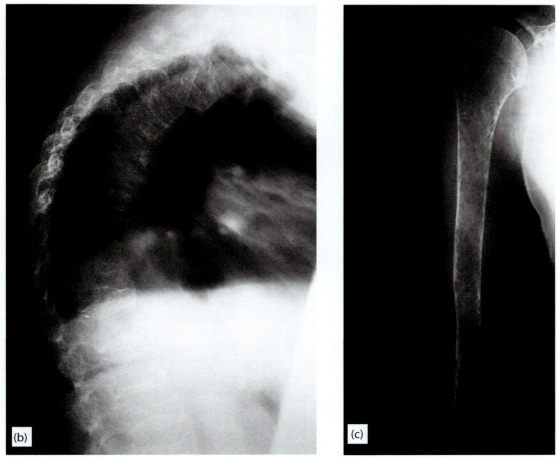

Figure 17.2 X-rays of (a) skull, (b) spine and (c) humerus, showing multiple lytic bone deposits of myeloma.

Haematological malignancy

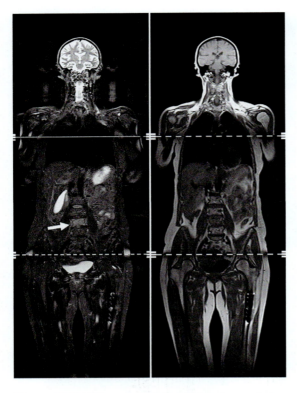

Figure 17.3 MRI scan of whole skeleton demonstrating lytic lesions of multiple myeloma in spine (arrowed) and surgical fixation of pathological fracture of the left femur.

blood urea, serum calcium, extent of bone lesions and level of paraprotein. The original classification was the Durie–Salmon staging system:

- *Stage 1*: Hb >10 g/dL
  - Calcium normal
  - Normal bone skeletal survey (or solitary plasmacytoma)
  - Low serum and urine paraprotein (serum IgG <6 g/dL; IgA <3 g/dL; urine <4 g/24 hr).
- *Stage 2*: Neither stage 1 nor stage 3
- *Stage 3*: Hb <8.5 g/dL
  - Calcium >12 mg/dL (3 mmol/l)
  - Multiple lytic bone lesions
  - High paraprotein levels (serum IgG >7 g/dL; IgA >5 g/dL; urine>12 g/24 hr)

There is a further subclassification into 'A' (normal renal function) or 'B' (raised serum creatinine).

This has now been superceded by the International Staging System:

- *Stage I*: β_2-microglobulin <3.5 mg/L and albumin ≥3.5 g/dL
- *Stage II*: Not R-ISS I or III
- *Stage III*: β_2-microglobulin ≥5.5 mg/L and either high LDH or high-risk chromosomal abnormalities by I-FISH (immunostaining fluorescence *in situ* hybridization) [defined as presence of deletion (17p) and/or translocation t(4;14) and/or translocation t(14;16)].

TREATMENT

Solitary lesions (true plasmacytomas) are treated with local radiotherapy alone.

Asymptomatic patients with no lytic bone lesions and normal renal function can be observed monitoring haemoglobin and paraprotein.

The remaining patients will require treatment with chemotherapy and, where indicated, radiotherapy to sites of painful bone lesions.

Four components to the treatment of myeloma can be identified:

- Induction
- Consolidation
- Maintenance
- Supportive

CHEMOTHERAPY FOR MYELOMA

The mainstay of initial induction chemotherapy is now a three-drug regime such as cyclophosphamide, bortezomib and dexamethasone; lenalidomide may be substituted for cyclophosphamide.

- Consolidation with autologous stem-cell transplant should then be offered to younger patients who are fit for the high-dose chemotherapy option; this will usually be those up to 65 years who have no other co-morbidities. Initial chemotherapy will comprise a combination of idarubicin and high-dose dexamethasone (Z-DEX) or cyclophosphamide, Adriamycin, vincristine and dexamethasone. Responding patients will then proceed to a stem-cell harvest and high-dose BEAM

(BCNU, etoposide, cytosine arabinoside, methyl prednisolone) chemotherapy followed by stem-cell reinfusion.
- Maintenance therapy will take the form of thalidomide, lenalidomide or bortezomib.
- Less intensive oral chemotherapy may be offered to older (>70 years) patients or those with other co-morbidities that would exclude them from a high-dose chemotherapy. The current schedule of choice is a combination of melphalan or cyclophosphamide, dexamethasone and thalidomide (MDT or CDT).

SUPPORTIVE TREATMENT

Alongside chemotherapy, management of the complications of myeloma will have a considerable impact on both the quality of life and the survival of the patient.

- Anaemia will require blood transfusion.
- Infections will require prompt treatment with appropriate antibiotics.
- Hypercalcaemia will require active hydration, diuresis and the use of bisphosphonates.
- Renal failure will require management of fluid balance and, in severe cases, dialysis, pending definitive chemotherapy, may be justified.
- Adjuvant bisphosphonate therapy (clodronate, pamidronate or zolendronate) has been shown to reduce the likelihood of complications such as pathological fracture owing to bone deposits and is given routinely.
- Pathological fracture will require internal fixation followed by local radiotherapy.
- Spinal canal compression will require steroids and urgent radiotherapy or surgical spinal stabilization.
- Active rehabilitation is also important as immobility is a further adverse prognostic factor.

RELAPSE TREATMENT

Treatment on relapse will depend on initial management. Further response induction should be attempted with bortezomib. Alternative approaches in patients having relapsed on bortezomid include one of the high-dose dexamethasone-based schedules (Z-DEX or CVAD) or further exposure to alkylating agent-based schedules with thalidomide or lenalidomide.

A second autograft procedure should be considered in those who achieve a second remission and have had a response duration of over 12 months from their first autograft. In young patients allogeneic transplant may be considered.

TUMOUR-RELATED COMPLICATIONS

These have been covered under the section 'Supportive treatment'.

TREATMENT-RELATED COMPLICATIONS

Chemotherapy will cause bone marrow depression and the blood count must be carefully monitored with aggressive treatment of neutropenic infections. This is particularly the case when high-dose therapy is given where there will be a period of 2–3 weeks when the patient is pancytopenic.

Steroid infusions can cause Cushingoid symptoms and, particularly in the elderly, fluid retention, causing cardiac failure.

PROGNOSIS

Between 2000 and 2010 there was an increase in 5-year relative survival in myeloma from around 30% to 40%. In younger patients having intensive therapy, median survivals of 4–5 years are now seen with 33% of patients now surviving more than 10 years.

Increasing age, poor renal function and a high β_2-microglobulin are associated with a poor prognosis with survival of less than 1 year.

Those with solitary plasmacytoma in a site other than bone, usually in the head and neck region, have the best prognosis with progression to myeloma being unusual; plasmacytoma in bone will progress to myeloma in 55% of patients with a further 10% developing multiple lesions confined to the skeleton.

Haematological malignancy

CASE HISTORY

MULTIPLE MYELOMA

A 68-year-old man presents to his GP with a 3-month history of increasing back pain. His GP elicits local tenderness in the thoracolumbar spine and sends him for an x-ray. This showed scattered lytic abnormalities in the vertebral bodies and it is commented that similar lesions are seen in adjacent ribs taken on the thoracic spine views. His GP proceeds to take blood for a full blood count, ESR, biochemical profile and paraproteins. A urine sample is tested at the local surgery and found to be positive for protein. A further sample is therefore sent to the pathology laboratory for detection of Bence–Jones proteins. In addition to this being positive he is found to have a paraprotein consisting of an immunoglobulin G with a level 48 g/L. His other tests show that he is mildly anaemic with a haemoglobin of 10.3 but his other blood count parameters are normal. His ESR is 97 mm/hr. His urea is marginally elevated at 7.5 with a serum creatinine of 160 µmol/L. Serum calcium and other biochemical parameters are normal. He is referred to the haemato-oncology clinic. Further investigations performed there include an FDG CT PET scan that shows scattered bone lesions, and his bone marrow is reported as consisting of 35% plasma cells. A formal diagnosis of multiple myeloma is confirmed.

He is started on treatment with bortezomib and dexamethasone. He finds this treatment is surprisingly easy to take but does note that he is feeling tired and has developed some tingling in his fingers and toes, which he was told are recognized side effects. He also attends every 3 weeks for intravenous zolendronate infusions.

His paraprotein level falls satisfactorily and after his third month of treatment it has reached 12 g/L. Over the next 2 months he continues with his treatment but no further change in the paraprotein level is seen and, his paraproteins having reached a plateau, chemotherapy is discontinued and he is started on maintenance therapy with oral lenalidomide. He also continues the 3-weekly zolendronate infusions.

He remains well for the next 8 months, seen occasionally in the clinic. A slow rise in his paraproteins is observed and, whilst out walking, he stumbles and develops severe pain in the right thigh; he is unable to weight bear and is brought to the accident and emergency department where an x-ray confirms a pathological fracture through a lytic area of myeloma in the femur. The orthopaedic team perform internal fixation with an intramedullary nail and he makes a good post-operative recovery, being mobile with sticks when he is discharged 2 weeks later. He is then referred to the radiotherapy department and a short 5-day course of radiotherapy is given to the femur covering the site of fracture.

He makes a good recovery but investigations in the haematology clinic reveal a further rise in the paraprotein to 46 g/L, a rising creatinine which has reached 230 µmol/L and a fall in his haemoglobin to 8.2 g/dL. His myeloma is clearly progressing and he is offered further chemotherapy with idarubicin and dexamethasone. Once again after 6 months of treatment his paraprotein stabilizes at around 15 g/L, he maintains his haemoglobin steady at around 10 g/dL and his renal function is stable with only mild impairment.

A paraprotein level measured 6 months later again starts to show a slight rise and when seen 2 months later he is complaining of some new back pain. X-rays show that he still has quite extensive lytic abnormalities in the bone. When seen at the end of the first month of restarting treatment his back pain is becoming more and more troublesome and he is referred for local radiotherapy. He attends the radiotherapy department and receives a single treatment to the thoracolumbar spine treating the painful area. That night he has quite troublesome nausea despite the dose of steroids and ondansetron given to him at the time of radiotherapy treatment. This, however, settles over the next 24 hours when he takes regular metoclopramide tablets. He notices little change in the pain over the first few days but after 10 days there has been some gradual improvement and 2 weeks later he is left with a mild ache but otherwise untroubled by the previous pain.

When seen in the clinic, however, 2 weeks later it is noted that his paraprotein is continuing to rise. He is offered further chemotherapy with a combination of cyclophosphamide, dexamethasone and thalidomide.

He remains well again for a period of 8 months. He returns to the clinic complaining of general malaise and lack of energy. It is found that his haemoglobin has fallen to 8.6 and his white cell count is only 2.9 with a neutrophil count of 1.2. His platelet count is 112. His paraprotein level has risen once more to 42 g/L. He is given a 3-unit blood transfusion. The role of further chemotherapy is discussed with him and he is told that it is unlikely he will get a long response to further treatment but he is anxious to try further alternatives and is entered into a clinical trial of an new agent, pomalidomide. After the first month his paraprotein and haemoglobin levels stabilized. After the third month of pomalidomide he reports swelling of his left calf. He is seen in the Acute Assessment Unit of his local hospital and Doppler ultrasound confirms an extensive deep venous thrombosis of the femoropopliteal veins, despite having been on prophylactic anticoagulants. This is a recognized complication of this class of drugs. He is admitted to the ward and an IVC filter is inserted.

The next week he stumbles whilst coming down stairs at home and has severe pain in the left hip following which he can no longer weight bear. An ambulance is called and he is admitted through the acute admissions unit. X-rays show that he has a pathological fracture of the left femur through a large lytic lesion. Following admission he develops a temperature and a productive cough. His blood count shows that, whilst the erythropoietin has maintained his haemoglobin, his white cell count has fallen with a neutrophil count of 0.9. He is started on intravenous antibiotics. His chest infection, however, progresses with signs of widespread pneumonia. Three days later he has become semiconscious and confused with widespread signs of bronchopneumonia on his chest x-ray. His serum creatinine has risen to 380 µmol/L. The role of further antibiotics is discussed with his family who agree that in this circumstance it is unlikely to improve the situation and they are discontinued. He lapses into unconsciousness and dies peacefully over the next 24 hours.

FURTHER READING

Alvarnas JC, Brown PA, Aoun P et al. Acute lymphoblastic leukemia, version 2.2015. *J Natl Compr Canc Netw*. 2015 Oct; 13(10): 1240–79

BMJ Best Practice: Acute lymphocytic leukaemia. https://bestpractice.bmj.com/topics/en-gb/273

BMJ Best Practice: Acute myelogenous leukaemia https://bestpractice.bmj.com/topics/en-gb/274

BMJ Best Practice: Chronic lymphocytic leukaemia https://bestpractice.bmj.com/topics/en-gb/275

BMJ Best Practice: Chronic myelogenous leukaemia https://bestpractice.bmj.com/topics/en-gb/276

Myeloma diagnosis and management https://www.nice.org.uk/guidance/ng35 (2016)

Radich JP, Deininger M, Abboud CN et al. Chronic myeloid leukemia, version 1.2019, NCCN clinical practice guidelines in oncology. *J Natl Compr Canc Netw*. 2018 Sep; 16(9): 1108–1135

Schuh AH, Parry-Jones N, Appleby N et al. Guideline for the treatment of chronic lymphocytic leukaemia: A British Society for Haematology guideline. *Br J Haematol*. 2018 Aug; 182(3): 344–359

Tallman MS, Wang ES, Altman JK et al. Acute myeloid leukemia, version 3.2019, NCCN clinical practice guidelines in oncology. *J Natl Compr Canc Netw*. 2019 Jun 1; 17(6): 721–749.

Tsang RW, Campbell BA, Goda JS et al. Radiation therapy for solitary plasmacytoma and multiple myeloma: Guidelines from the International Lymphoma Radiation Oncology Group. *Int J Radiat Oncol Biol Phys*. 2018; 101(4): 794–808.

SELF-ASSESSMENT QUESTIONS

1. Which of the following is true of acute lymphoblastic leukaemia (ALL)?
   a. It is most common in girls over 5 years of age
   b. It is increased in incidence in Down syndrome
   c. The T-cell type may exhibit the t(12;21)(p13;q22) translocation
   d. Exhibits Philadelphia chromosome when it develops in CLL
   e. Is characterized by cells which stain positive with Sudan black

2. Which three of the following are common presenting features of ALL?
   a. Anaemia
   b. Gum hypertrophy
   c. Purpura
   d. Peripheral neuropathy

Haematological malignancy

   e. Erythema nodosum
   f. Fever
   g. Diarrhoea

3. Which of the following is true of the treatment of ALL?
   a. Induction treatment will include cranial irradiation
   b. Vincristine and prednisolone are used in induction
   c. Consolidation will be given with bone marrow transplant
   d. There is no role for maintenance treatment once remission is achieved
   e. Testicular irradiation will cause impotence

4. Which of the following is true of acute myeloid leukaemia (AML)?
   a. It accounts for 50% of childhood leukaemias
   b. The common form is the M3 subtype
   c. Involvement of soft tissues is less common than in ALL
   d. Disseminated intravascular coagulation occurs in the M1 subtype
   e. The presence of *11q23* gene rearrangement is seen after etoposide

5. In the treatment of AML, which of the following is true?
   a. Induction is usually with vincristine, prednisolone and daunorubicin
   b. Consolidation includes bone marrow transplant for high-risk cases
   c. Intrathecal methotrexate is an important component of induction
   d. Response increases with age beyond 40 years
   e. AML secondary to myelodysplasia has a better prognosis than de novo

6. Which of the following is true of chronic granulocytic leukaemia (CML)?
   a. The incidence increases with age
   b. Translocation from chromosome 9 to 22 is seen in 80% of patients
   c. Massive hepatomegaly is characteristic
   d. There may be preceding myelofibrosis
   e. The blood film will show an excess of neutrophils

7. Which three of the following are true of the treatment of CML?
   a. Imatinib mesylate is an inhibitor of tyrosine kinase
   b. Patients with hyperviscosity may require leukapheresis
   c. Intrathecal methotrexate is used in induction
   d. Interferon is used to improve the response rates to chemotherapy
   e. Up to 15% of patients will never require treatment
   f. Thrombocytosis is a poor prognostic feature
   g. Blast crisis should be treated as an acute leukaemia

8. Which of the following is characteristic of chronic lymphocytic leukaemia (CLL)?
   a. Gum hypertrophy
   b. Joint pains
   c. Massive splenomegaly
   d. Neutrophilia
   e. Painless lymphadenopathy

9. Which of the following is true in the treatment of CLL?
   a. Induction therapy is the same as for acute lymphoblastic leukaemia
   b. Many patients require no active treatment
   c. Imatinib mesylate has improved the outcome of this disease
   d. Leucophoresis may be required for hyperviscosity
   e. Consolidation is with maintenance rituximab

10. Which of the following is true of multiple myeloma?
    a. Hypercalcaemia is a diagnostic criterion
    b. Paraproteinaemia is present in all cases
    c. Bence–Jones protein is found in serum
    d. The marrow having >10% plasma cells is a diagnostic criterion
    e. It is usually asymptomatic

11. Which three of the following apply to the treatment of myeloma?
    a. Thalidomide is a useful drug
    b. Pathological fracture is best treated with radiotherapy

c. Transfusion is contraindicated owing to hyperviscosity
d. Autologous bone marrow transplant is used in younger patients
e. Bisphosphonates reduce the incidence of pathological fracture
f. Rituximab improves the response to chemotherapy
g. Bortezomib is a monoclonal antibody against plasma cell receptors

12. Which three of the following are poor prognostic factors in myeloma?
    a. Raised serum IL-6
    b. High β_2-microglobulin
    c. Extraskeletal plasmacytoma
    d. Serum creatinine >350 µmol/L
    e. Hyponatraemia
    f. Circulating plasma cells
    g. Haemoglobin <10 g/dL

Paediatric cancer

Malignant tumours are rare in children, with an incidence of just over 1,800 cases per year. The greatest incidence is under the age of 5 years when around half of all the paediatric cancers are diagnosed. Childhood cancer is the most common cause of death in the age groups up to 14 years. Leukaemias account for around 30% of cancer deaths in children and central nervous system (CNS) tumours for 30%. This differs from adults with relatively more leukaemias and lymphomas and fewer solid epithelial cancers. The general distribution is illustrated in Table 18.1.

Overall, the outlook for paediatric malignancy is far better than that for adults, with an overall cure rate of over 80%. Around 40%–50% will require radiotherapy and because of the high cure rate there is now increasing emphasis on the long-term effects of treatment, in particular the influence of chemotherapy and radiotherapy on growth and both physical and intellectual development.

Table 18.1 Frequency and type of common paediatric cancers

Cancer	Incidence (%)
Leukaemia	30
CNS tumours	20
Bone and soft tissue	15
Lymphoma	10
Neuroblastoma	7
Nephroblastoma (Wilms')	7
Others	11

LEUKAEMIA

Leukaemias in childhood are predominantly acute lymphoblastic leukaemia which accounts for 80%; acute myeloblastic leukaemias occur less frequently. Chronic leukaemia, although recognized, is extremely rare. Details of these conditions have been covered in Chapter 17.

CENTRAL NERVOUS SYSTEM TUMOURS

Around 70% of childhood CNS tumours are astrocytomas, predominantly low grade, the management of which has been covered in Chapter 12; of the remainder, the most common are CNS embryonal tumours. Medulloblastoma is the most common of these, accounting for 15%–20% of the total.

MEDULLOBLASTOMA

EPIDEMIOLOGY

Medulloblastomas are most common in children under 5 year of age and occur in twice as many boys as girls.

AETIOLOGY

There are no recognized aetiological factors in the development of this tumour other than the small proportion, estimated around 2%, which have an inherited component developing within the context of Gorlin syndrome.

Paediatric cancer

PATHOLOGY

Medulloblastoma is a CNS embryonal tumour which typically arises in the posterior fossa. This type of tumour can also arise in the pineal region (pineal blastomas) and supratentorial regions.

Local growth can result in obstruction of the fourth ventricle or aqueduct causing secondary hydrocephalus. A characteristic feature of this tumour is its propensity to seed throughout the neuroaxis so that meningeal deposits are found at any site both within the skull and down the spinal cord.

Blood-borne metastases have been described, particularly in bone, but these are rare.

Microscopically, the cells are derived from precursors of neuronal tissue and have a characteristic appearance likened to short carrots, forming circles or rosettes.

Cytogenetically, around 50% have a deletion of the short arm of chromosome 17, and up to 18% have an abnormality of the short arm of chromosome 9, which is also implicated in Gorlin syndrome.

SYMPTOMS

In children, CNS tumours can have an insidious onset with irritability and failure to achieve appropriate milestones. Children or their parents might complain of specific difficulties with walking or headache. Spinal disease can cause nerve root pains and arm or leg weakness.

SIGNS

Posterior fossa tumours can cause specific signs of cerebellar dysfunction with incoordination, ataxic gait and scanning dysarthria. There might also be lower cranial nerve signs.

Spinal involvement will cause weakness of limbs and sensory changes, particularly the development of nerve root pains.

Hydrocephalus, causing raised intracranial pressure, can in a young child result in bulging of the fontanelle and increased head circumference.

DIFFERENTIAL DIAGNOSIS

Other tumours of the posterior fossa should be considered, of which the most common is a low-grade astrocytoma. Other rarer tumours include ependymoma and germ cell tumours.

INVESTIGATIONS

This includes routine tests such as a full blood count and biochemical screening.

CT scan

The tumour will be seen on CT scan, which should be enhanced with intravenous contrast. CT will also demonstrate any degree of hydrocephalus.

Magnetic resonance imaging

This is superior to CT in imaging the posterior fossa (Figure 18.1). Some form of spinal imaging is

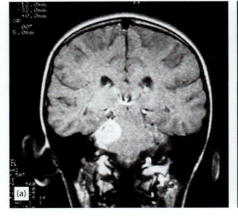
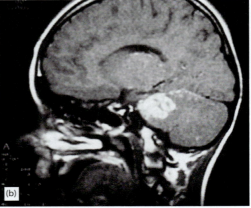

Figure 18.1 MRI showing medulloblastoma arising in posterior cranial fossa: (a) coronal and (b) sagittal views.

Central nervous system tumours

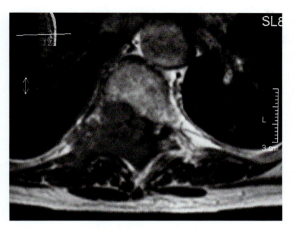

Figure 18.2 MRI demonstrating spinal metastases from medulloblastoma.

essential to complete the staging process. In the past, this has required a myelogram but this can now be replaced by MRI scan as demonstrated in Figure 18.2.

STAGING

There is no TNM staging for medulloblastoma, although various other staging systems have been proposed. Patients can be divided by certain prognostic factors into two groups:

- *Good risk*: Age >3 years; posterior fossa tumour with no dissemination; total excision or <1.5 cm³ residual tumour post-operatively; non-large cell/anaplastic, non-MYC/MYCN amplified
- *Poor risk*: Defined by any one of the following criteria: age <3 years, primary site outside posterior fossa; metastatic disease; metastatic disease and/or localized large-cell/anaplastic and/or MYC/MYCN amplified tumour subtotal resection, i.e. >1.5 cm³ residual tumour

TREATMENT

Initial treatment following the diagnosis of a posterior fossa tumour will be surgery. Surgery has three roles in the management of this tumour:

- To confirm the histological diagnosis from resected tissue
- To remove all visible tumour if technically possible
- To relieve hydrocephalus if present by the insertion of a ventriculoperitoneal shunt

Following surgery, post-operative radiotherapy will be given. This involves treatment of the whole craniospinal axis, i.e. the whole brain and spinal column down to the level of S2 where the thecal sac terminates. A boost to the primary site of tumour is also given.

There may also be some benefit from chemotherapy for poor-risk patients as defined earlier.

TUMOUR-RELATED COMPLICATIONS

Obstructive hydrocephalus may occur. There can be permanent neurological deficits, in particular incoordination and ataxia. Spinal disease can result in permanent limb weakness.

TREATMENT-RELATED COMPLICATIONS

Immediate post-operative complications include meningitis and transient loss of speech (cerebellar mutism). Ventriculoperitoneal shunts may become infected or blocked requiring surgical revision. Craniospinal irradiation can cause significant bone marrow depression, particularly in those patients receiving chemotherapy. Late effects of this treatment include impaired growth, particularly of the spine, resulting in a disproportionate reduction in sitting height compared with standing height. The ovaries are usually included in the sacral radiation field and, unless they are surgically placed outside the irradiated area (oophoropexy), sterility will occur.

Radiation to the pituitary gland which will be within the whole brain volume can result in varying degrees of hypopituitarism requiring appropriate replacement therapy. Late results of whole brain irradiation include long-term neurocognitive effects with a reduction in IQ scores, greatest with younger age at the time of irradiation.

Despite these concerns, many patients achieve good results and function normally within society.

Paediatric cancer

PROGNOSIS

The overall long-term cure rate using the preceding treatment strategies is around 50%.

RARE TUMOURS

EPENDYMOMAS

These account for around 8% of childhood brain tumours. When occurring in the posterior fossa, they behave in a manner very similar to medulloblastomas and the principles of treatment are the same. Cure rates are also similar.

BONE AND SOFT-TISSUE TUMOURS

The common bone tumours in children are osteosarcoma and Ewing sarcoma; both are discussed in Chapter 15.

The common soft-tissue tumour to occur in children is the embryonal rhabdomyosarcoma. This differs significantly from the alveolar form, which occurs particularly in adolescents, and pleomorphic forms of rhabdomyosarcoma found in adults.

RHABDOMYOSARCOMA (EMBRYONAL TYPE)

EPIDEMIOLOGY

These tumours are usually seen in the first 5 years of life and two-thirds are seen in children under 10 years of age. There is an overall incidence of 3 per million children under 15 years of age in the United Kingdom. They arise in any site, the most common being the head and neck region and the genitourinary tract.

AETIOLOGY

There are a number of rare inherited syndromes associated with rhabdomyosarcoma including Li–Fraumeni and neurofibromatosis type 1 but in most cases no specific aetiological factors are identified.

PATHOLOGY

Approximately, one-third arises in the head and neck region, one-third in the genitourinary tract and a quarter in the soft tissues of the trunk or extremities. The orbit is also a relatively frequent site, accounting for 10% of the total.

Macroscopically, they appear as pink fleshy masses and proliferative forms are likened to a bunch of grapes ('sarcoma botryoides').

Microscopically, they are embryonal cells rich in glycogen and within which myofibrils can be demonstrated. Immunohistochemistry will be positive for desmin, myoglobin, myo-D1 and muscle-specific actin. The embryonal subtype is distinct from the alveolar rhabdomyosarcoma of adults, although this type can be seen in older children and adolescents.

A specific chromosome deletion has been identified at chromosome 11p15 associated with embryonal type distinct from the other subtypes of rhabdomyosarcoma. Other associated genetic mutations include point mutations in the *N-ras* and *K-ras* oncogenes. The presence of one of the PAX3/7-FOX01 fusion genes is associated with a worse prognosis.

NATURAL HISTORY

The natural history of this form of rhabdomyosarcoma is for rapid local growth with infiltration along tissue planes and early blood-borne metastases. Around one in five patients will have bone marrow infiltration at presentation and 15%–20% will have evidence of distant metastases. Lymph node spread also occurs, particularly in those tumours arising in the genitourinary tract and limbs.

SYMPTOMS

Presenting symptoms depend on the site of origin. Many arise as rapidly enlarging but painless masses. Other local symptoms can be present including nasal obstruction and epistaxis from the nasopharynx, haematuria from the urinary tract and vaginal bleeding from the vagina or uterus. Orbital tumours can cause local discomfort and blurred or double vision.

SIGNS

Clinical signs will go along with the presenting symptoms. There might be an obvious mass visible. Vaginal tumours can present with a fleshy mass of 'botryoid' tumour at the introitus. Orbital tumours will cause proptosis and ophthalmoplegia.

DIFFERENTIAL DIAGNOSIS

In childhood, there are few other tumours that are likely to arise in similar sites to rhabdomyosarcoma. Other causes of presenting symptoms such as epistaxis or haematuria in the absence of an obvious mass should be sought.

INVESTIGATIONS

Routine tests such as full blood count and biochemistry may well be normal.

CT scan and MRI

CT scan or MRI of the affected site will be valuable in delineating the extent of local tumour most accurately.

CT of the chest, abdomen and pelvis or CT PET scan is important to identify potential sites of metastases.

Bone marrow examination

Bone marrow examination should be performed in view of the high incidence of marrow involvement.

Biopsy

A full examination of the affected site under anaesthetic with biopsy of the tumour is essential to confirm the diagnosis.

Lumbar puncture to examine CSF is indicated for parameningeal tumours to exclude meningeal disease.

STAGING

TNM staging is used and is based on post-surgical status:

- T1: Tumour limited to the site of the origin with microscopic margins of excision clear
- T2: Tumour extending beyond the site of the origin but complete microscopic clearance of tumour
- T3: Tumour extending beyond the site of the origin with incomplete excision
- N0: Regional nodes negative
- N1: Regional nodes involved
- M0: No metastases
- M1: Distant metastases

In practice, group staging as used by the Intergroup Rhabdomyosarcoma Studies (IRS) may be of more value:

- *Stage I*: Localized disease completely resected
- *Stage II*:
  - A: Localized disease with residual microscopic disease
  - B: Node involvement completely resected
  - C: Node involvement with microscopic residual disease
- *Stage III*: Incomplete resection or biopsy only
- *Stage IV*: Distant metastases at diagnosis

Around 50% of patients will be stage III at diagnosis and 20% will present with metastases.

TREATMENT

Radical treatment

Chemotherapy

Chemotherapy is given to all cases; treatment is based on the overall risk grouping for each patient: low, standard, high, very high or metastatic.

Low-risk disease is treated with eight cycles of vincristine and actinomycin D (VA), while all other risk groups receive nine cycles of chemotherapy; standard risk groups are treated with initial ifosfamide, vincristine and actinomycin D (IVA) then with VA; high-risk group receives IVA alone. Good risk patients, which includes stage I orbital and paratesticular tumours, receive vincristine and actinomycin D alone. In advanced disease, additional agents can be used such as topotecan or irinotecan.

One or two courses are given followed by definitive surgery or radiotherapy and then chemotherapy is continued for a period of up to 1 year.

Surgery

This is the treatment of choice in the absence of advanced distant metastases. For urogenital, truncal and limb rhabdomyosarcoma, wide resection is usually performed.

Radiotherapy

This is used for inoperable tumours such as orbit and nasopharynx, delivering doses of around 50 Gy in 5 weeks. Pelvic rhabdomyosarcoma affecting the bladder, prostate or vagina may be treated with brachytherapy to minimize radiation dose to the pelvic bones and in girls to the ovaries whilst preserving the organ affected.

Proton therapy is chosen for many children to reduce radiation exposure to surrounding organs.

Palliative treatment

For recurrent disseminated disease, a course of palliative chemotherapy or radiotherapy could be valuable in minimizing symptoms. Second-line chemotherapy using drugs such as ifosfamide and etoposide might achieve good responses, although further relapse is usual. Local recurrence, particularly in patients with the botryoid type of tumour, should be treated actively as there is a high salvage rate in this group.

TUMOUR-RELATED COMPLICATIONS

These will depend on the site. Urogenital tumours can permanently affect renal, urinary and reproductive function, and orbital tumours can affect sight.

TREATMENT-RELATED COMPLICATIONS

Chemotherapy using VAC can cause nausea, vomiting and alopecia during the period of administration. In the longer term peripheral neuropathy from vincristine can persist.

Radical surgery sometimes has late sequelae depending on the type of procedure. There are obvious effects of cystectomy or hysterectomy for urogenital tumours.

Radical radiotherapy can have late sequelae also, in particular growth impairment in the treated area. In a young child, this can result in quite marked disfigurement if significant asymmetry develops, as may be the case following, for example, orbit irradiation. Inclusion of pelvic organs may result in infertility when the gonads receive radiation. Second malignancy many years later is an ongoing concern.

PROGNOSIS

The overall prognosis for embryonal rhabdomyosarcoma confined to the site of origin is good with cure rates of around 80%. Once metastatic, the outlook is poor with less than 20% surviving.

Age, stage and site are important predictors of cure. The best prognoses are associated with tumours of the orbit, paratesticular region and vagina. Poor prognosis sites are parameningeal, prostate and perineum. Patients with metastatic disease aged <10 years have a significantly better outcome than older patients.

LYMPHOMA

Both Hodgkin disease and non-Hodgkin lymphoma occur in children. While they obey the general rules discussed in Chapter 16, there are certain features of paediatric lymphomas which should be considered.

NON-HODGKIN LYMPHOMA

NHL in children is usually a high-grade nodal disease with a particular propensity for diffuse lymphoblastic or undifferentiated tumours, and also T-cell lymphomas associated with a mediastinal mass. Low-grade NHL is rare in children.

Treatment usually involves combination chemotherapy and, for extensive high-grade disease, bone marrow transplant can be considered. Local radiotherapy can also be given in reduced doses of 25–30 Gy.

HODGKIN DISEASE

Hodgkin disease is relatively more common in boys than in girls, which is in contrast to a more even sex distribution in adults. Lymphocyte-predominant histology is relatively more common and the less favourable lymphocyte-depleted form uncommon.

Treatment is based on the same principles as in adult Hodgkin disease but with even greater emphasis on minimizing late effects. For this reason, chemotherapy is often preferred for relatively early disease, avoiding the local growth problems after radiotherapy. Schedules containing vincristine, procarbazine, prednisolone and Adriamycin (OPPA) and OEPA, which substitutes etoposide for procarbazine, combined with localized radiotherapy, have been highly successful. Where irradiation is used, lower doses of around 20–30 Gy are given compared with 30–35 Gy in adults.

NEUROBLASTOMA

EPIDEMIOLOGY

Neuroblastoma is the commonest solid extracranial tumour in children; 50% occur before the age of 2 years and 80% under 5 years. It has an annual incidence of 8 per million in the United Kingdom and is slightly more common in boys than in girls. There is some geographical variation: it is rare in Africa compared with Europe and the United States.

AETIOLOGY

There is an association with von Recklinghausen disease (multiple neurofibromatosis) and colonic aganglionosis, but most cases have no recognizable causal factor. There is some evidence that it arises as a congenital anomaly and cases in utero have been reported.

Specific chromosome abnormalities have been identified in neuroblastoma, including amplification of the *N-myc* oncogene, deletions affecting chromosome 1 and gain of the long arm of chromosome 17 (17q).

PATHOLOGY

Two-thirds of neuroblastomas are intra-abdominal tumours, of which 60% occur in the adrenal and 40% at other sites related to the sympathetic chain. The remaining one-third are divided between the chest, pelvis and the head and neck region. In a small number of these tumours, widespread metastatic disease may be present with no recognizable primary site.

Macroscopically, the tumour is usually encapsulated but soft and friable, containing areas of haemorrhage, necrosis, cystic degeneration and calcification.

Microscopically, there is a spectrum of appearances depending on the degree of differentiation. Typically, it is composed of densely packed, small round cells which can form rosettes. In the more differentiated forms neurofibrils and ganglionic elements and granule-containing chromaffin cells can be seen.

NATURAL HISTORY

Local infiltration of surrounding tissues is seen.

Regional lymph nodes can be involved but the predominant pattern of metastases is by early blood-borne dissemination with around two-thirds of children having widespread disease at presentation, affecting in particular bone and liver. Lung metastases are relatively rare.

Spontaneous maturation and regression may occur, typically in young children <12 months presenting with abdominal disease. Post-mortem studies suggest a much higher incidence of asymptomatic tumours in patients dying from unrelated conditions than in the general population.

SYMPTOMS

These will depend on the site and age at presentation.

Abdominal tumours, which are the most common, will present with abdominal discomfort and bowel or urinary obstruction.

In the head and neck a painless mass may be the first manifestation.

There may also be fever, anorexia, malaise and weight loss.

Metastatic disease can cause the first symptoms, particularly bone pain from bone metastases.

Excessive catecholamine production from the tumour cells causes flushing, palpitations, diarrhoea and headache.

Rarely in utero it presents with pre-eclampsia in the mother.

SIGNS

These may include:

- A palpable mass
- Intrathoracic tumours, causing venous obstruction with dilated neck veins, plethora and oedema
- Catecholamine secretion, causing hypertension.

There are rare neurological syndromes associated with neuroblastoma, in particular an acute cerebellar disturbance (opsomyoclonus) characterized by truncal ataxia and rapid random eye movements (so-called 'dancing feet', 'dancing eyes').

DIFFERENTIAL DIAGNOSIS

A palpable mass must be distinguished from other types of tumour. In the abdomen, this will include Wilms' tumour and in the neck a lymph node from lymphoma.

The differential diagnosis of a small round cell tumour in bone includes not only neuroblastoma but also rhabdomyosarcoma, Ewing sarcoma and lymphoma. A benign counterpart, ganglioneuroma, and the transitional tumour, ganglioneuroblastoma, might also have similar pathological appearances.

INVESTIGATIONS

Routine blood tests can be unremarkable but extensive bone metastases can cause pancytopenia and there could also be obstructive renal impairment.

RADIOGRAPHY

X-ray of the tumour can demonstrate speckled calcification within it.

CT SCAN OR MRI

CT scan or MRI is needed for more accurate definition of the tumour.

CT of the chest, abdomen and pelvis or CT PET is important to identify sites of metastatic disease.

BIOPSY

Biopsy of the accessible tumour to confirm the diagnosis, ploidy and cytogenetics should be undertaken to give additional prognostic information.

BONE MARROW EXAMINATION

This examination is important because of the high incidence of bone metastases.

URINE TESTS

Twenty-four-hour urine collections will be made to measure catecholamines such as vanillylmandelic acid (VMA) and homovanillylmandelic acid (HVA), the ratio of the two having prognostic importance. Other peptides such as vasoactive intestinal peptide (VIP) might also be raised.

OTHER TESTS

Because many of the tumours will contain cells synthesizing catecholamines from their precursors, a labelled precursor called meta-iodobenzyl guanidine (mIBG) may be used as a tracer in scanning labelled with radioactive iodine. This also has therapeutic uses.

Serum levels of neurone-specific enolase (NSE), ferritin and ganglioside GD2 have prognostic value.

STAGING

Stage 1: The tumour can be removed completely during surgery. Lymph nodes attached to the tumour removed during surgery may or may not contain cancer, but other lymph nodes near the tumour do not.
Stage 2A: The tumour is located only in the area it started and cannot be completely removed during surgery. Nearby lymph nodes do not contain cancer.
Stage 2B: The tumour is located only in the area where it started and may or may not be completely removed during surgery, but nearby lymph nodes do contain cancer.
Stage 3: The tumour cannot be removed with surgery. It has spread to regional lymph nodes (lymph

nodes near the tumour) or other areas near the tumour, but not to other parts of the body.

Stage 4: The original tumour has spread to distant lymph nodes (lymph nodes in other parts of the body), bones, bone marrow, liver, skin, and/or other organs, except for those listed in stage 4S.

Stage 4S: The original tumour is located only where it started (as in stage 1, 2A, or 2B), and it has spread only to the skin, liver, and/or bone marrow, in infants younger than 12 months. The spread to the bone marrow is minimal; usually less than 10% of cells examined show cancer.

A risk stratification to aid management decisions is as follows.

Low-risk neuroblastoma

Stage 1 disease
Stage 2A or 2B disease, >50% of the tumour surgically removed, except for a child with MYCN amplification
Stage 4S disease, no MYCN amplification, favourable histopathology and hyperdiploidy

Intermediate-risk neuroblastoma

Stage 2A or 2B disease, no MYCN amplification with <50% of the tumour removed with surgery
Stage 3 disease in children younger than 18 months, no MYCN amplification
Stage 3 disease in children older than 18 months, no MYCN amplification and favourable histopathology
Stage 4 disease in children younger than 12 months, no MYCN amplification
Stage 4 disease in children aged 12–18 months, no MYCN amplification, hyperdiploidy and favourable histology
Stage 4S disease, no MYCN amplification, unfavourable histopathology and/or diploidy

High-risk neuroblastoma

Stage 2A or 2B disease with MYCN amplification
Stage 3 disease with MYCN amplification
Stage 3 disease in children aged 18 months or older, no MYCN amplification and unfavourable histopathology
Stage 4 disease in children <12 months with MYCN amplification

Stage 4 disease in children aged 12–18 months with MYCN amplification, and/or diploidy and/or unfavourable histology
Stage 4 disease in children ≥18 months
Stage 4S disease and MYCN amplification

TREATMENT

Treatment is tailored according to the risk assignment.

Low-risk disease will be treated with surgery alone.

Low-risk stage 4S disease can be managed by observation or single agent vincristine if there is no spontaneous regression.

Intermediate-risk disease receives surgery and chemotherapy. Commonly used drugs are cisplatin or carboplatin, cyclophosphamide, doxorubicin and etoposide.

High-risk disease will be treated primarily by chemotherapy using more intensive schedules. Consolidation using high-dose chemotherapy and peripheral blood stem cell rescue to restore bone marrow function may be considered.

A further approach uses targeted radiation using iodine-131-labelled mIBG, which is actively concentrated in cells synthesizing catecholamines.

PALLIATIVE TREATMENT

Local radiotherapy for painful bone metastases or large tumour masses can be given.

TUMOUR-RELATED COMPLICATIONS

Mediastinal, renal or intestinal obstruction can occur depending on primary site. Excess catecholamine secretion can cause hypertension and tachycardia with arrhythmias. Diarrhoea occurs if vasoactive intestinal peptide (VIP) is produced.

TREATMENT-RELATED COMPLICATIONS

Intensive chemotherapy regimens result in profound bone marrow suppression with the risk of neutropenic sepsis.

PROGNOSIS

The prognosis for localized neuroblastoma is good with virtually all patients with stage 1 disease and 80% of those with stage 2 cured. Stage 4S also has a good outlook with cure rates approaching 80%. In contrast, older patients with metastatic disease have a very poor prognosis with long-term survival between 10% and 40%. Important prognostic factors are hyperploidy conferring a good prognosis and diploidy or *N-myc* expression predicting a poor outcome.

NEPHROBLASTOMA (WILMS' TUMOUR)

EPIDEMIOLOGY

Wilms' tumour (WT) is a tumour of young children with a peak incidence between 1 and 3 years and the majority occurring before the age of 5 years. It is relatively rare with around 80 cases per year in the United Kingdom. There is equal distribution between boys and girls.

AETIOLOGY

WT is familial in 1%–2% of cases and there is marked racial variation with an incidence of 2.5 per million in Chinese children to 10.9 per million in African American children.

There is an association with certain rare congenital abnormalities including Beckwith–Wiedemann syndrome, WAGR syndrome when associated with aniridia, Denys–Drash syndrome, hemi-hypertrophy, Bloom syndrome and other abnormalities of the urogenital tract. Trisomy 18 is another associated disorder and a deletion on the short arm of chromosome 11 (11p13) is seen in around one-third of cases of WT as well as certain other abnormalities of the genitourinary system such as hypospadias and cryptorchidism. The gene that causes aniridia is also located close to this position on chromosome 11. This has led to the identification of the *WT1* gene associated with WT; this encodes a transcription factor critical for normal kidney development.

Other deletions in WT are seen on chromosomes 16 and 1p.

Genetic linkage studies have identified two loci on chromosomes 17 and 19, *FWT1* and *FWT2*. Loss of heterozygosity at either of these sites conveys a relatively poor prognosis.

PATHOLOGY

The tumour arises in the kidney and 5% are bilateral. It can be lobular and is surrounded by a pseudocapsule as it compresses surrounding tissue. There might be areas of haemorrhage, necrosis and cyst formation.

Microscopically, there is often considerable variety within the tumour with areas of primitive mesenchymal cells, which can show differentiation into fat, muscle or cartilage within which are the areas of recognizable embryonal glomerular and renal tubular elements.

Certain microscopic features are of prognostic importance. Anaplastic areas are associated with a worse prognosis, particularly if there are diffuse rather than focal areas of anaplastic change, and are found in around 5% of cases. Subtypes previously-labelled sarcomatous and clear cell are now thought to be distinct entities rather than variants of WT and also have a poor prognosis.

NATURAL HISTORY

Local invasion from the renal parenchyma into the renal pelvis and renal vein will occur. Lymph node involvement is relatively infrequent.

Blood-borne metastases are the usual means of spread beyond the kidney, the most common distant site being the lungs.

SYMPTOMS

Abdominal pain is the most common presenting feature.

Haematuria occurs in about 20% and a similar proportion can have unexplained fevers. There may be weight loss or anorexia.

Pulmonary metastases can cause cough, haemoptysis or dyspnoea.

SIGNS

The majority have a palpable abdominal mass at presentation which can be entirely asymptomatic. Hypertension can be present but is relatively unusual.

DIFFERENTIAL DIAGNOSIS

Abdominal neuroblastoma can also present with a large abdominal mass but is usually associated with greater systemic upset and bone metastases rather than lung metastases.

INVESTIGATIONS

BLOOD TESTS

A full blood count might show anaemia and urea and electrolytes can be disturbed.

URINE TESTS

Urinalysis can show both blood and protein in the urine.

RADIOGRAPHY

CT of chest abdomen and pelvis will define the primary tumour and also identify potential metastatic sites as shown in Figure 18.3.

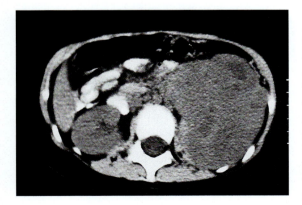

Figure 18.3 CT scan demonstrating large renal mass in nephroblastoma.

OTHER TESTS

The primary tumour will also be seen on abdominal ultrasound.

STAGING

The largest group investigating Wilms' tumour is the National Wilms' Tumour Study Group in the United States and their staging system is commonly reported:

- *Stage 1*: Tumour completely excised and retained within capsule
- *Stage 2*: Tumour completely excised but extending beyond capsule
- *Stage 3*: Tumour incompletely excised but no blood-borne metastases
- *Stage 4*: Blood-borne distant metastases
- *Stage 5*: Bilateral tumours

They may be further classified into risk groups as follows:

- *Very-low risk*: <2 years of age, <550 g tumour weight, stage I, any loss of heterozygosity (LOH) status
- *Low risk*: Any age or tumour weight, stage I or II, but no LOH at 1p and 16q
- *Standard risk*: Stage I tumours >550 g with LOH at 1p and 16q, or stage II with LOH or stage III/IV with no LOH
- *High risk*: Stage III or IV with LOH at 1p and 16q

Around 5% will present with bilateral tumours and a second tumour develops in the contralateral kidney in up to 3%.

TREATMENT

All stages will initially be treated with 4 weeks of chemotherapy using vincristine and actinomycin D. This will be followed by surgery; laparotomy and radical resection of the tumour is performed, which will usually entail a nephro-ureterectomy and regional node dissection. An important feature of the operation should be mobilization and careful inspection of the contralateral kidney in view of the significant incidence of bilateral tumours. If there are bilateral tumours then every effort will be made to spare some renal tissue in the kidney having the smaller tumour to provide some residual renal function.

Post-operative radiotherapy or chemotherapy are used as follows:

- Where histology shows no anaplastic elements:
  - Stage 1 and 2 disease is given a short course (usually over 18 weeks) of vincristine with actinomycin D.
  - Stages 3 and 4 are given chemotherapy using vincristine, actinomycin D and Adriamycin with radiotherapy to the renal bed delivering 20–30 Gy in 3–4 weeks.
- Where histology shows anaplastic tumour:
  - Stage 1 disease is given a short course of vincristine with actinomycin D.
  - Stages 2, 3 and 4 are treated with more intensive chemotherapy using vincristine, Adriamycin, etoposide and cyclophosphamide followed by radiotherapy to the renal bed and also metastatic sites.
  - Stage 5 disease is a special and more difficult case. Initial chemotherapy will be given to achieve tumour shrinkage and allow surgery with the intent of performing nephron-sparing surgery or partial nephrectomy. Post-operative treatment will then continue as previously described.

PALLIATIVE TREATMENT

This can take the form of chemotherapy or local radiotherapy to symptomatic disease. High-dose chemotherapy with bone marrow rescue has been used but may be no better than alternative alternating chemotherapy regimens using ifosfamide, etoposide and carboplatin. Around 50% of patients might be salvaged after recurrence. For chemotherapy-resistant lung disease low-dose whole lung irradiation can be given, delivering 10–12 Gy in seven or eight small fractions.

TUMOUR-RELATED COMPLICATIONS

Most survivors will have normal renal function, the incidence of renal failure being 1% or less.

TREATMENT-RELATED COMPLICATIONS

Radiotherapy to the renal bed will include the lumbar vertebrae and there will therefore be growth retardation in this area. Because of this it is extremely important that the radiotherapist includes the entire width of the vertebral body to avoid a scoliotic deformity owing to differential growth across the vertebral body.

Immediate side effects of chemotherapy include nausea, vomiting and alopecia. In the longer term, vincristine can be associated with a peripheral neuropathy, actinomycin D with liver dysfunction and Adriamycin with dose-related cardiomyopathy.

PROGNOSIS

Wilms' tumour is both radio- and chemosensitive and the prognosis for localized disease is therefore very good with 80%–90% of patients with stage 1 or 2 disease being cured. There are a number of important prognostic features including anaplasia, aneuploidy, lymph node or hepatic metastases and intravascular tumour thrombus, and loss of heterozygosity (LOH) at 1p and 16q; however, even those presenting with distant metastases (stage 4) have a cure rate of over 70%.

RARE TUMOURS

The rhabdoid tumour of kidney is highly malignant metastasizing widely to lungs and CNS in particular. Clear cell sarcoma of the kidney also disseminates widely and both have a far worse prognosis than WT.

OTHER TUMOURS

LANGERHANS' CELL HISTIOCYTOSIS

This is a complex condition arising from a proliferation of histiocytes. Three distinct forms are recognized:

- Letterer–Siwe disease
- Hand–Schüller–Christian disease
- Eosinophilic granuloma

Letterer–Siwe disease affects infants and is usually rapidly fatal owing to widespread infiltration of liver, spleen, skin and lymph nodes with proliferating histiocytes.

Hand–Schüller–Christian disease occurs at any age with a less fulminant course and is once again characterized by widespread infiltration of histiocytes which in this case is characterized by intracellular accumulation of lipid. Bones in particular are affected and patients survive for many years, although most ultimately succumb. It can be treated using drug combinations such as VAC (vincristine, Adriamycin or actinomycin D and cyclophosphamide).

Eosinophilic granuloma is the least aggressive form of the disease and is usually localized, presenting as solitary lytic bone lesions. Deposits around the pituitary are a recognized cause of diabetes insipidus. They are characterized by accumulations of lipid-filled histiocytes, eosinophils and giant cells. They can regress spontaneously. If symptomatic they respond well to low doses of irradiation.

RETINOBLASTOMA

This is a rare tumour present in around 1 in 20,000 live births in the United Kingdom and usually presents in the first 2 years of life. There are two distinct forms: hereditary bilateral or multifocal tumours, 40% of which are characterized by germline mutations in the retinoblastoma gene, and non-hereditary unifocal or unilateral tumours.

The retinoblastoma gene is located on chromosome 13q,14 and was one of the first tumour-suppressor genes to be identified.

Retinoblastoma presents with reduced vision, characteristic white pupils or strabismus. As the tumour occludes fluid drainage within the eye secondary glaucoma can develop. The diagnosis is confirmed on examination of both eyes under anaesthetic as shown in Figure 18.4.

Small tumours can be treated by light coagulation using a xenon arc laser or cryotherapy. Larger tumours can be treated with neoadjuvant chemotherapy using carboplatin, vincristine and etoposide followed by radiotherapy, which can be delivered either by placing over the tumour cobalt discs or with external beam treatment where most of the eye has

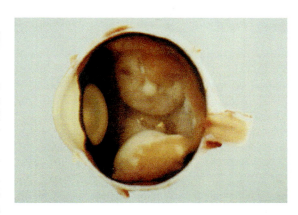

Figure 18.4 Lateral section of eyeball showing extensive primary retinoblastoma.

to be included. Enucleation is avoided but could be necessary if the optic nerve is invaded.

Most tumours are cured using this approach with preservation of vision.

Genetic counselling is an important feature of further management; the risk of retinoblastoma developing in children of a patient with the hereditary bilateral form of the tumour is 45%; it is only 2.5% for those with unilateral non-hereditary tumours.

GERM CELL TUMOURS

Teratomas present in the first 5 years. The majority are benign but 20% or so will be malignant. The common sites are the ovary and the sacrococcygeal region but they are also found in the mediastinum, neck, nasopharynx, retroperitoneum or brain.

The management of these tumours is essentially that of germ cell tumours in the adult. Initial treatment will be surgical removal where possible followed by appropriate adjuvant chemotherapy using combinations such as BEP (bleomycin, etoposide and cisplatin). Local radiotherapy is considered where surgical excision is not feasible, as in the brain. Overall, the prognosis, as in adult germ cell tumours, is good.

FURTHER READING

BMJ best practice: Neuroblastoma https://bestpractice.bmj.com/topics/en-gb/1305.
BMJ best practice: Wilms tumour https://bestpractice.bmj.com/topics/en-us/934.

Cairo MS, Beishuizen A. Childhood, adolescent and young adult non-Hodgkin lymphoma: Current perspectives. *Br J Haematol*. 2019; 185(6): 1021–1042.

Pollack IF, Agnihotri S, Broniscer A. Childhood brain tumors: Current management, biological insights, and future directions. *J Neurosurg Pediatr*. 2019; 23(3): 261–273.

Skapek SX, Ferrari A, Gupta AA et al. Rhabdomyosarcoma. *Nat Rev Dis Primers*. 2019; 5(1): 1.

SELF-ASSESSMENT QUESTIONS

1. Which of the following is true of childhood cancer?
   a. Acute leukaemia causes one-third of childhood cancer deaths
   b. The peak incidence is in the 5–10-year age group
   c. The most common solid tumour is nephroblastoma
   d. It is more common in lower socioeconomic groups
   e. After trauma it is the second most common cause of death up to the age of 15 years

2. Which three of the following apply to medulloblastoma?
   a. It is a primitive neuroectodermal tumour (PNET)
   b. It occurs in the posterior fossa of the skull
   c. It is related to hypoxic birth injury
   d. It is most common over 5 years of age
   e. It disseminates to distant blood-borne sites at an early stage
   f. It can be cured by radical surgery
   g. Seeding along the craniospinal axis is characteristic

3. Which of the following is true of bone and soft-tissue tumours in children?
   a. The most common bone tumour is chondrosarcoma
   b. Ewing sarcoma is usually extraskeletal in children
   c. Osteosarcoma typically affects the limb girdles
   d. Embryonal rhabdomyosarcoma is the common form in children
   e. The prognosis is worse in children than adults

4. Which of the following is true of rhabdomyosarcoma in childhood?
   a. Initial surgery may be curative
   b. They typically arise in the limbs
   c. Urogenital tumours commonly seed to the CNS
   d. Chemotherapy containing vincristine will be given to all patients
   e. Over 50% have metastases at presentation

5. Which three of the following are true of neuroblastoma?
   a. The majority are intra-abdominal
   b. Most present in the first 2 years of life
   c. It may be associated with the retinoblastoma gene
   d. Stage IVS usually requires no treatment
   e. Catecholamines are detectable in the urine
   f. CNS prophylaxis is required after induction treatment
   g. Lung metastases are relatively common

6. Which of the following is true of nephroblastoma?
   a. It arises from the suprarenal gland
   b. Lymph node metastases are common
   c. It is bilateral in 5% of cases
   d. It is more common in trisomy 21
   e. The majority occur between 5 and 10 years of age

7. Which of the following is true of the treatment of nephroblastoma?
   a. Initial treatment is with chemotherapy
   b. Chemotherapy is followed by radiotherapy to the involved side
   c. Nephro-ureterectomy is the usual operation
   d. Chemotherapy is reserved for anaplastic tumours
   e. Radiotherapy should avoid as much of the vertebra as possible

8. Which three of the following are true of retinoblastoma?
   a. Hereditary forms account for 40%
   b. Enucleation is the treatment of choice
   c. Meningeal infiltration is common
   d. Survival beyond 5 years is unusual
   e. Lung metastases are common
   f. The retinoblastoma gene is a tumour-suppressor gene
   g. Genetic counselling is important in management

9. Which of the following is true of germ cell tumours in children?
   a. The testis is the common site in boys
   b. The majority are malignant teratomas
   c. They are common in the sacrococcygeal region
   d. Initial treatment will be with BEP chemotherapy
   e. Benign teratomas are best managed with local radiotherapy

10. Which of the following is true of Langerhans' cell histiocytosis?
    a. The most aggressive form is Hand–Schüller–Christian disease
    b. Letterer–Siwe disease may regress spontaneously
    c. They may transform into a histiocytic lymphoma
    d. Eosinophilic granuloma is usually a solitary lytic bone lesion
    e. More than one form may be present at initial diagnosis

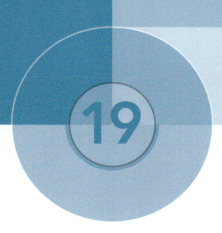

Skin cancer

The skin is the largest organ in the body. Its large surface area and location make it particularly vulnerable to environmental carcinogens. Recent cultural, economic and environmental changes have resulted in many more people being exposed to high levels of ultraviolet radiation. As this is the main risk factor for developing skin cancer, many more cases can be expected in the decades to come.

SQUAMOUS AND BASAL CELL CARCINOMA

EPIDEMIOLOGY

Each year in the United Kingdom there are 140,000 cases of non-melanomatous skin cancer, 80,000 cases in men and 60,000 cases in women, and leading to a total of over 1300 deaths per annum, 1% of all cancer deaths. In the last two decades the incidence has risen 147%. Basal cell carcinoma (BCC) is twice as common as squamous cell carcinoma (SCC). The peak incidence is at over 90 age group and it is exceptional in the under-40s in whom an underlying predisposition can usually be identified, e.g. Gorlin syndrome or arsenic exposure. It is more common in white people living in a sunny climate, particularly South Africa and Australia, the incidence increasing with proximity to the equator. It is uncommon dark-skinned races.

AETIOLOGY

Radiation: Non-ionizing ultraviolet radiation is the most important cause accounting for the geographical and racial distribution of skin cancers. They are therefore most frequent on sun-exposed areas of the body.

Ionizing radiation usually in relation to previous radiotherapy can lead to skin cancer in sites of irradiation. Radiation-induced cancers were a particular problem to the pioneering radiologists who used to calibrate their x-ray machines by exposing their hands to a dose sufficient to cause erythema of the skin.

Chemical carcinogens: Tar and soot are rich in aromatic hydrocarbons. SCC of the scrotum was described in nineteenth-century chimney sweeps where soot had become trapped in the rugose skin of the scrotum. Similarly, occupational exposure to tar and bitumen can lead to tumours on the exposed skin, and mineral oils were the cause of SCC described in yarn workers which they used to lubricate the spinning mules.

Arsenic is a potent cause of skin cancers but a history of exposure is not common. It will be associated with multiple BCCs and SCCs. It was once used as a 'tonic' and is found in some pesticides.

Chronic inflammation: SCC has been described arising in chronic varicose ulcers, burn scars, cutaneous TB, sinuses from chronic osteomyelitis, and epidermolysis bullosa.

Genetic predisposition: Gorlin syndrome is a very rare, dominantly inherited syndrome predisposing to multiple BCCs and should be considered in all cases arising in those under 40 years of age. Palmar pits are characteristic but other features include bifid ribs, a calcified falx cerebri, frontal bossing of the skull and mandibular cysts.

Xeroderma pigmentosum is even rarer, recessively inherited, and patients inevitably develop multiple BCCs and SCCs at a very young age.

Chronic immunosuppression: Patients having prolonged immunosuppressive therapy after organ transplant recipients are associated with an increased incidence of BCC and SCC.

PATHOLOGY

Macroscopically, these tumours arise typically on sun-exposed skin such as the scalp, nose, ears, periorbital tissues and dorsum of hand. BCC is very rare in nonhair-bearing skin such as the palms and soles. They are frequently multiple, with evidence of solar damage in surrounding skin such as keratoses. An invasive SCC can arise in an area of *in situ* carcinoma such as Bowen disease. SCCs are usually well circumscribed, appearing as nodules which may have central ulceration or ulcers with raised, everted, nodular edges (Figure 19.1). A BCC can appear predominantly nodular, ulcerating or mixed. A morphoeic BCC is typically flat and infiltrating. The surface of a BCC may have telangiectasia and raised edges which have a characteristic 'pearly' appearance (Figure 19.2).

They vary greatly in rate of growth, some, particularly BCCs, persisting unnoticed for many years, others growing rapidly over a period of several months. Large, neglected tumours (Figures 19.3 and 19.4) are accompanied by local tissue destruction and secondary infection. Both BCCs and SCCs can occur concurrently in the same patient.

Microscopically, local invasion, often for some distance beyond their macroscopic margins, is common. The cell of origin of a BCC is uncertain, but thought

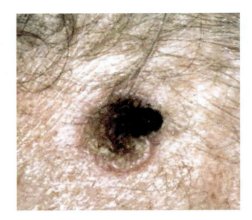

Figure 19.1 A typical ulcerating squamous carcinoma on the forehead with raised 'pearly' edge and central ulceration.

to be a basal cell of a hair follicle giving rise to small dark-staining cells. SCCs arise from keratinocytes, are well differentiated, demonstrate intercellular bridges on electron microscopy and produce keratin seen as 'keratin pearls'. Sometimes the appearances are those of a mixed 'basisquamous' tumour.

NATURAL HISTORY

Both types of tumour are characterized by local infiltration of the surrounding skin and normal tissues lying deep into or adjacent to the skin leading to their eventual destruction. This behavior resulting in the destruction of the surrounding tissue has led to BCCs often being referred to as 'rodent ulcers'.

About 5% of SCCs and less than 0.1% of BCCs spread to the regional lymph nodes (Figure 19.5).

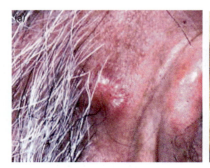
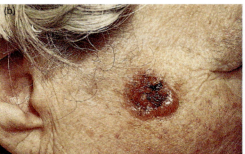

Figure 19.2 Basal cell carcinoma. (a) Common nodular variant; note raised edges with taelangiectasia. (b) Ulcerating variant.

Squamous and basal cell carcinoma

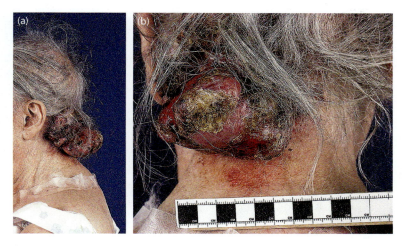

Figure 19.3 Basal cell carcinoma. This lesion had been neglected for 20 years and covered by a headscarf. Surgical excision was curative. (a) Side view. (b) Rear view.

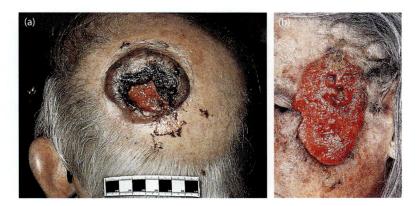

Figure 19.4 Squamous carcinoma. (a) Arising from the skin overlying the vertex of the skull. Such tumours may penetrate into the skull and involve the underlying brain. (b) Large plaque of tumour arising from temple.

Blood-borne spread is rare for SCCs and virtually unknown for BCCs. Lung and bone are the most common sites of metastatic spread.

SYMPTOMS

The patient is usually asymptomatic, the lesion being noticed at a routine medical examination, or the patient might complain of a skin lesion which is causing concern or cosmetic defect. Ulcerating lesions can bleed spontaneously if traumatized and irritation is a common complaint, although pain is exceptional usually reflecting local infiltration and tissue damage.

SIGNS

Careful inspection under a bright light with a magnifying glass is recommended as it is the most accurate way of defining the macroscopic extent of the tumour, which may be much greater than naked eye inspection would suggest. Telangiectasia suggests a BCC. Otherwise, it is difficult to distinguish an SCC from a BCC by appearance alone. The tumour can be tethered or fixed to underlying tissues depending on the depth of invasion. There can be destruction of the surrounding tissues and secondary infection of the tumour. Regional lymph nodes should be examined in all cases.

Skin cancer

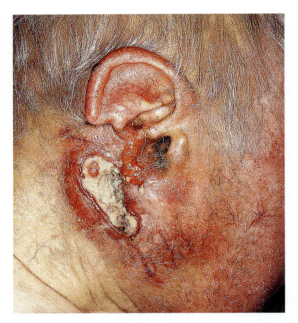

Figure 19.5 Nodal relapse of squamous carcinoma. This man had originally undergone surgery for a carcinoma arising from the pinna. There is now invasion and ulceration of skin overlying an enlarged lymph node.

DIFFERENTIAL DIAGNOSIS

This includes:

- Keratoacanthoma
- Solar keratosis
- Bowen disease

Keratoacanthoma is a benign lesion. It can grow very rapidly to form a large conical lesion with a characteristic central pit filled with keratin. It never spreads beyond the skin and usually resolves spontaneously within several weeks. Solar keratosis is a benign lesion seen in sun-damaged skin. It is usually a hyperkeratotic plaque with no evidence of nodularity, ulceration or invasion of the adjacent tissues.

INVESTIGATIONS

It is essential to obtain a tissue diagnosis in all cases prior to treatment.

SKIN SCRAPING CYTOLOGY

This is the least traumatic means of obtaining a sample for analysis. A scalpel is used to scratch the surface of the tumour until the skin begins to bleed lightly, and the debris smeared onto a microscope slide. In conjunction with interpretation by a skilled cytopathologist, it is a sensitive test and can give a result within hours, but equivocal or obviously inconsistent results mean that a biopsy is necessary.

INCISION BIOPSY

A wedge of tissue is removed, with care taken to include representative tumour and surrounding normal skin. This is usually performed when the lesion is too extensive to be treated with surgery.

EXCISION BIOPSY

This is best for small lesions that can be easily excised as it provides an accurate histological diagnosis and can be curative if microscopically complete.

FINE-NEEDLE ASPIRATION (FNA) OF ANY ENLARGED REGIONAL LYMPH NODES

Enlarged lymph nodes can be sampled by FNA to confirm malignancy.

RADIOLOGICAL INVESTIGATIONS

For larger, fixed or deeply invasive tumours CT or MRI should be performed prior to any treatment.

STAGING

The AJCC staging system is the most widely used:

- *Stage 0*: Carcinoma *in situ*, confined to the epidermis
- *Stage I*: <2 cm with no spread beyond skin
- *Stage II*: >2 cm with no spread beyond skin, or any size with two or more or the following:
  - Invasion into the lower dermis or subcutis
  - Neural invasion
  - Tumours on the ear or a hair-bearing lip

- *Stage III*: Involvement of facial bones or one nearby lymph node, but not to other organs
- *Stage IV*: Any size with spread to one or more lymph nodes >3 cm or distant metastases

TREATMENT

Both surgery and radiotherapy achieve local control in about 95% of cases. The choice is dependent on the anatomical site, size of lesion, convenience and previous treatment.

SURGERY

This is the treatment of choice for:
- Very large tumours involving bone (radiotherapy would have a reduced local control and risk of osteonecrosis)
- Scalp lesions (where radiotherapy would produce an area of permanent alopecia)
- Tumours in regions that do not tolerate radiotherapy well, e.g. skin overlying lower third of tibia and the back
- Tumours of the upper eyelid where radiotherapy scarring could cause repeated trauma to the cornea
- Local recurrences after radiotherapy (Figure 19.6) or arising in previously irradiated skin
- Younger patients in whom the late cutaneous effects of radiotherapy will have longer to become manifest

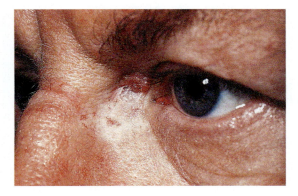

Figure 19.6 Recurrent basal cell carcinoma. This lesion has arisen at the edge of a previous radiation field. Such recurrences are best treated surgically.

Excision is usually performed under local anaesthetic, although large lesions requiring a skin graft or flap reconstruction can be removed under general anaesthetic. Facial lesions are best dealt with by a plastic surgeon to optimize the cosmetic result. Complete macroscopic and microscopic excision will be curative for SCC and BCC and so a margin of macroscopically normal skin of up to 10 mm (depending on size of tumour, cytological type and how well circumscribed it is) should be taken away en bloc.

Surgery is the treatment of choice for cases with involved regional lymph nodes when a block dissection is indicated. Overall, local control rates of 95% or more are to be expected after excision alone.

RADIOTHERAPY

Radiotherapy is equivalent to surgery in terms of local control and is better for:

- Tumours at sites where surgery would lead to an inferior cosmetic result, e.g. nasolabial fold
- Tumours at sites where surgery would lead to an inferior functional result, e.g. lower eyelid (Figure 19.7)

Superficial x-rays or electrons are used to limit irradiation of subcutaneous tissues. Treatment can be given as a large single fraction or a course of daily treatment over 2–6 weeks. Large single doses are preferred for patients with small tumours who would find travelling difficult due to age or infirmity, but this approach gives an inferior cosmetic outcome.

- Post-operative radiotherapy is indicated where surgical excision is incomplete and to nodal areas if there is extracapsular extension on microscopy of lymph nodes removed at surgery.

Inoperable nodes should also be treated with radiotherapy which may be followed by surgery if there is sufficient response.

CHEMOTHERAPY

Topical 5-fluorouracil can cause complete regression of Bowen disease (squamous carcinoma *in situ*) and small, flat BCCs/SCCs, but has to be applied regularly, is inconvenient and requires careful follow up. It is not routinely used.

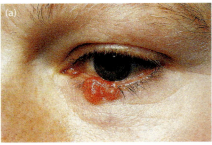
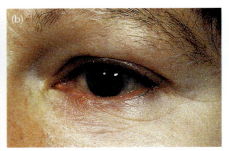

Figure 19.7 Basal cell carcinoma arising from the lower eyelid in a young woman (a) before treatment and (b) after radiotherapy. Note the permanent loss of eyelashes along the lower eyelid.

Advanced or metastatic SCC may respond to systemic chemotherapy but response rates are disappointing.

Defects in the hedgehog signalling pathway, a group of proteins involved in regulation of cell growth, are found in over 90% of sporadic BCCs. This has been a target for new drug development. Vismodegib is the first of these to be used clinically in BCCs unsuitable for surgery or radiotherapy or the rare cases of metastases. Response rates of 65% are reported.

CRYOTHERAPY

Liquid nitrogen topically is very effective for small superficial tumours. It is usually administered by a dermatologist, who will have the greatest expertise.

CURETTAGE

Suitable for small (≤1 cm), well-circumscribed and superficial tumours. However, there is a higher risk of local recurrence as the margins are more likely not to be free of tumour.

TUMOUR-RELATED COMPLICATIONS

Local tissue destruction will cause loss of function, disfigurement and predispose to secondary infection and bleeding. Secondary infection will lead to discharge and discomfort and can predispose to delayed healing after surgery or radiotherapy.

TREATMENT-RELATED COMPLICATIONS

After radiotherapy an acute skin reaction is inevitable, characterized by erythema, hyperpigmentation, itching, dry desquamation and in some cases moist desquamation. (Figure 19.8). This begins after 10–14 days of treatment and resolves within 2–4 weeks of completing radiotherapy. Occasionally, healing of a large area of skin can take many months. Chronic

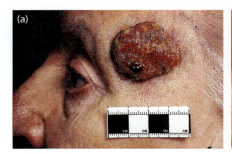
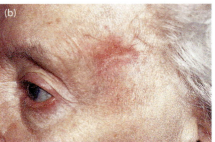

Figure 19.8 (a) Large squamous carcinoma at presentation; (b) 12 weeks after radiotherapy.

Melanoma

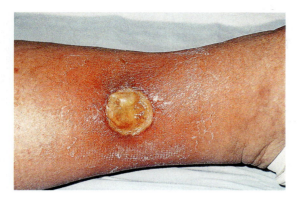

Figure 19.9 Necrosis after radiotherapy for a basal cell carcinoma arising from the skin of the lower calf region.

radionecrosis is a rare complication and may require skin grafting (Figure 19.9).

PROGNOSIS

It is unusual for a patient to die from non-melanoma skin cancer. Local control should be expected in over 95%, with most recurrences being successfully salvaged by further local treatment.

SCREENING/PREVENTION

The risks of ultraviolet radiation need to be appreciated, particularly by children and young adults. Avoidance of direct sun exposure and use of sunblocks is recommended in sunny climates. Patients with a past history of skin cancer are at risk of developing other cancers subsequently and benefit from surveillance and instructions regarding the early signs of a new tumour.

MELANOMA

This is a more serious form of skin cancer arising from the melanocytes of the skin but is curable if detected and treated at an early stage.

EPIDEMIOLOGY

Each year in the United Kingdom there are 16,000 cases of melanoma, approximately evenly distributed between men and women, leading to a total of 2400 deaths per annum, 1% of the total. There has been a doubling in incidence over the last two decades, more so in men than women with an ongoing increased forecast over the next two decades. It is one of the few cancers that has a significant impact on young adults, 22% arising in the under-40s, although rates are highest in the 85–90 age group. The geographical and racial distribution is similar to that of non-melanomatous skin cancer. Malignant melanoma does occasionally arise in dark-skinned people but is 10 times less common than in white people living a similar lifestyle. Severe sunburn (and therefore skin type) and childhood UV exposure are high-risk factors.

AETIOLOGY

Ultraviolet radiation is the main causative factor, sun exposure being very important in determining risk, particularly during childhood. Additional risk factors include blond or red hair colour, and intense episodic sun exposure, particularly in those who tan poorly and burn easily. The vast majority of naevi confer no additional risk of melanoma, although individuals with large numbers (>100) are at increased risk. Dysplastic naevi can be congenital and are usually large lesions with irregular pigment and an irregular edge. Affected individuals should be watched very closely.

PATHOLOGY

The site distribution in men and women differs as shown in Figure 19.10. Mucosal melanoma is rare and described in the upper aerodigestive tract, anus and vagina. Melanoma of the choroid of the eye is also described as the pigment cells which is homologous with those of the skin.

Macroscopically, melanoma is typically brown or black in colour due to increased melanin production by the melanocytes, frequently with irregularity of pigment (Figure 19.11). Amelanotic tumours are seen in about 5% of cases. They can be nodular or flat and seen to be spreading along the superficial layers of the skin. Fifty percent are superficial spreading melanomas and have a more favourable prognosis than

Skin cancer

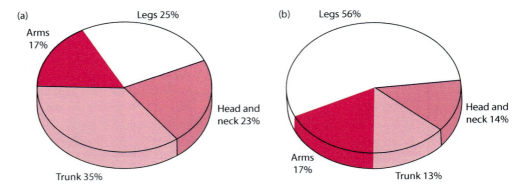

Figure 19.10 Site distribution of malignant melanoma in (a) males and (b) females.

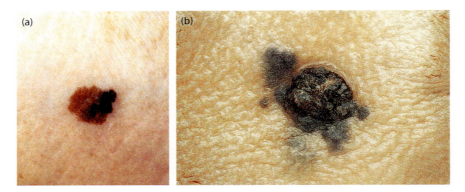

Figure 19.11 Malignant melanoma. Note the irregular edge, uneven pigmentation in both examples. (a) Superficial spreading melanoma. (b) Nodular melanoma.

nodular types, which have an early vertical growth phase. In advanced cases there can be associated ulceration or satellite lesions on the adjacent skin.

Microscopically, the tumour is composed of melanocytes that invade along the superficial layers of the skin and penetrate the basement membrane into the deeper layers of the dermis. The cells characteristically stain for S100, melan A and HMB45 reflecting their origin from neural crest cells. Diagnosis may be confirmed with positivity for MiTF1 and SOX10. A lymphocytic infiltrate is common, reflecting a host cellular immune response.

NATURAL HISTORY

Melanoma can remain in a superficial spreading phase for many months before it grows into the papillary dermis, reticular dermis and subcutaneous fat.

Nodular melanomas tend to spread into the dermis at an early stage, which accounts for their poorer prognosis. Permeation of the dermal lymphatics sometimes leads to satellite nodules adjacent to the main bulk of disease (Figure 19.12).

Regional lymph nodes can be involved when the melanoma invades the deeper layers of the skin.

Melanoma can spread widely. Lung, bone (Figure 19.13), brain and skin metastases are the most common and it is one of the few extra-abdominal tumours to spread to the bowel and its mesentery. Primary melanoma of the choroid of the eye has a propensity to spread to the liver.

SYMPTOMS

Presentation is usually with a pigmented skin lesion. Changes in a preceding naevus or appearance of a

Melanoma

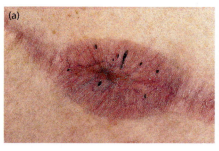
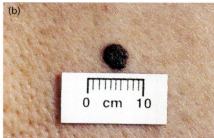

Figure 19.12 In-transit metastases from melanoma. (a) Spread radiating from site of original skin lesion. (b) In-transit metastasis in skin some 20 cm away.

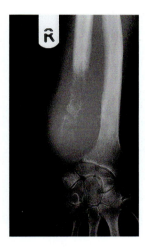

Figure 19.13 Bone metastasis from melanoma. There is significant bone destruction at a site that is less frequently affected by other solid tumours.

new pigmented lesion frequently go unnoticed, particularly if on the back.

Changes in pigmentation, itching or bleeding are suspicious and should be evaluated in a specialist pigmented lesion clinic.

SIGNS

The melanoma will usually be on a sun-exposed area. The degree and pattern of pigmentation is variable but is characteristically irregular, particularly at the edge of the lesion. Ulceration is a poor prognostic feature.

Regional lymph nodes should always be palpated for enlargement, which may be due either to tumour infiltration or in reaction to the tumour/secondary infection.

There can be signs of distant metastases such as hepatomegaly, pleural effusion/collapse/consolidation, or focal neurological signs. Patients with a heavy burden of metastases have been described as having a slate grey complexion from increased circulating melanin released by the tumour cells. Skin metastases have a typical blue/black colour (Figure 19.14).

DIFFERENTIAL DIAGNOSIS

Benign pigmented skin lesions need to be distinguished from melanoma, including benign naevi, seborrhoeic warts, dermatofibromata and pigmented BCC/SCC.

Lentigo maligna (Hutchinson's melanotic freckle) typically occurs in the elderly on the face as a large, slow-growing, superficial, pigmented and irregular lesion, which represents a melanoma *in situ*, with the potential to become invasive.

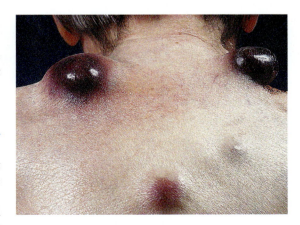

Figure 19.14 Multiple cutaneous metastases from malignant melanoma. Note the characteristic pigmentation of the lesions reflecting their origin.

INVESTIGATIONS

EXCISION BIOPSY

This is preferable to incision biopsy as it will provide a large specimen for detailed histological analysis and remove the lesion in toto. It is mandatory for any atypical pigmented lesion. Only a small macroscopic margin of normal skin is taken.

FINE-NEEDLE ASPIRATION (FNA) OF ANY ENLARGED REGIONAL LYMPH NODES

This should differentiate between reactive and metastatic enlargement.

EXCLUSION OF METASTATIC DISEASE

CT of chest, abdomen and pelvis and in those at high risk of metastatic disease, e.g. deeply invasive (4 mm or deeper) lesions, lymph-node positive cases, a brain scan should be included in the staging investigations.

STAGING

Clark's levels measure the depth in relation to histological landmarks:

- *Level I*: Confined to the lamina propria
- *Level II*: Reaches the papillary dermis
- *Level III*: Reaches the papillary/reticular dermis
- *Level IV*: Reaches the reticular dermis
- *Level V*: Reaches subcutaneous fat

The Breslow thickness measures absolute depth in millimetres and is the distance of the deepest malignant cell from the stratum granulosum classified as follows:

- <0.75 mm
- 0.76–1.50 mm
- 1.51–4.0 mm
- >4.0 mm

The TNM staging incorporates both Clark's level and Breslow thickness.

TREATMENT

SURGERY

This is usually curative for early localized lesions, a wide excision down to subcutaneous fat being necessary including a margin of macroscopically normal skin, the size of which is dependent on the depth (if known). A centimetre of clearance for every millimetre of depth (clinical estimate or from result of previous excision biopsy) up to a maximum of 2 cm is adequate and re-excision is necessary if the margins are not clear microscopically. A skin graft or vascularized skin flap might be needed to close the defect if too large to heal by itself. In the case of subungual melanoma, amputation of the digit is performed.

Sentinel lymph-node mapping (see Chapters 4 and 8) is performed and if positive formal regional lymph-node dissection is indicated.

Surgery also has a role in the management of distant metastatic relapses. If limited to one anatomical site, resection should be considered. This can result in successful salvage and long-term remission.

RADIOTHERAPY

Melanomas are considered relatively radio-resistant tumours. The treatment technique is similar to that used for other skin tumours.

In the rare case of melanoma of the choroid, very high doses of radiation administered using radioactive plaques sutures temporarily on the outer eyeball adjacent to the tumour sewn to the eye are curative in a high proportion. Otherwise, radiotherapy has little role as a curative treatment, being used when the patient refuses surgery or the tumour is inoperable, e.g. some mucosal melanomas. Low doses of radiation are valuable in palliating pain from skeletal metastases and focal, symptomatic metastases elsewhere.

SYSTEMIC TREATMENT

Significant advances have been made in recent years with the development of MAP kinase pathway inhibitors such as vemurafenib and immune modulating drugs such as ipilimumab acting on the CTLV-4 pathway targeting the CD8 lymphocyte population or pembrolizumab targeting the PD1-L pathway regulating immunogenic T cells. These drugs have replaced conventional chemotherapy and older immunotherapies such as interferon.

Staining for mutant BRAF, a downstream molecule in the MAP kinase is now important in deciding whether one of these agents is appropriate. A weaker association with CTLV-4 or PD-1 L activation is seen for the immune modulators. In BRAF positive patients it is unclear whether treatment should be started with a MAP kinase inhibitor or an immunomodulator. Resistance to drugs such as vemurafenib develops within a few months but initial response rates tend to be higher. Most patients with metastatic disease will in practice receive both types of drug sequentially and current trials are seeking to determine whether combination therapy is superior.

TUMOUR-RELATED COMPLICATIONS

Secondary infection is an uncommon complication, predisposing to local discomfort, discharge and bleeding. Uncontrolled nodal disease may lead to lymphatic obstruction and lymphoedema of a limb.

TREATMENT-RELATED COMPLICATIONS

Wide local excision and extensive lymph-node dissection can have a major cosmetic impact and cause lymphoedema. Immunotherapy can cause significant toxicity including immune pneumonitis, colitis and ileitis. High-dose steroids alongside supportive therapy will be required in more severe cases.

PROGNOSIS

Poor prognostic factors correlate with the risk of developing distant metastases and include:

- Deep Clarke's level
- Deep Breslow thickness (5-year survivals for lesions <1.5, 1.5–3.5 and >3.5 mm are approximately 90%, 70% and 40% respectively)
- Ulceration
- Mucosal melanoma versus cutaneous (detected earlier)
- Nodular melanoma versus superficial spreading (longer horizontal growth phase)
- Male sex
- Age >50 years

Overall, 5-year survival is 50%–%60 for men and 70%–%80 for women.

The outlook for patients with metastatic disease has improved considerably since the use of new drugs, MAP kinase inhibitors and immunomodulators. Median survival of 24–30 months can now be expected.

SCREENING/PREVENTION

As far as melanoma is concerned, early detection during the horizontal growth phase is essential. Education of community physicians and other healthcare professionals is important in facilitating this. People should be encouraged to visit their general practitioner or specialist dermatology clinic for an opinion if a pigmented lesion:

- Increases in size
- Changes shape or colour, particularly if pigmentation becomes irregular
- Develops an inflammation at its edge
- Itches
- Bleeds or crusts

Regular photographs of dysplastic naevi will aid early diagnosis of malignant change and screening of other family members should be undertaken if they have similar lesions.

Four out of five melanomas are preventable. Health education is again vital to inform people to:

- Avoid visible sunburn, e.g. avoiding midday sun by seeking shade, use of sunscreen creams and clothing to protect skin
- Take measures to protect skin of children
- Take care to avoid excessive UV exposure in Northern Europe and not just when overseas
- Take extra care if involved in outdoor occupations and/or leisure pursuits

Skin cancer

> **CASE HISTORY**
>
> A 34-year-old woman with a fair complexion presents to her GP with a mole on her right calf. This had been present for at least 10 years but over the last 6 months had enlarged in diameter, become more nodular, irregularly pigmented and itchy. She is referred to a fast-track pigmented lesion clinic.
>
> Clinical examination reveals a pigmented lesion 1 cm in diameter suspicious for a melanoma. A detailed survey of the rest of the skin shows 20–30 benign naevi randomly distributed over the trunk and upper limbs. There is no popliteal, inguinal or femoral lymphadenopathy. There is no hepatomegaly. There are no other signs of disseminated malignancy.
>
> Excision biopsy confirms a nodular melanoma with strong S100 immunostaining, 12 mm in diameter with a Breslow thickness of 4 mm. The margins of excision are clear but by <1 mm at the superior and a lateral margin. She therefore undergoes a further wide excision and split skin graft to attain skin closure. Histology reveals a few residual nests of melanoma cells but the margins of excision are confirmed to be clear by 5 mm or more at all points. Baseline staging CT scan of the thorax and abdomen shows no evidence of visceral disease.
>
> Four years after diagnosis, she notices a lump in the right groin. Fine-needle aspiration confirms melanoma cells. Further CT scan shows no evidence of metastatic disease and no iliac lymphadenopathy. She therefore undergoes a radical groin lymph-node dissection yielding three involved nodes.
>
> Despite occasional swelling of the right lower leg, she remains well 8 years after diagnosis. She and her GP keep the other naevi under regular surveillance and she always avoids excessive sun exposure.

There is some evidence in at-risk populations that use of a powerful sunscreen can reduce the incidence of solar keratoses, the precursor lesion for cutaneous squamous carcinoma. Chemoprevention programmes using isotretinoin or β-carotene have to date been ineffective.

METASTASES

The skin is frequently the site of distant metastases in patients with advanced cancer, particularly from breast and lung primaries (Figure 19.15), usually presenting as one or more well-circumscribed subcutaneous nodules. They can be asymptomatic, cause irritation or fungate. If the diagnosis is in doubt, fine-needle aspiration for cytology, incision or excision biopsy provides the definitive diagnosis. Symptomatic lesions can be treated by any of the usual local or systemic cancer therapies to which the primary tumour is sensitive.

RARE TUMOURS

MYCOSIS FUNGOIDES

This is a cutaneous T-cell lymphoma with a peak incidence at 30–50 years. It has a predilection for body creases, buttocks and face and is initially non-specific, resembling chronic eczema or psoriasis. This stage can last for several years before progression to plaques that are well demarcated, erythematous, sometimes itchy lesions. The plaque stage progresses to the tumour stage consisting of erythematous nodules arising in the plaques or in normal skin. Erythroderma is described when the whole skin is affected, and Sézary syndrome when abnormal lymphocytes are seen in the peripheral blood (see Chapter 16). Treatment options include phototherapy with UV light, steroids, radiotherapy either locally or to the whole skin, topical or systemic chemotherapy, retinoids and interferon. The clinical course is protracted and many will die of unrelated causes.

NON-HODGKIN LYMPHOMA

B-cell non-Hodgkin lymphoma may also affect the skin.

KAPOSI SARCOMA

This arises from vascular endothelial cells and is characteristically found in patients with HIV infection although sporadic cases also occur.

MERKEL CELL CARCINOMA

The mean age at diagnosis is 65–70 years and it presents as a solitary lesion, most frequent on head and

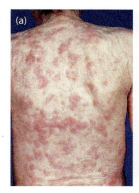 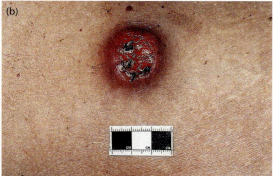

Figure 19.15 Cutaneous metastases from breast cancer. (a) Generalized rash. The skin infiltration was intensely irritating. (b) Solitary lesion. Note the dark areas corresponding to diathermy used to treat bleeding.

neck in sun-damaged skin. It arises from neuroendocrine cells and is locally aggressive, spreading to regional lymph nodes and to distant sites. Even with combined wide local excision and post-operative radiotherapy, over one-third will recur locally and about half will eventually die from their disease.

HIDRADENOCARCINOMA

This is a carcinoma arising from the sweat glands.

SARCOMA

These arise from the soft tissues of the skin and include leiomyosarcoma, liposarcoma, malignant fibrous histiocytoma and angiosarcoma.

FURTHER READING

BMJ Best Practice: Overview of skin cancer. https://bestpractice.bmj.com/topics/en-gb/267

BMJ Best Practice: Basal cell carcinoma. https://best-practice.bmj.com/topics/en-gb/269

BMJ Best Practice: Squamous cell carcinoma of the skin. https://bestpractice.bmj.com/topics/en-gb/270

BMJ Best Practice: Melanoma. https://bestpractice.bmj.com/topics/en-gb/268

Coit DG, Thompson JA, Albertini MR et al. Cutaneous Melanoma, Version 2.2019, NCCN Clinical Practice Guidelines in Oncology. *J Natl Compr Canc Netw.* 2019; 17(4): 367–402.

Peris K, Fargnoli MC, Garbe C et al. Diagnosis and treatment of basal cell carcinoma: European consensus-based interdisciplinary guidelines. *Eur J Cancer.* 2019; 118: 10–34.

SELF-ASSESSMENT QUESTIONS

1. Which one of the following is true about skin cancer?
   a. Only seen in the elderly
   b. Never occurs in dark-skinned races
   c. It is the commonest form of malignant disease
   d. Only caused by exposure to ultraviolet radiation
   e. With better public awareness the incidence is decreasing

2. Which three of the following are the recognized causes of skin cancer?
   a. Immunosuppression
   b. Strychnine
   c. Chronic skin ulceration
   d. Gorlin syndrome
   e. Phosphorus
   f. Microwaves
   g. Sarcoidosis

3. Which three of the following statements apply to basal cell carcinoma of the skin?
   a. Most commonly seen on legs
   b. Less common than squamous carcinoma

Skin cancer

    c. Usually slow growing
    d. Only metastasize after many years
    e. Lymph-node spread is common
    f. Highly sensitive to radiotherapy
    g. Can be treated by cryotherapy

4. Which three of the following statements apply to squamous cell carcinoma of the skin?
    a. More common than malignant melanoma
    b. Usually well differentiated
    c. Rarely arise on hair-bearing skin
    d. 10% will have evidence of lymph-node spread
    e. Much higher rate of cure compared with non-cutaneous squamous carcinoma
    f. Produce melanin
    g. May metastasize to the lungs

5. Which three of the following statements apply to malignant melanoma?
    a. Usually pigmented
    b. More common than squamous carcinoma
    c. Spreads to regional lymph nodes
    d. Higher mortality rate than other forms of skin cancer
    e. Can be treated by cryotherapy
    f. Highly sensitive to radiotherapy
    g. Resistant to immunotherapy

6. Which three of the following are typical signs of melanoma?
    a. Hyperkeratosis
    b. Irregular pigmentation
    c. Spontaneous regression of a mole
    d. Itching
    e. Sun damage in surrounding skin
    f. Bleeding
    g. Secondary infection

7. Which one of the following is not a prognostic factor for melanoma?
    a. Mucosal origin
    b. Intensity of pigmentation
    c. Depth of invasion
    d. Thickness of lesion
    e. Ulceration

8. Which three of the following statements apply to Merkel cell carcinoma?
    a. Signet ring cells are characteristic
    b. More frequent in head and neck area
    c. Affects older age group than melanoma
    d. Higher risk of local recurrence than other forms of skin cancer
    e. Usually pigmented
    f. Treated with cryotherapy
    g. More common than melanoma

Carcinoma of unknown primary

Some patients present with metastatic cancer but with no evidence of the site of origin, e.g. presenting with enlarged cervical lymph node(s), bone metastases or pulmonary metastases on chest x-ray. Their management can be a difficult problem, the oncologist having to determine whether the patient has a curable tumour such as a teratoma or lymphoma, one that can benefit from systemic therapy (e.g. a hormone-responsive cancer such as the breast or prostate cancer), or one where treatment would not be justified.

The following definitions have been introduced to help define the status of a patient presenting without a clear primary origin and to lead to a logical and rapid process of coming to a diagnosis and management plan and many cancer pathways have structured pathways such that these patients are discussed at a specific CUP (carcinoma of unknown primary) multidisciplinary meeting.

Malignancy of undefined primary origin (MUO) – Metastatic malignancy identified on the basis of a limited number of tests, without an obvious primary site, before comprehensive investigation or histology. This applies to any potential histological type.

Provisional carcinoma of unknown primary (provisional CUP) origin – Metastatic epithelial or neuroendocrine malignancy identified on the basis of histology or cytology, with no primary site detected despite a selected initial screen of investigations, before possible review and possible further specialized investigations.

Confirmed carcinoma of unknown primary origin (confirmed CUP) – Metastatic epithelial or neuroendocrine malignancy identified on the basis of final histology, with no primary site detected despite a selected initial screen of investigations, review and further specialized investigations as appropriate, CUP accounts for 3%–5% of all malignancies.

A detailed history may yield important clues. Questions should be aimed at eliciting symptoms of the underlying primary neoplasm, judging its time course and rate of progression, as well as gauging the performance status of the patient. The presence of 'B' symptoms could suggest an underlying lymphoma. The possibility (albeit rare) of choriocarcinoma should be considered in a young woman with a recent history of pregnancy. The development of breast tenderness in a young male can suggest an underlying trophoblastic germ cell tumour.

A detailed physical examination should include the skin, oral cavity, thyroid, breasts, peripheral lymph node groups (cervical chains, Waldeyer's ring, supraclavicular fossae, axillae and groins), spleen, rectum including prostate and testes in males, and pelvic examination in females. If the patient has presented with lymphadenopathy, the region that drains to those nodes should be examined thoroughly. For example, inguinal lymphadenopathy should prompt a thorough survey of both lower limbs, perianal region and anal canal, penis and scrotum in males, vulva and vagina in females. Some women will present with adenocarcinoma in one or more axillary lymph nodes and this should trigger breast-specific imaging to exclude an occult ipsilateral breast primary.

Carcinoma of unknown primary

DIFFERENTIAL DIAGNOSIS

The most likely primary sites vary with histology (Table 20.1). The common solid tumours (lung, breast, colorectal, prostate, pancreas) should be considered. Anaplastic tumours are mainly poorly differentiated carcinomas, the rest being undifferentiated teratomas, lymphoma, melanoma (particularly amelanotic variant), sarcomas and neuroendocrine tumours.

INVESTIGATIONS

Patients with distant metastases should not undergo exhaustive investigation in the relentless search for a primary that is ultimately unlikely to be curable and where local treatment of the primary will not be justified. For those with distant metastases, localization of the primary tumour site is unlikely to affect materially the diagnosis or immediate management. However, histological typing of the tumour will influence the assessment of prognosis and the type of systemic therapy chosen.

BIOPSY

A balance has to be struck between the need to confirm the histological diagnosis, how it will affect ultimate management and what treatment is reasonable for the patient to undergo. The general principle is to obtain an adequate piece of tissue from a representative part of the tumour that is not necrotic. This should ensure sufficient tissue for immunocytochemistry so that an accurate analysis is possible. If several sites of bulk disease are accessible, the safest and least traumatic route of access should be followed. A needle biopsy is usually the optimum means of getting enough tissue to perform the required histological testing. The lesion for biopsy might need to be localized using CT or ultrasound depending on its anatomical location and accessibility.

IMMUNOCYTOCHEMISTRY

Some tissues have staining characteristics depending on their embryological origin and constituent cells:

- *Germ cell tumour*: α-Fetoprotein (AFP) β-human chorionic gonadotropin (HCG)
- *Prostate cancer*: Prostate-specific antigen (PSA)
- *Colorectal cancer*: Carcinoembryonic antigen (CEA) and CK2 +ve, CK20 +ve, CK7 −ve
- *Lung cancer*: TTF1 +ve, CK7 +ve
- *Ovary cancer*: CA125, CK7 +ve, CK20 +ve
- *Breast cancer*: Oestrogen/progesterone receptors, CA15-3, vimentin, desmin +ve
- *Pancreatic cancer*: CA 19-9
- *Lymphoma*: Leucocyte common antigen, CD45, CD20, CD79a (B cell), CD5 (T-cell)
- *Melanoma*: S100, HMB45, vimentin, desmin +ve
- *Sarcoma*: S100, HMB45, vimentin, desmin +ve
- *Neuroendocrine*: Neurone-specific enolase (NSE), chromogranin, synaptophysin +ve, vimentin, desmin±

CYTOGENETIC STUDIES

These are of value in tumours arising in children and adolescents as many tumours have characteristic chromosomal abnormalities, e.g. translocations in Ewing sarcoma (t11;22), rhabdomyosarcoma (t2;13), non-Hodgkin lymphoma (NHL) (t8;14). Extragonadal germ cell tumours can have abnormalities of

Table 20.1 Most likely sites of primary carcinomas according to histology

Histological type	Most likely sites of primary
Adenocarcinoma	Lung
	GI tract (stomach, colon, pancreas)
	Breast
	Prostate
	Ovary
	Kidney
Squamous carcinoma	Lung
	Head and neck
Small cell carcinoma	Lung

chromosome 12. These are of less value in adult solid tumours.

Recent advances in genomic studies have led to the development of a test whereby fixed tissue is analysed using gene microarrays and matched against a tissue bank of different tumours to cross reference it and thereby identify a likely site of origin (CupPrint® test). This is commercially available but expensive, and it is still unclear whether such tests effect overall survival in these patients.

POLYMERASE CHAIN REACTION

The PCR detection of Epstein–Barr virus genome can suggest an occult nasopharyngeal primary or NHL.

RADIOLOGICAL INVESTIGATIONS

CT scan of the thorax, abdomen and pelvis not only allows a detailed radiological survey of a number of possible sites of origin of metastases that are clinically impalpable (e.g. pancreas, ovaries), but also allows full staging, which is of prognostic value and of use in planning treatment. An isotope bone scan is useful to assess the skeleton for staging purposes. Bilateral mammography should be considered in women with adenocarcinoma of unknown primary to exclude an occult breast primary that would be amenable to aggressive locoregional therapy or hormone manipulation. A transrectal ultrasound should be considered if the prostate feels suspicious or the PSA is elevated, and if clinically indicated, will facilitate a needle core biopsy of the prostate under direct vision. A transvaginal ultrasound is useful in evaluating the lower female genital tract. A whole body PET survey sometimes discloses the location of an occult primary cancer amidst known metastatic disease (Figure 20.1). A PET scan is indicated in a patient who presents with neck nodes and no obvious primary on pan-endoscopy, as it may help in identifying an occult primary head and neck cancer.

BLOOD TESTS

Serum tumour marker assays can be useful for giving a clue as to the likely origin of the metastases and therefore allow a more focused approach to

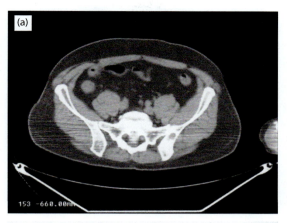

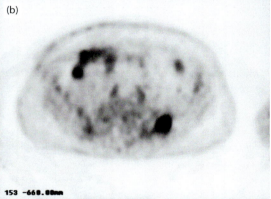

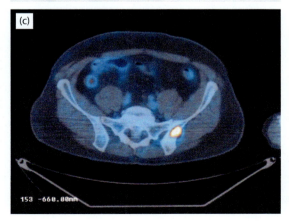

Figure 20.1 Whole body PET survey. The patient presented with bone metastases. (a) CT study. (b) Corresponding PET image. There are several areas of focal uptake. (c) Fusion PET/CT image. This confirms uptake in the pelvic bone posteriorly. Importantly, it suggests a hypermetabolic, rounded density within the right side of the pelvis, which turned out to be a primary colon cancer.

Carcinoma of unknown primary

investigations. A normal PSA test makes carcinoma of the prostate unlikely. A very high CEA can suggest a gastrointestinal primary and CA19-9 upper gastrointestinal malignancy such as pancreas. CA15-3 and CA125 should be measured in women presenting with adenocarcinoma of unknown primary to exclude carcinoma of the breast and ovary, respectively. Young adults presenting with undifferentiated cancers should have blood taken for AFP and HCG to exclude a trophoblastic germ cell tumour. In an urgent situation, a urinary pregnancy test is a crude way of checking for excess HCG levels in a male. Such tumour markers should be considered and ordered appropriately rather than being a blanket screen.

OTHER INVESTIGATIONS

Patients presenting with squamous carcinoma in lymph nodes draining the head and neck region must be referred to an ENT surgeon for an endoscopy of the upper aerodigestive tract (especially nasopharynx, tonsils, posterior third of tongue, supraglottic larynx and pyriform fossa) as the patient could still have a curable occult primary cancer.

MANAGEMENT

The problem is usually one of systemic disease at the outset and so it is logical to consider some form of systemic therapy. The patient should be managed according to their age, general condition, site and stage of disease and symptomatology. In cases of widespread distant metastases in a patient with a very poor performance status, local treatment directed towards symptom relief is likely to be most appropriate as the patient will be incurable and unlikely to gain from chemotherapy. Conversely, the patient should be treated with curative intent if there are distant metastases and the tumour is particularly chemosensitive (e.g. teratoma, lymphoma) or if there are regional lymph node metastases from a tumour that could be cured by aggressive locoregional therapy, e.g. in the head and neck or breast. For this reason, women presenting with isolated axillary lymphadenopathy containing adenocarcinoma and no other primary site should be assumed to have an occult carcinoma of the breast and treated accordingly. A young person presenting with a rapidly enlarging mediastinal mass or retroperitoneal mass and a biopsy showing poorly differentiated tumour cells and negative lymphocyte markers should be suspected as having a non-gonadal germ cell tumour, and treated accordingly with a cisplatin chemotherapy regime, even if serum AFP and HCG levels are not elevated.

Most patients fall between these two extreme ends of the spectrum, in which case systemic therapy can be employed to maximize the symptom-free interval with the expectation that this may in turn lead to a prolongation of survival. Hormonal therapy should be initiated in selected tumours, e.g. prostate cancer and breast cancer. Chemotherapy is frequently used in good performance status patients. For those where the primary tumour origin is found or suspected from biopsy, the regimens specific for that disease are most appropriate. For those where it is impractical to obtain a histological diagnosis, it is rational to select several drugs that cover the most common solid tumours, e.g. an anthracycline, an alkylating agent, 5FU and/or platinum derivative.

PROGNOSIS

Tumours which present in this way are those which will have a strong propensity to spread widely before the primary discloses its presence, and hence have an innately worse prognosis. The prognosis is poor, with a median survival of approximately 3–4 months in most studies and less than 25% and 10% of patients alive at 1 and 5 years, respectively. Male gender, increasing number of involved organ sites, adenocarcinoma histology and hepatic involvement are all unfavourable prognostic factors. Only the few with lymphoma or a germ cell tumour stand a higher chance of cure.

Unfortunately, the site of the primary tumour might never be found during life. A post-mortem examination can be very instructive for the clinicians and relieve uncertainty for the next of kin, although even then the primary origin can prove elusive.

Self-assessment questions

CASE HISTORY

CARCINOMA OF UNKNOWN PRIMARY

A previously fit 51-year-old woman is well until she joins a gym. Following a quadriceps toning exercise, she develops persistent discomfort in the right thigh. This persists for 2 weeks despite the use of a topical anti-inflammatory gel. She was climbing a flight of stairs when she hears a loud 'crack', and collapses with severe acute pain in the thigh. She is taken to the accident and emergency department where a plain radiograph confirms a transverse fracture of the femoral midshaft. There is some lysis of the cortex either side of the fracture suggesting a pre-existing condition, which had led to bone absorption. The diagnosis of a pathological fracture is made, the radiologist confirming that there is almost certainly a metastasis at this site. She is referred to an orthopaedic surgeon and undergoes an emergency open reduction and internal fixation. A specimen is sent for histology and this shows normal connective tissue and bone infiltrated with undifferentiated cancer cells which do not stain with a panel of immunohistochemical stains.

Post-operatively, she is referred to an oncologist. A full history fails to reveal any symptoms of an underlying malignant process and therefore does not give any clue as to the likely underlying cause. She has had a recent normal cervical smear and her first screening mammogram was unremarkable. A detailed physical examination reveals a hard, solitary 1.5 cm lymph node in the left supraclavicular fossa. There is no abnormality within the breasts or axillae and all other lymph node groups are normal. The thyroid is unremarkable and there is no mucosal abnormality within the oral cavity and oropharynx. The chest is clear and there is no hepatomegaly. Digital examination of the rectum and vaginal examination are normal. There are a few benign naevi but no obvious cutaneous manifestation of primary or secondary malignancy.

Full blood count is normal. Liver function tests show a moderate elevation of both γ-glutamyltransferase and alkaline phosphatase at 125 and 340 U/L, respectively. The serum calcium corrected for the serum albumin is 3.2 mmol/L (normal range 2.1–2.6 mmol/L). Fine-needle aspiration of the supraclavicular lymph node reveals adenocarcinoma cells, which are both CEA negative and oestrogen receptor negative. Bilateral mammography is normal. Chest x-ray is clear but CT scan shows low volume bilateral lung metastases and multiple liver metastases. Isotope bone scan confirms increased isotope uptake at the site of recent bone surgery and in the dorsal spine, lumbar spine and contralateral humerus. Plain radiographs are obtained of the latter, which confirm that this area is not at risk of imminent fracture and therefore does not require prophylactic internal fixation. The CA15-3, CA125, thyroglobulin and CEA tumour markers are all within the normal range. Taking account of the extent of metastatic disease, it is not felt appropriate to investigate the gastrointestinal tract for an occult primary.

In view of the presentation and asymptomatic hypercalcaemia, she is encouraged to maintain a high fluid intake and commenced on infusions of disodium pamidronate 90 mg 4 weekly. A short course of radiotherapy is delivered to the fracture site to consolidate the surgical fixation. Bearing in mind her good performance status and extent of disease, having discussed the option of best supportive care with chemotherapy kept in reserve for symptomatic progression, an indwelling venous catheter is inserted and chemotherapy is started with continuously infused 5-FU and 3-weekly boluses of epirubicin and cisplatin. Restaging after three cycles shows stable disease but after six there is evidence of progression within the thorax and liver. Repeat physical examination at this point reveals an ill-defined 2 cm lump within the left breast. Core biopsy confirms adenocarcinoma cells with staining characteristics similar to those obtained from the original lymph node. The tumour is HER2 negative. Her chemotherapy is changed to taxotere and she attains a good partial response which is sustained for 4 months. At second relapse, she fails to respond to further chemotherapy and dies of her disease. The certified cause of death is metastatic breast cancer.

FURTHER READING

Fizazi K, Greco FA, Pavlidis N, Daugaard G, Oien K, Pentheroudakis G. ESMO Guidelines Committee. Cancers of unknown primary site: ESMO Clinical Practice Guidelines for diagnosis, treatment and follow-up. *Ann Oncol*. 2015; 26 (Suppl 5): v133–v138. http://www.cancer.gov/cancertopics/pdq/treatment/unknownprimary/health professional/

SELF-ASSESSMENT QUESTIONS

1. Which three of the following are true for carcinoma of unknown primary?
   a. It is an uncommon clinical scenario
   b. The primary cancer is found in most cases after investigation
   c. Biopsy is mandatory
   d. Treatment is withheld until the primary tumour is identified

Carcinoma of unknown primary

  e. Tissue immunohistochemistry is useful
  f. Investigation is futile
  g. Most cases will lead to the death of the patient

2. Which three of the following are true associations?
  a. CK20 and bowel cancer
  b. TTF-1 and lung cancer
  c. CA15-3 and ovarian cancer
  d. S100 and melanoma
  e. CA125 and pancreatic cancer
  f. CD117 and lymphoma
  g. Calcitonin and lung cancer

Oncological emergencies

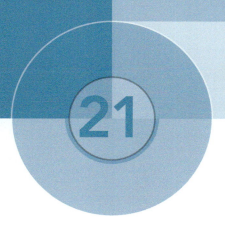

There are few conditions in the management of malignant disease that are true emergencies. However, it is important to identify those patients in whom urgent treatment is required. The following conditions can be associated with rapid deterioration and even death, and should be considered situations requiring urgent management:

- Hypercalcaemia
- Spinal cord or cauda equina compression
- Superior vena cava obstruction
- Neutropenic sepsis
- Tumour lysis syndrome
- Toxicities related to immunotherapy

HYPERCALCAEMIA

Malignant hypercalcaemia is the most common cause of a raised serum calcium in oncology patient. It is associated in particular with lung cancer, breast cancer, prostatic cancer and myeloma. It is generally found in patients with disseminated metastatic disease and is an indicator of poor prognosis.

AETIOLOGY

There is increasing evidence that hypercalcaemia associated with malignancy is due principally to the effects of chemical agents released by the tumour, which disturb the normal mechanisms of calcium balance. A number of these have now been identified that act as osteoclast-activating factors (OAFs) and include parathyroid hormone-like peptides, prostaglandins, interleukins and transforming growth factor β (TGFβ). They result in osteoclast activation and mobilization of calcium from bones.

SYMPTOMS

These include anorexia, nausea, vomiting, constipation, confusion, polyuria, thirst, polydipsia and bone pains.

SIGNS

There are usually no specific physical signs. The patient might appear drowsy and have signs of confusion or dehydration.

DIFFERENTIAL DIAGNOSIS

Other causes of similar symptoms including polyuria, polydipsia and confusion that should be considered include diabetes mellitus, cerebral metastases, hepatic failure, renal failure and neutropenic sepsis.

INVESTIGATIONS

The diagnosis is confirmed by measuring the serum calcium. It is important to correct the total level of serum albumin which is often low in patients with advanced malignant disease. The simple correction is to add 0.02 mmol/L to the serum calcium level for every g/dL of albumin below 40 g/dL, which is the conventional standardization level. For example, a reading of calcium at 2.3 mmol/L with an albumin of 30 g/dL gives a corrected serum albumin of 2.5 mmol/L. The normal range after correction is between 2.1 and 2.6 mmol/L but symptoms are not often seen until the level reaches 3.0 mmol/L or above. It is now usual for modern laboratories to report both actual and corrected calcium levels.

TREATMENT

There are two components to the treatment of malignant hypercalcaemia:

- Correction of dehydration and establishing good urine flow. An intravenous infusion of normal saline giving 1 L every 6 hours should be started. Careful attention to fluid balance is essential, particularly in the elderly who may easily become fluid overloaded. Frusemide can be added which, in addition to acting as a diuretic, also promotes urinary excretion of calcium. Thiazides should be avoided as they increase calcium reabsorption.
- Specific therapy to reduce calcium levels using intravenous zolendronate once good urine flow has been established. Other bisphosphonates such as pamidronate or ibandranate are also effective.

Although rapid correction of serum calcium is often possible with the previously mentioned approach, rebound hypercalcaemia is common unless regular bisphosphonate infusions are continued at 3–4 weekly intervals.

The ultimate prognosis for malignant hypercalcaemia is poor with most patients surviving for only a few months, succumbing to either refractory hypercalcaemia or the effects of widespread malignancy.

SPINAL CORD AND CAUDA EQUINA COMPRESSION

This condition arises most commonly as a result of extradural tumour. It may complicate most malignancies but most common are carcinoma of the lung, breast and prostate. It should be treated as an emergency because the outcome in terms of final neurological disability is determined by the speed of diagnosis and neurological function at the time of starting treatment.

AETIOLOGY

Extradural metastases are usually a result of blood-borne dissemination. Less often paravertebral tumour or tumour within the vertebral body can infiltrate directly into the spinal canal.

SYMPTOMS

Spinal cord compression presents with neurological symptoms of weakness and reduced or altered sensation below the site of cord damage. This is accompanied by constipation and hesitancy in micturition leading to urinary retention.

Cauda equina compression similarly presents with weakness and sphincter disturbance. The sensory disturbance can be of reduced or altered sensation but nerve root pain affecting the lumbosacral segments is also seen.

SIGNS

Spinal cord compression causes a spastic paraparesis, or if it affects the cervical spine, quadriparesis, with a cut-off of sensory changes corresponding to the anatomical level of the compression – a sensory level. In contrast, cauda equina compression will result in a flaccid paraparesis with loss of sensation in a dermatome pattern affecting the lumbosacral segments (the lower limbs and buttocks). Reflexes are increased with extensor plantars in cord compression whilst, with cauda equina compression, reflexes are reduced or lost with flexor plantar responses.

Sphincter function might be disturbed and, with cauda equina compression, a distended bladder might be palpable and anal tone will be lax.

DIFFERENTIAL DIAGNOSIS

This includes intrinsic spinal cord tumours and paraneoplastic neuropathies. Transverse myelitis will give a clinical picture similar to cord compression and, in cancer patients, could be due to viral infection and rarely as a side effect of chemotherapy or radiotherapy. Other unrelated causes include prolapsed intervertebral disc, subacute combined degeneration of the cord and a parasagittal intracranial tumour.

Spinal cord and cauda equina compression

Acute onset of symptoms should raise suspicion of vertebral artery occlusion and cord infarction.

INVESTIGATIONS

Urgent investigations are required to confirm the diagnosis. Plain x-rays of the spine can demonstrate associated vertebral disease but urgent MRI of the whole spine is essential and will give the definitive diagnosis as shown in Figure 21.1. If MRI is contraindicated, e.g. those with a pacemaker or metal fragments, then CT imaging should be used and combined with a myelogram if required. Since multiple levels of cord involvement will be found in a third of patients the entire spine should be imaged.

TREATMENT

If spinal cord compression is the first manifestation of malignancy, then cytology or histology is obtained. If no primary site is apparent after a CT scan of the chest, abdomen and pelvis then a needle biopsy of the tumour at the site of spinal cord compression should be performed under CT guidance.

In the presence of a known histologically confirmed malignancy, treatment should proceed immediately as follows:

- All patients should start on high-dose steroids using dexamethasone 4 mg qds with, if necessary, prophylactic omeprazole or lansoprazole. Urine should be monitored for sugar, many patients having borderline glucose tolerance.
- Definitive treatment with surgery or radiotherapy should be given:
    - Patients with spinal instability should all be reviewed by a spinal surgeon.
    - Those with localized cord compression, having primary breast cancer with good performance status and no evidence of active metastases elsewhere have better outcomes with primary surgery and post-operative radiotherapy than with primary radiotherapy alone.
    - Most of the remaining patients should receive urgent local radiotherapy starting on the same day as the diagnosis is made. A dose ranging from of 8 Gy in 1 treatment to 30 Gy over 2 weeks will usually be prescribed, depending on the diagnosis and prognosis. For many patients with advanced disease, 8 Gy in a single dose will be effective in maintaining and improving neurological function whilst minimizing treatment.
- Certain patients may be more appropriately treated with chemotherapy, in particular those with lymphoma, small-cell lung cancer and germ cell tumours who have not been previously treated.
- In addition, appropriate general measures should continue. Patients with sphincter disturbance might require catheterization and analgesia should be given as necessary.
- Active physiotherapy and rehabilitation is a further important component of the management to optimize the chances of neurological recovery.

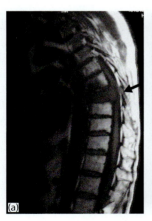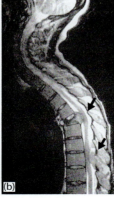

Figure 21.1 MRIs demonstrating (a) metastatic spinal canal compression owing to direct infiltration from a bone metastasis, (b) upper level: vertebral collapse and lower level: an extradural metastasis.

PROGNOSIS

Survival following cord compression is defined by the underlying condition and the performance status of the patient. It is often a reflection of disseminated disease and average survivals are usually measured in only a few months from diagnosis.

339

Oncological emergencies

The prognosis for neurological recovery is dependent almost entirely on the speed of diagnosis and instigation of treatment. Of patients who are mobile at the start of treatment, the majority (85%) will walk after treatment. In contrast, fewer than 15% of paraplegic patients will regain useful neurological function despite intensive treatment. For this reason, there should be a high index of suspicion for this condition, particularly in patients known to have metastatic disease, with urgent referral to a specialist centre for treatment.

SUPERIOR VENA CAVA OBSTRUCTION

Superior vena cava obstruction (SVCO) is typically due to a large mediastinal tumour mass causing obstruction to venous return to the right side of the heart, and is often associated with other symptoms of mediastinal compression including dysphagia and stridor.

AETIOLOGY

Any tumour involving the mediastinum could be the cause. The most common cause is carcinoma of the bronchus (80% of cases). In young patients, in particular, it is important to consider malignant lymphomas and germ cell tumours. Rarely a thymic tumour or retrosternal thyroid tumour can be the cause.

Post-mortem studies suggest that in most patients, although mechanical obstruction to venous flow may be the first event, thrombosis within the large veins inevitably follows, although emboli are almost unknown.

SYMPTOMS

Dyspnoea, stridor or dysphagia can be presenting symptoms. Intracranial venous congestion can cause headache or confusion. There might also be swelling of the face, neck and arms.

SIGNS

Oedema of the face, neck and arms can be apparent with fixed engorged jugular veins and dilatation of superficial skin veins over the chest, neck, face and upper limbs. There might be obvious respiratory distress or stridor. A tumour mass might be palpable arising out of the mediastinum in the supraclavicular fossae. Papilloedema can be present on fundoscopy.

INVESTIGATIONS

A chest x-ray will usually demonstrate a mediastinal mass, which will be better defined on CT scanning. Unless a diagnosis of malignancy has already been made, it is important to obtain a tissue diagnosis if at all possible. Other readily accessible disease sites should be sought such as a peripheral lymph node. If the mediastinum is the only site of disease, then a needle biopsy under CT control will usually be possible. More invasive approaches are usually avoided because of the theoretical risk of excessive haemorrhage from the area of raised venous pressure.

TREATMENT

Immediate treatment should take the form of high-dose steroids with dexamethasone 4 mg qds. Initial management should include consideration of vascular stenting, which is the most effective means of overcoming the venous obstruction in the early stages of SVCO and will result in immediate restoration of blood flow, as shown in Figure 21.2. The use of anticoagulation or antiplatelet therapy should be considered.

Definitive treatment will be either radiotherapy or chemotherapy. Where a diagnosis of lymphoma or germ cell tumour is made, further staging investigations should be completed as soon as possible followed by immediate chemotherapy. In small-cell lung cancer chemotherapy may also be the treatment of choice unless there has been previous exposure to chemotherapy or the patient is elderly or frail. All other patients should receive a course of radiotherapy to the mediastinum.

PROGNOSIS

The prognosis of SVCO depends on the underlying condition and in itself this is not a poor prognostic factor. For this reason, it is important to identify patients with lymphoma and germ cell tumour so that correct radical treatment can be given despite the acute nature of their presentation.

Superior vena cava obstruction

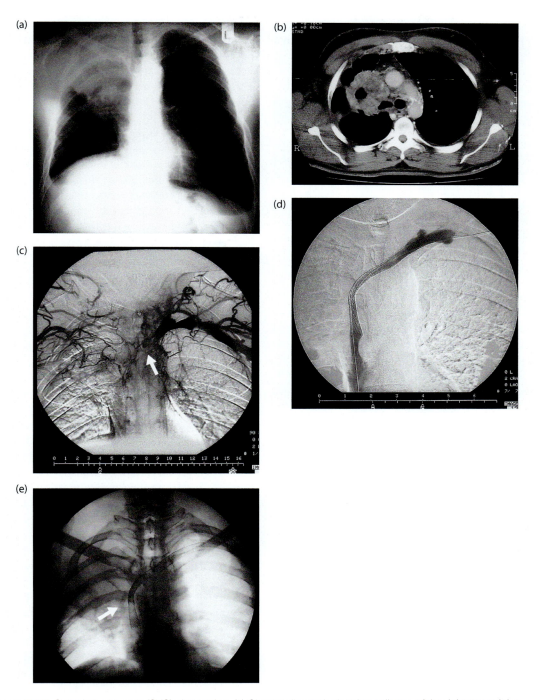

Figure 21.2 Superior vena cava (SVC) obstruction. (a) Chest radiograph showing collapse of the right upper lobe. (b) CT image of the same patient showing a soft tissue mass in the medial segment of the right upper lobe. It is impinging on the SVC. (c) SVC venogram. The left brachiocephalic vein is patent. Blood flow is obstructed at the SVC. (d) Flow in SVC restored. (e) SVC stent *in situ*.

Oncological emergencies

Most patients will benefit symptomatically from local treatment although recurrence of symptoms can occur at a later date.

NEUTROPENIC SEPSIS

Neutropenic sepsis is a major hazard and the principal cause of treatment-related death associated with the use of cancer chemotherapy. However, if promptly identified and aggressively treated, most episodes can be successfully controlled. Centres delivering chemotherapy will have a clearly defined neutropenic sepsis policy to ensure that all staff are familiar with the management of patients presenting with fever and neutropenia.

AETIOLOGY

Neutropenia will occur after most chemotherapy and may also be a problem when radiotherapy encompasses large volumes of bone marrow, e.g. long spinal fields or large pelvic fields. Bone marrow infiltration by tumour is a further cause. Life-threatening infection is most likely to occur when the total neutrophil count falls below $1.0 \times 10^9/L$. Host organisms in the bowel or skin are the major cause of infection. The presence of a central venous line is a further risk factor. The common pathogens are Gram-negative bacteria such as *Escherichia coli*, *Klebsiella* and *Pseudomonas* and Gram-positive organisms including *Staphylococcus aureus*, *Staphylococcus epidermidis* and *Streptococcus faecalis*. Less often the organism may be an anaerobe, *Pneumocystis carinii*, cytomegalovirus or a fungal infection.

SYMPTOMS

The patient might be initially asymptomatic or have non-specific symptoms such as malaise and anorexia. Specific symptoms related to a site of infection can include dysuria, cough or sore throat.

SIGNS

Any fever over 38.5°C in a patient with $<1.0 \times 10^9/L$ neutrophils should be considered due to systemic infection even in the absence of any other positive findings. There might be specific signs of infection in the oropharynx or chest. Sites of intravenous catheters should be carefully inspected for erythema or discharge. In more severe cases, there could be obvious septicaemic shock with hypotension and tachycardia.

INVESTIGATIONS

Any patient who is at risk of neutropenia and found to be febrile requires an urgent blood count. If a low neutrophil count is confirmed, blood cultures (peripheral and from a central venous access device if present), a midstream urine, throat swab and chest x-ray are required together with swabs from other clinically relevant sites, such as a catheter or cannula site, and collection of sputum if produced.

TREATMENT

Intravenous antibiotics should be instigated as a matter of urgency – a target of administration of intravenous antibiotic within 1 hour of a patient presenting with symptoms is a recognized standard. The results of cultures should not be awaited as life-threatening septicaemia can develop if there is any delay. The precise antibiotic combination to be used will be guided by individual hospital antibiotic policies but will take the form of broad-spectrum cover against both Gram-negative and -positive organisms. Typical combinations are an aminoglycoside with an extended spectrum penicillin, e.g. gentamicin or amikacin and carbenicillin, ticarcillin or piperacillin. Alternatively, a single-agent cephalosporin, such as ceftazidime or cefotaxime, can be used. If the fever does not settle after 48 hours and there have been no positive results from culture, then it might be necessary to add metronidazole for anaerobic organisms or amphotericin for fungi. If there is clinical evidence for *Pneumocystis* then treatment with high-dose co-trimoxazole will be required.

Granulocyte colony-stimulating factor (G-CSF) may be useful both initially to speed recovery of neutrophil count and subsequently to prevent further recurrence of neutropenia if chemotherapy is to be continued.

Once the results of cultures become available, then antibiotics can be adjusted appropriately. They should be continued for at least 5 days or for 48 hours after the fever has settled, whichever is the longer period.

Persistent fever in patients having a central intravenous line suggests colonization of the line and will require removal of that line to eradicate the source of infection.

If the patients are at high risk of infection then antibiotic prophylaxis is recommended. This includes those with leukaemia and lymphoma undergoing intensive chemotherapy. Co-trimoxazole, fluconazole and aciclovir are commonly used.

TUMOUR LYSIS SYNDROME

This is a syndrome arising as a result of rapid breakdown of large numbers of cells, usually at instigation of chemotherapy for a highly sensitive tumour such as lymphoma or leukaemia. There is an extensive metabolic disturbance characterized by hyperkalaemia, hyperuricaemia, hyperphosphataemia and hypocalcaemia.

If clinically significant, the syndrome presents as acute renal failure or acute cardiac arrhythmias with the risk of sudden death.

TREATMENT

Tumour lysis should be anticipated in any patient with a bulky lymphoma or leukaemia who is about to undergo chemotherapy. Preventative measures should be instigated prior to chemotherapy with 24 hours of prehydration ensuring good renal output and urine flow, and oral allopurinol should be started to prevent hyperuricaemia.

Rasburicase is an enzyme which oxidizes uric acid to allantoin, thereby resulting in rapid clearance of uric acid. It is indicated in patients with a high risk of tumour lysis providing greater protection against tumour lysis syndrome than allopurinol. It is particularly indicated in those with acute leukaemias, Burkitt lymphoma, chemosensitive paediatric tumours and other groups with renal impairment. It should be given prior to chemotherapy and daily for up to 7 days.

In patients who develop metabolic disturbances after chemotherapy, intravenous hydration should be continued. Alkalinization of urine with sodium bicarbonate can increase tubular excretion of potassium and phosphate. Specific measures to reduce very high levels of potassium might be required using insulin and glucose in order to prevent cardiac arrhythmias. In the most severe cases, particularly, if renal function deteriorates, then dialysis may be required.

PROGNOSIS

In most cases, the metabolic sequelae of tumour lysis should be predictable and preventable. Where metabolic disturbance does occur, prompt treatment is usually successful and the effects are usually self-limiting with resolution within 5–7 days of chemotherapy.

TOXICITIES RELATED TO IMMUNOTHERAPY AGENTS

The use of these agents is increasing in several disease sites and the management of side effects in a timely manner is essential. The most commonly used agents currently are the monoclonal antibodies pembrolizumab, nivolumab and ipilimumab.

These agents can affect one or multiple organs and systems.

- *GI*: Diarrhoea, anorexia, hepatitis, pancreatitis
- *Endocrine*: Pituitary function, adrenal function, diabetes
- *Lung*: Pneumonitis and interstitial lung disease
- *Skin*: From mild maculopapular rash to a severe rash or development of Stevens–Johnson syndrome, toxic epidermal necrolysis
- *Neurological*: Encephalitis, Guillain–Barre syndrome
- *Renal*: Autoimmune nephritic or nephrotic syndromes
- *Haematology*: Haemolytic or aplastic anaemia, idiopathic thrombocytopenic purpura

The oncologist managing the patient must be informed and expert advice from the appropriate physician sought as an emergency. The patient will often require admission to hospital and the use of high-dose steroids (prednisolone or methyl prednisolone) and management of specific symptoms (see Table 21.1).

Table 21.1 Manifestations of toxicity associated with immunomodulating drugs

Side effect	Grade	Signs/symptoms	Tests	Management
Diarrhoea	Mild	<4 loose stools, no pain or bleeding	Review diet Stool culture	Increase fluid intake Loperamide Oncologist informed
	Moderate	Cramping abdominal pain, blood or mucus	Stool culture CT chest and abdomen	Admit patient IV methylprednisolone Oncology and gastroenterology review If no improvement manage as per severe
	Severe	Diarrhoea with electrolyte disturbance, abdominal pain, low BP	Stool culture CT chest and abdomen	Admit patient IV methylprednisolone Oncology and gastroenterology review Infliximab therapy may be required
Endocrine	Moderate	Headache, fatigue, pituitary hormone abnormalities	Pituitary blood tests; cortisol, ACTH, TFT, LH and FSH, prolactin and testosterone in men and oestradiol in women MRI brain and pituitary	IV methylprednisolone Oncology and endocrinology review Thyroxine replacement if low
	Severe	Collapse Adrenal crisis New onset diabetes	Blood glucose Arterial blood gases	Insulin if diabetic ketoacidosis Urgent endocrine and oncology review
Hepatitis	Moderate	AST or ALT <5xULN Bilirubin <3xULN	Monitor LFTs HBsAg	Monitor patient Oncology review
	Severe	AST or ALT >5xULN Bilirubin >3xULN	Daily LFTs and INR Viral serology Liver US	IV methylprednisolone Urgent hepatology and oncology review Consider mycophenolate

(Continued)

Table 21.1 (Continued) Manifestations of toxicity associated with immunomodulating drugs

Side effect	Grade	Signs/symptoms	Tests	Management
Pneumonitis and interstitial lung disease		Shortness of breath, cough, hypoxia, pyrexia	CXR CT PA	If pneumonitis – IV methylprednisolone Urgent respiratory and oncology review
Skin	Mild	Rash	Document extent (medical photograph)	Topical emollients and steroids and antihistamine
	Severe	>50% body rash Stevens–Johnsons Toxic epidermal necrolysis	Document extent (medical photograph)	IV methylprednisolone Urgent dermatology and oncology review
Neurological	Severe	Guillain–Barre syndrome Myasthenia gravis Meningitis/encephalitis		Urgent neurology and oncology review IV methyprednisolone
Renal	Severe	Nephritis and nephrotic	Review medication Rehydration Renal assessment and US	Rehydration Renal and oncology review
Haematology	Severe	Haemolytic anaemia Aplastic anaemia Idiopathic thrombocytopenic purpura		Admit Haematology and oncology review IV methylprednisolone

Oncological emergencies

FURTHER READING

1. National Collaborating Centre for Cancer. *Neutropenic Sepsis: Prevention and Management of Neutropenic Sepsis in Cancer Patients*. National Institute for Health and Clinical Excellence (UK), London, 2012.
2. Metastatic spinal cord compression. National Institute for Health and Clinical Excellence (UK), February 2019. https://pathways.nice.org.uk/pathways/metastatic-spinal-cord-compression
3. Friedman CF, Proverbs-Singh TA, Postow MA. Treatment of the immune-related adverse effects of immune checkpoint inhibitors: A review. *JAMA Oncol*. 2016; 2(10): 1346–1353.
4. Wagner J, Arora S. Oncologic metabolic emergencies. *Hematol Oncol Clin North Am*. 2017; 31(6): 941–957.

SELF-ASSESSMENT QUESTIONS

1. Which of the following is true of malignant hypercalcaemia?
   a. It is a complication of lytic bone metastases
   b. It presents with diarrhoea
   c. The serum level of calcium should be corrected for the total protein
   d. Osteoclast-activating factors are important in its aetiology
   e. It is frequently a poor prognostic sign

2. Which three of the following are true in the management of hypercalcaemia?
   a. Most patients will have fluid retention requiring diuretics
   b. Patients should be put on a low calcium diet immediately
   c. Bisphosphonates are the drug of choice
   d. Management will frequently require repeated bisphosphonate usage
   e. Treatment of the underlying malignancy will be helpful
   f. Insulin and glucose will reduce the calcium rapidly in an emergency

3. Which of the following is true of spinal cord and cauda equina compression?
   a. It is usually due to tumour metastases within the spinal cord
   b. Most cases have a sudden onset of neurological disability
   c. Hemiplegia is the most common motor deficit
   d. Typically back pain is absent
   e. Recovery is related to the speed of initiation of treatment

4. Which three of the following are true in the management of cord compression?
   a. An urgent CT scan is essential for diagnosis
   b. High-dose steroids are started once the diagnosis is suspected
   c. Treatment should be deferred where there is no known primary tumour
   d. Surgery is indicated for spinal collapse or instability
   e. Catheterization should be avoided to encourage bladder training
   f. Urgent radiotherapy is the treatment of choice for most cases
   g. Around 50% of paraplegic patients will regain independent mobility

5. Which three of the following are true of superior vena cava obstruction?
   a. Lung cancer is the most common cause
   b. Widespread peripheral oedema will result
   c. Headache is a common presenting symptom
   d. Urgent embolectomy is indicated
   e. Most cases will resolve with heparin
   f. Superior vena cava stents are the treatment of choice
   g. Chemotherapy is contraindicated

6. Which of the following are common pathogens in neutropenic sepsis?
   a. *E. coli*
   b. *Clostridium difficile*
   c. *Pseudomonas aeruginosa*
   d. *Helicobacter pylori*
   e. Herpes zoster

Self-assessment questions

7. Which three of the following are true of the treatment of neutropenic sepsis?
   a. Intravenous antibiotics should be given despite no site of infection being found
   b. Urgent rehydration is required
   c. High-dose steroids should be started with antibiotics
   d. Inotropes may be required for hypotension
   e. Most patients can be managed as outpatients
   f. GCSF should be given to speed bone marrow recovery

8. Which of the following is true of antibiotic use in neutropenic sepsis?
   a. Gentamicin alone is adequate for most patients
   b. If fever persists after 48 hours, metronidazole should be added
   c. The antibiotic of choice for initial use is cefuroxime
   d. Antibiotics should not be started until culture results are available
   e. If there is evidence of *Pneumocystis* infection, rifampicin should be added

9. In the treatment of which of the following does tumour lysis syndrome most likely occur?
   a. Small-cell lung cancer
   b. Follicular lymphoma
   c. Testicular seminoma
   d. Mycosis fungoides
   e. Burkitt lymphoma

10. Which three of the following are seen in tumour lysis syndrome?
    a. Hypercalcaemia
    b. Hyperphosphataemia
    c. Renal failure
    d. Hyperkalaemia
    e. Hepatic failure
    f. Hypouricaemia

11. In the management of severe diarrhoea after nivolumab which of the following should be considered:
    a. Oral dexamethasone
    b. IV methylprednisolone
    c. Vancomycin
    d. Infliximab
    e. Salazopyrine

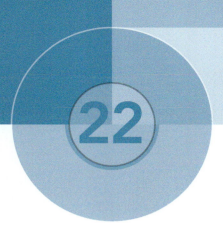

Palliative care

22

Medical care of a cancer patient does not stop when there is no curative treatment to offer and indeed over 50% of cancer treatments are palliative. In this area lie many of the greatest challenges in patient care – controlling pain, dyspnoea, vomiting, haemorrhage and other tumour-related symptoms.

PAIN CONTROL

Cancer pain is a chronic pain distinct from that associated with acute events such as trauma, postoperative pain or a toothache. An important feature for its management is that it will often be associated with a significant emotional component alongside the physical cause of pain. Most cancer patients have associated anxiety, fear, depression and anger, which will modulate their perception of pain and attention to these features will be of equal importance to the use of analgesic drugs. Three components to the pain of advanced cancer have been described:

- Physical
- Emotional
- Spiritual

Careful evaluation of pain is important in this group of patients in order that treatment can be directed to the principal underlying cause. The measurement of pain on an objective scale is of value, particularly in monitoring response to treatment. The use of a 10-point scale is common, sometimes in the form of a visual analogue scale, i.e. a 10 cm line on which the patient is asked to place a mark representing the severity of their pain as shown in Figure 22.1.

Another important principle in the management of pain in this setting is that few patients will have a single cause of pain, the average will have three or four individual pains identified and in some circumstances several more. Such pains may be interrelated, and around one-quarter might not be directly due to the cancer but reflect pre-existing pathology, e.g. osteoarthritis, or be associated pains from the effects of treatment interventions. The overall picture for an individual patient can therefore be quite complex. Assessment and monitoring can be helped by the use of a 'pain diagram' alongside the use of pain scores as shown in Figure 22.1.

The incidence of pain in patients with advanced cancer is between 70% and 80%. This can be effectively controlled in most cases by the application of simple rules governing the use of analgesics and related drugs:

1. Make a precise diagnosis of the cause of pain, e.g. whether a bone metastasis or nerve root pain.
2. Remember that many patients will have more than one pain and that pre-existing causes of pain such as arthritis will still be important.
3. Prescribe analgesics regularly, not as required, to prevent pain rather than wait for pain to return before the next dose.
4. Use and be familiar with a small number of drugs based on the analgesic ladder shown in Figure 22.2.
5. Consider specific cancer treatments, e.g. radiotherapy for bone pain whenever appropriate.

Palliative care

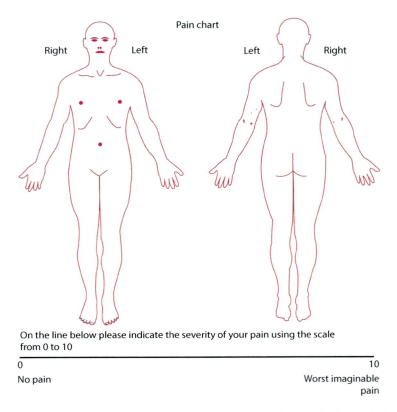

Figure 22.1 Pain assessment chart showing pain diagram on which the patient is asked to mark sites of pain, and 10 cm visual analogue scale (VAS) on which the patient is asked to mark severity of pain (0 = no pain, 10 = worst imaginable pain).

6. Establish realistic aims and expectations; not all patients will experience complete pain relief within a full range of activity and this should be made clear. Three levels of pain relief are described:

   - Pain free at night
   - Pain free sitting at rest
   - Pain free on movement

   Whilst the first two of these should be expected by most patients, pain control for movement-related pain is often much more difficult to achieve without limitation to movement.
7. Continually reassess the response to treatment and be prepared to modify regimens as the patient's condition evolves.

The use of analgesics in this situation should be based on a simple three-step analgesic ladder progressively escalating the potency of drug used. Alongside this, it is important to consider more specific causes of pain that may respond to additional treatment, for example radiotherapy for bone metastases.

LEVEL I ANALGESICS

Although these are freely available non-prescription drugs, of the patients who have not experienced regular analgesics around 20% will achieve good pain control simply by starting regular level I analgesics. Paracetamol and ibuprofen are the drugs of choice, available 'over the counter' in many countries, but nonetheless highly effective drugs when given on a regular basis. Paracetamol has the advantage of a very low incidence of side effects whilst ibuprofen or a similar non-steroidal anti-inflammatory drug

Pain control

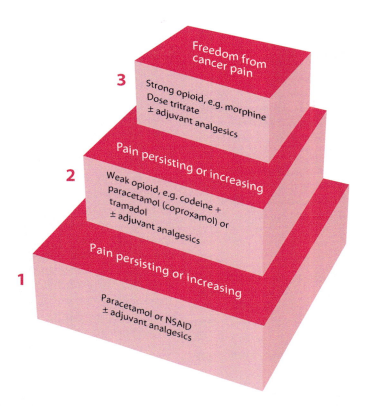

Figure 22.2 The analgesic ladder.

(NSAID) might be better where an anti-inflammatory action is required, although it is associated with gastrointestinal side effects, particularly in the elderly.

LEVEL II ANALGESICS

When level I analgesics are no longer effective, the next step is to use regular level II analgesics. These drugs are weak opioids, i.e. they act by binding to the same opioid receptors as morphine but are less potent. Because of this, however, they tend to have a similar side-effect profile, in particular being associated with nausea and constipation. The drugs available in this group are:

- Codeine, given as codeine phosphate 4–6 hourly
- Dihydrocodeine, a derivative of codeine
- Combination formulations of the aforementioned with paracetamol (co-codamol or codydramol)
- Tramadol, a synthetic opioid

There is no evidence to suggest that any one of the aforementioned is superior in the treatment of cancer pain; choice will be based on availability, patient tolerance and physician preference.

LEVEL III ANALGESICS

MORPHINE

Morphine should be used when the pain is no longer responsive to a level II analgesic. The following principles apply to the use of morphine in this setting:

1. Start treatment with regular administration. This may be achieved with a low dose of controlled-release tablets with regular breakthrough medication or 4-hourly morphine solution or tablets. The use of regular 4-hourly administration is much more flexible for dose titration. A double dose may be given at bedtime to avoid waking in the night.

2. Start a regular laxative with morphine, such as co-danthramer.
3. Start or be prepared to introduce a regular anti-emetic such as haloperidol.
4. Slowly increase the dose from an initial 10 mg 4 hourly until pain control is achieved. Initially the dose can be doubled every 24–48 hours; beyond 60 mg, increments of 50% will be better tolerated.
5. Warn the patient that during introduction and dose titration, they could feel drowsy and this will improve once they are on a stable dose.
6. Reassure the patient that addiction does not occur in this setting.

Parenteral opioids

Injection of opioid drugs such as morphine does not make them more potent when equivalent doses are given and should be considered only when oral or rectal administration is not possible. Remember that because of its greater bioavailability when injected, the oral dose should be approximately halved to give an equivalent analgesic action.

Controlled-release morphine

Morphine tablets give a 12- or 24-hourly release of morphine, and are generally preferred by patients once their dose requirements have been defined. Conversion from one morphine preparation to the other is simple as they are equivalent and a 12-hourly dose can therefore be given as a single controlled-release tablet or divided into three doses of immediate-release morphine at 4-hourly intervals.

If pain recurs then the cause should be investigated. Immediate-release morphine tablets or liquid should be given in addition to controlled-release tablets for 'breakthrough pain'. It is important to remember that the breakthrough dose should reflect the 12-hourly dose, i.e. be equivalent to a further 4-hourly dose so that a patient on 30 mg 12 hourly will require 10 mg breakthrough doses, but another taking 120 mg 12 hourly will require 30 mg breakthrough doses.

Spinal opioids

Epidural or intrathecal administration, usually of diamorphine, can have a place in patients with very high morphine requirements or who are resistant to oral medication.

ALTERNATIVES TO MORPHINE

Whilst morphine is universally available and accepted as the level III analgesic of choice, some patients will have unacceptable side effects, in particular drowsiness, hallucinations, confusion and constipation. In this setting, alternatives to morphine should be considered.

Fentanyl

This is a highly potent opioid drug with a short half-life. It is available in the form of skin patches allowing continuous transdermal absorption. This may have advantages over morphine in patients experiencing limiting side effects or in whom oral administration is difficult. A single patch will provide analgesia for 72 hours at a time and a dose of 25 µg/hr gives equivalent analgesia to a 24-hour morphine dose of approximately 100 mg. If necessary, breakthrough morphine doses can be combined with the use of fentanyl patches and, because of the delay in immediate absorption, the previous full dose of morphine should be continued for the first 24 hours after starting fentanyl patches to avoid withdrawal symptoms.

Sublingual or buccal fentanyl is rapidly absorbed and several formulations are available. These can be used for difficult incident or breakthrough pain to give additional pain relief over the background analgesia from regular opioid, for example when dressings need to be changed or for pain on movement.

Hydromorphone

This is a synthetic strong opioid, similar to morphine but in some patients better tolerated. It is therefore a useful alternative to morphine when side effects intrude. It is available in the same oral formulations as morphine but, because it is more potent, a dose reduction is needed, with 1.5 mg hydromorphone giving equivalent analgesia to 10 mg morphine.

Oxycodone

This is another alternative strong opioid. It has for many years been available as a suppository, but is now also produced as an oral drug in both immediate-release and controlled-release formulations. With hydromorphone it represents a suitable alternative to morphine for patients who cannot tolerate morphine because of limiting side effects, although since it is also a strong opioid a similar spectrum of unwanted effects are to be expected with both these drugs, in particular nausea and constipation. The use of these drugs should therefore follow guidelines similar to those for morphine with the accompanying use of regular prophylactic laxatives and anti-emetics.

Diamorphine (diacetyl morphine)

This is preferred for injections because of its greater solubility. Otherwise it has no advantages and is converted to morphine rapidly on passing through the liver.

OPIOIDS IN RENAL FAILURE

Morphine is converted in the liver to morphine 3 glucuronide and morphine 6 glucuronide, the latter being a potent analgesic. In renal failure, there is an accumulation of the morphine glucuronides resulting in significant toxicity. Morphine is therefore contraindicated in patients with impaired renal function.

Oxycodone and fentanyl are not metabolized in the same way and can be given safely in renal failure.

MORPHINE-RESISTANT PAIN

Whilst the previously mentioned approach will work well for most patients, there is undoubtedly a group of patients whose pain is not sensitive to morphine or other opioid drugs. It is important to recognize these patients and not submit them to ever-increasing doses of morphine for no benefit. In particular, musculoskeletal pains and neurogenic pains fall under this category. A further group of patients has been identified whose pain has been described as 'morphine irrelevant pain'. This refers to those in whom the overriding aetiology of their pain is due to an affective or spiritual component.

Therefore, in patients who, after dose titration to 40 or 60 mg morphine 4 hourly, are reporting no pain reduction with medication, it is important to reconsider the further use of morphine and explore alternative approaches with adjuvant analgesics, non-drug treatments or specific treatment such as local radiotherapy. A small group of patients can be identified who have true 'morphine resistance'. This has been attributed to an adaptive central response resulting in 'wind up', with altered perception of painful and non-painful stimuli (hyperalgesia and allodynia). This is thought to be mediated by a specific neurotransmitter, N-methyl-D-aspartate (NMDA). Specific NMDA inhibitor drugs are available including methadone and ketamine. Methadone dosage is often difficult to titrate and ketamine can be associated with significant psychotomimetic side effects. Such measures should be considered only under careful supervision in a specialist pain unit.

ADJUVANT ANALGESICS

This includes all drugs that do not have intrinsic analgesic activity but in specific situations will help in pain relief.

Non-steroidal anti-inflammatory drugs (NSAIDs)

These are useful in bone pain and soft tissue infiltration by tumour. They include drugs such as aspirin, ibuprofen or naproxen and can be adequately used alone as step I analgesics in some patients. Their main disadvantage is their association with gastritis and gastrointestinal haemorrhage. The risk is least with ibuprofen and greatest with ketorolac. If there is a previous history of dyspepsia or proven peptic ulceration, then particular care is required and concomitant use of a protective drug such as omeprazole, lansoprazole or misoprostol is recommended. They are also contraindicated in patients with renal impairment and significant asthma.

Steroids

These are of value in nerve root pain, raised intracranial pressure, hepatomegaly and soft tissue infiltration. Dexamethasone might be more convenient than prednisolone but both are effective in moderate doses, e.g. dexamethasone 4 mg twice daily or prednisolone 20–40 mg daily. There may be the added advantage of increased well-being experienced by many patients on taking steroids, but care should be taken not to induce steroid-related side effects, in particular fluid retention, restlessness and insomnia. The latter can be avoided by taking single early morning doses.

Bisphosphonates

Both zolendronate and ibandranate can be effective in metastatic bone pain even in the absence of hypercalcaemia. Oral absorption is variable and oral formulations are often not well tolerated; many patients are therefore better served by intermittent intravenous infusions. Hypocalcaemia and transient fever during administration can occur and adequate renal function is important. Serum calcium and creatinine should therefore be monitored prior to each administration. A rare complication of prolonged use is mandibular necrosis.

Anxiolytic drugs

Small doses of drugs such as diazepam or lorazepam might be required where anxiety is either a major component of pain or a debilitating condition in its own right. In the terminal phase patients often become restless and agitated and then midazolam given by subcutaneous infusion is effective.

Antidepressants

These could be required for some patients who are significantly depressed and can also be of value for neuropathic pain. Evidence for a role in neuropathic pain is greatest for amitriptyline, whereas, if a true antidepressant effect is sought, newer drugs with selective serotonin uptake inhibitor activity such as fluoxetine, paroxetine and sertraline may be preferable.

Muscle relaxants

Baclofen can be of value where muscle spasm is a significant component of pain, for example in paraplegia or pain associated with underlying bone or soft tissue metastases.

Anticonvulsants

Pain from peripheral nerve damage, either from tumour infiltration or other associated conditions, for example herpes zoster, can be particularly difficult to control and is often not very responsive to pure analgesics. It is typically a burning or stabbing pain within the affected dermatome. Alongside amitriptyline, gabapentin and pregabalin have emerged as the most useful drug in neuropathic pain largely replacing older drugs such as carbamazepine, sodium valproate or clonazepam, although objectively they each appear effective.

SPECIFIC CANCER TREATMENTS FOR PAIN CONTROL

For local pain from a growing and infiltrating tumour, specific therapy aimed at a reduction in tumour bulk and growth arrest is often the most effective approach.

RADIOTHERAPY

This is highly effective for metastatic bone pain and also of value in relieving headache from raised intracranial pressure due to primary or metastatic intracranial tumours. In this setting, it is important to select those patients with good performance status whose symptoms cannot otherwise be controlled with medication or those in whom medication such as morphine and steroids causes troublesome side effects.

In other situations where tumour is invading nerve roots or plexuses, as with an apical lung tumour invading the brachial plexus or presacral rectal tumour invading the lumbosacral plexus, radiotherapy is indicated for pain control.

CHEMOTHERAPY

In sensitive tumours, such as small-cell lung cancer, breast cancer and myeloma, chemotherapy can be of value for both bone and soft tissue pain where tumour infiltration is the main cause of pain. Despite only modest objective activity, chemotherapy is often associated with improvements in quality of life including pain and mobility scores. Some of the examples include cisplatin and gemcitabine in non-small cell lung cancer, taxotere in hormone-resistant prostate cancer and gemcitabine in pancreatic cancer. Again careful patient selection is required to optimize benefits and avoid unnecessary treatment in the face of disease that will inexorably progress.

OTHER PAIN TREATMENTS

Pain can have many components. The pain associated with malignant disease can have a major affective (emotional) component, and neuropathic pain and incident movement-related pain can present major challenges. In such pain analgesics and adjuvant drugs are often not successful alone. Alternative non-drug treatments can be very effective in selected patients, which include:

- *Transcutaneous electrical nerve stimulation (TENS)*: Sometimes particularly valuable for neuropathic pains
- *Specific nerve blocks*: Sometimes dramatically successful in selected cases
- Neurosurgical procedures such as cordotomy, rhizotomy or thalotomy
- *Massage*: Including the use of heat and cold on painful and tender areas
- *Acupuncture*: It can be particularly successful for difficult neuropathic pains
- *Relaxation and techniques such as aromatherapy*: They may also have a place in alleviating distress related to advanced malignancy

OTHER SYMPTOMS

Many symptoms other than pain can affect the patient with advanced cancer. These include anorexia, nausea and vomiting, constipation, sore mouth, confusion, cough and dyspnoea. Management should focus on the basic principle of diagnosing the precise cause of each symptom based on which the most effective treatment can be devised.

Common patterns are seen. In particular, many symptoms can be attributable to biochemical disturbance, and simple investigations including blood urea, creatinine and electrolytes, liver function tests and serum calcium may provide the cause for specific problems. It is always important to take a full and detailed drug history, since many of the problems encountered will be related to medication. Renal and hepatic dysfunction will also influence drug handling, and a change in these can suddenly destabilize a previously satisfactory drug schedule, a particular issue with morphine in renal impairment as discussed earlier.

ANOREXIA

This may have many causes, often interrelated, including:

- Anxiety
- Nausea
- Pain
- Liver metastases
- Sore mouth
- Uraemia

Specific treatment for each of these could be required, alongside which appetite can be stimulated by the use of low-dose steroids such as dexamethasone 4 mg daily or prednisolone 10–20 mg daily. An alternative is a progestogen such as medroxyprogesterone or megestrol which has the advantage of fewer steroid side effects.

It is important to have clear goals and realistic expectations. Patients with advanced cancer do not typically regain the weight lost prior to diagnosis and there is no evidence that specific dietary approaches will prolong life at this stage. Often considerable anxiety and tension develop between patients and those caring for them who, with the best possible motives, wish to see them eating heartily. Small, perhaps more frequent, meals with the emphasis on patient enjoyment and avoiding dehydration rather than high calorie intake is a preferable approach.

NAUSEA AND VOMITING

This can be a side effect of many drugs used in advanced cancer, in particular morphine. Other potential causes include:

- Mechanical bowel obstruction
- Hepatic metastases
- Uraemia
- Hypercalcaemia
- Cerebral metastases

A biochemical profile should be taken as the initial step in management with correction, where possible, of any biochemical disturbance. In addition, anti-emetic drugs will be required. Many drugs are available; choice for any individual should be based on the cause of nausea and the drug's site of action as illustrated in Table 22.1.

If there is no clear individual cause, then treatment should be started with metoclopramide 10 mg 4–6 hourly, haloperidol 1.5–3 mg nocte or cyclizine 50 mg 8 hourly. A similar principle of regular medication to prevent symptoms rather than 'as required' medication applies to the use of anti-emetics as to

Table 22.1 Anti-emetic drugs in advanced cancer

Site of action	Drugs	Indication
Vomiting centre	Cyclizine	Can be useful in all causes as this is the final common pathway for vomiting reflex
Chemoreceptor trigger	Prochlorperazine Chlorpromazine Haloperidol Metoclopramide Domperidone Ondansetron	Drug-induced Metabolic, e.g. hypercalcaemia, uraemia, hepatic Metastases
Peripheral	Metoclopramide Domperidone Ondansetron	Gastric stasis

analgesics. Often patients end up on a cocktail of three or four drugs and it is important to evaluate carefully the response to each and discontinue them if there is no clear benefit.

Patients with nausea and particularly those who are already vomiting might have difficulty in taking oral medication which may, if anything, simply provide an additional stimulus to emesis. In this situation, rectal administration using domperidone or prochlorperazine suppositories or buccal prochlorperazine can be helpful. Alternatively, subcutaneous administration, the infusion often also incorporating analgesics, can be used; metoclopramide, cyclizine and haloperidol are all compatible in this setting.

CONSTIPATION

Constipation and fear of constipation is often a major concern to patients and should be actively managed to avoid the situation where effective medication such as opioid analgesia is refused because of this. Constipation can be a side effect of drugs, in particular morphine and other opioids, or related to dehydration, hypercalcaemia or mechanical compression of the bowel from intra-abdominal or pelvic tumour. Good hydration and, where appropriate, a diet containing fruit and other fibre should be encouraged. Fruit juices are often welcome when solid food is no longer taken.

Laxatives should be given regularly to all patients receiving opioid medication. Co-danthramer, which has a combination of a bowel stimulant and faecal softener, is useful for opioid-related constipation and the dose can be titrated to the patient's requirements. Alternatives such as senna formulations, bisacodyl, docusate, osmotic salts, and lubricants, such as liquid paraffin, are also effective. Whilst oral agents are in general preferable in stubborn constipation, glycerine suppositories or phosphate enemas might be necessary to break a difficult cycle, particularly when preventive measures have not been used.

Methylnaltrexone is a specific μ-opioid receptor antagonist in the bowel and effective in difficult cases of opioid-induced constipation. If required subcutaneous injection could be given under the supervision of a physician as it may cause acute diarrhoea.

SORE MOUTH

This may be due to dryness of the oral cavity as a side effect of drugs, including morphine and phenothiazine anti-emetics, radiotherapy to the mouth, mucositis related to chemotherapy or candidiasis.

Oropharyngeal candidiasis can cause severe symptoms in these patients and should be treated actively with topical nystatin or amphotericin and, for persistent cases, oral ketoconazole. Regular mouthwashes, sucking ice cubes, carbonated drinks or ascorbic acid are also recommended.

CONFUSION

This can be one of the most difficult symptoms to deal with. There is often an identifiable precipitating cause which may include:

- Medication, e.g. morphine
- Hepatic failure

- Renal failure
- Hypercalcaemia
- Hypoxia
- Infection
- Cerebral metastases

Specific attention to the aforementioned can be supplemented with mild sedation using low doses of a benzodiazepine or, in more severe disturbance with hallucinations, haloperidol might be required in the acute phase. However, drugs should not take the place of sympathetic psychological support and reassurance counteracting the cycle of misinterpretation and overreaction which builds up.

COUGH AND DYSPNOEA

This is commonly the result of progressive intrathoracic tumour causing bronchial irritation or obstruction, lung collapse, lung metastases or pleural effusion. Chest infections are also common in this group of patients.

Alongside specific management of these problems, for example aspiration of effusion and antibiotics for overt infection, cough sedatives based on codeine linctus could be tried. When this is unsuccessful, morphine in doses of 10–20 mg 4 hourly can be effective. Steroids can be of value in diffuse lung infiltration with metastases or lymphangitis carcinomatosa.

THE DYING PATIENT

Inevitably, there will come a time when death is imminent. This may require changes in medication to minimize the physical distress for both the patient and relatives. The following points should be considered.

PLACE OF DEATH

Surveys suggest that the majority of patients would prefer to die in their own home. Only a small minority of patients die in a specialist palliative care setting such as a hospice and many die in a general hospital ward. When it is clear that the terminal course of the disease is approaching, the patient and their carers should have the opportunity to discuss the anticipated course of events and the place they would choose to die. The extent to which this is possible will depend on the individual patient, their wish to freely discuss such issues and to take part in such decisions. It is often a greater burden for the family of the patient who may worry about their ability to care for them at home, whilst having misgivings about the care available in local institutions. This is a particular concern where the patient expresses a strong wish to die at home but may live with only one elderly spouse whose physical capacity to provide the care required is limited. It is therefore important to identify the level of support that may be required for each individual, to have realistic plans for their care and to enable them to die in the surroundings in which they and their family are most comfortable.

MEDICATION FOR THE DYING PATIENT

Diminishing levels of consciousness will require a switch from oral medication. It is rarely necessary to give drugs intravenously or intramuscularly and the subcutaneous route should be chosen. If the patient is expected to succumb within a day or so, intermittent injections can be acceptable, but it is often easier and less traumatic to set up a continuous infusion pump. Diamorphine or morphine can be given by this route (remember to reduce the oral dose by 50%) and, if anti-emetics are required, haloperidol or metoclopramide can be added to the infusion. Alternatively, these can be given in suppository form.

AGITATION AND RESTLESSNESS

Terminal agitation and restlessness can develop. This is best treated by haloperidol, levopromazine or midazolam in the subcutaneous infusion.

RESPIRATION

Pooling of secretions can make respiration unpleasantly noisy and uncomfortable. This is best controlled with subcutaneous hyoscine in doses of 0.2–0.4 mg or glycopyrronium 0.6–1.2 mg by subcutaneous infusion. Levopromazine is also a useful

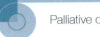

Palliative care

drug in this setting, compatible with subcutaneous infusions and, as a phenothiazine, it also has anti-emetic actions if required.

REASSESSMENT OF MEDICATION

Many patients continue to be left on large numbers of oral medications, most of which are irrelevant in these final hours. It is important therefore to review carefully all medication and in general most routine oral medical treatments such as antihypertensives, statins, anti-inflammatory drugs and laxatives can be discontinued without causing distress to the patient or hastening death.

ACUTE HAEMORRHAGE

Acute deaths are unusual in oncology but rarely a tumour can erode a large enough blood vessel to cause acute haemorrhage. The typical sites for this are the carotid artery in the neck, femoral artery in the groin or an intrapulmonary vessel. These are inevitably terminal events and can cause considerable distress. Sedation with parenteral diamorphine and local pressure to control blood loss should be administered. A dark-coloured blanket is also of great value in masking the dramatic loss of blood.

RESUSCITATION

It is always distressing following a chronic illness with inevitable death for the patient in the final moments to be subjected to inappropriate resuscitation procedures. It is important therefore that clear policies regarding resuscitation are given to those caring for the patient, arrived at only after full discussion with the patient and their family.

END OF LIFE MEDICATION: ANTICIPATORY PRESCRIBING

It is now common to supply 'just in case' medication packs for patients who are dying in their own home so that they are available if distressing symptoms arise, which include for example injectable diamorphine, levomepromazine, midazolam and glycopyrronium.

FURTHER READING

Cherney N, Fallon MT, Kassa S, Portenoy RK, Currow DC (eds.). *Oxford Textbook of Palliative Medicine*. 5th ed. Oxford University Press, Oxford, 2015.
NICE Care of dying adults in the last days of life. NG31 2016. https://www.nice.org.uk/guidance/ng31
Twycross RG, Wilcock A, Toller CS. *Symptom Control in Advanced Cancer*. 4th ed. Blackwell, Oxford, 2009.
WHO Guidelines for the pharmacological and radiotherapeutic management of cancer pain in adults and adolescents. January 2019 https://www.who.int/ncds/management/palliative-care/cancer-pain-guidelines/en/

SELF-ASSESSMENT QUESTIONS

1. Which of the following is true of cancer pain?
   a. It is usually traced to a single physical cause
   b. It is affected by emotional responses to cancer
   c. It is constant day and night
   d. Treatment is based on principles similar to postoperative pain
   e. It is difficult to assess accurately

2. Which three of the following apply to managing cancer pain?
   a. Analgesics should be given 'as required'
   b. Radiotherapy can play an important role
   c. A wide range of analgesics should be available
   d. Treatment might need to be changed regularly
   e. Different treatments may be required for individual pains
   f. Relief of daytime pain is the first goal
   g. Once pain is controlled, medication should be reduced

3. Which three of the following apply to the analgesic ladder?
   a. Non-steroidal anti-inflammatory drugs may be used as step 1

b. Tramadol is a useful level II analgesic
   c. Paracetamol is avoided as chronic use causes hepatic damage
   d. Severe pain will require level III analgesics
   e. Codeine is the most effective level I analgesic
   f. Morphine should be given only in the last weeks of life
   g. Level 2 analgesics should be discontinued when morphine is started

4. Which of the following is true of morphine use in cancer pain?
   a. Controlled-release formulations are best avoided
   b. Laxatives should be routinely prescribed with morphine
   c. Initially it can be introduced 'as required'
   d. Regular administration every 6 hours is most effective
   e. Regular anti-emetics are rarely required

5. Which of the following is a useful alternative to oral morphine in cancer pain?
   a. Sublingual buprenorphine
   b. Oral pethidine
   c. Oral tramadol
   d. Transcutaneous fentanyl
   e. Oral diamorphine

6. Which three of the following are useful adjuvant analgesics in cancer pain?
   a. Paracetamol
   b. Salbutamol
   c. Flucloxacillin
   d. Vitamin E
   e. Gabapentin
   f. Tamsulosin
   g. Methotrimeprazine

7. Which of the following is used in the treatment of anorexia?
   a. Acupuncture
   b. Diazepam
   c. Oravite
   d. Megestrol
   e. Methtrimeprazine

8. Which three of the following causes nausea and vomiting in advanced cancer?
   a. Hypercalcaemia
   b. Hyperuricaemia
   c. Cisplatin
   d. Renal failure
   e. Candidiasis
   f. Ascites
   g. Acoustic neuroma

9. Which of the following is true of constipation in advanced cancer?
   a. It may be due to renal failure
   b. Most patients respond to dietary changes
   c. Hyperuricaemia should be actively treated
   d. It will often respond to diuresis
   e. Patients on opioids will require daily laxatives

10. Which of the following is true in the dying patient?
    a. Regular meals should be maintained for as long as possible
    b. Sedation should be avoided
    c. Drugs and fluids are best given intravenously
    d. Analgesia can often be reduced
    e. Subcutaneous midazolam is used for terminal agitation

Appendix 1: Worldwide cancer burden – males and females

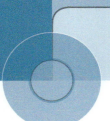

Incidence		Deaths	
Lung	2093876	Lung	1761007
Breast	2088849	Colorectum	880792
Colorectum	1849518	Stomach	782685
Prostate	1276106	Liver	781631
Stomach	1033701	Breast	626679
Liver	841080	Oesophagus	508585
Oesophagus	572034	Pancreas	432242
Cervix uteri	569847	Prostate	358989
Thyroid	567233	Cervix uteri	311365
Bladder	549393	Leukaemia	309006
Non-Hodgkin lymphoma	509590	Non-Hodgkin lymphoma	248724
Pancreas	458918	Brain,CNS	241037
Leukaemia	437033	Bladder	199922
Kidney	403262	Ovary	184799
Corpus uteri	382069	Lip,oral cavity	177384
Lip, oral cavity	354864	Kidney	175098
Brain,CNS	296851	Gallbladder	165087
Ovary	295414	Multiple myeloma	106105
Melanoma of skin	287723	Larynx	94771
Gallbladder	219420	Corpus uteri	89929
Larynx	177422	Nasopharynx	72987
Multiple myeloma	159985	Melanoma of skin	60712
Nasopharynx	129079	Oropharynx	51005
Oropharynx	92887	Thyroid	41071
Hypopharynx	80608	Hypopharynx	34984
Hodgkin lymphoma	79990	Hodgkin lymphoma	26167
Testis	71105	Mesothelioma	25576
Salivary glands	52799	Salivary glands	22176
Vulva	44235	Kaposi sarcoma	19902
Kaposi sarcoma	41799	Vulva	15222
Penis	34475	Penis	15138
Mesothelioma	30443	Testis	9507
Vagina	17600	Vagina	8062

Total numbers of cases excluding non-melanoma skin cancer
Derived from Globoscan data 2018: http://gco.iarc.fr/today/home

Appendix 2: Worldwide cancer burden – males

Incidence		Deaths	
Lung	1368524	Lung	1184947
Prostate	1276106	Liver	548375
Colorectum	1026215	Stomach	513555
Stomach	683754	Colorectum	484224
Liver	596574	Prostate	358989
Bladder	424082	Oesophagus	357190
Oesophagus	399699	Pancreas	226910
Non-Hodgkin lymphoma	284713	Leukaemia	179518
Kidney	254507	Bladder	148270
Leukaemia	249454	Non-Hodgkin lymphoma	145969
Lip,oral cavity	246420	Brain,CNS	135843
Pancreas	243033	Lip,oral cavity	119693
Brain,CNS	162534	Kidney	113822
Larynx	154977	Larynx	81806
Melanoma of skin	150698	Gallbladder	70168
Thyroid	130889	Multiple myeloma	58825
Gallbladder	97396	Nasopharynx	54280
Nasopharynx	93416	Oropharynx	42116
Multiple myeloma	89897	Melanoma of skin	34831
Oropharynx	74472	Hypopharynx	29415
Testis	71105	Mesothelioma	18332
Hypopharynx	67496	Hodgkin lymphoma	15770
Hodgkin lymphoma	46559	Thyroid	15557
Penis	34475	Penis	15138
Salivary glands	29256	Salivary glands	13440
Kaposi sarcoma	28248	Kaposi sarcoma	13117
Mesothelioma	21662	Testis	9507

Total numbers of cases excluding non-melanoma skin cancer
Derived from Globoscan data 2018: http://gco.iarc.fr/today/home

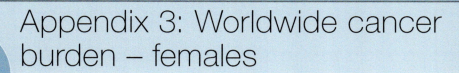

Appendix 3: Worldwide cancer burden – females

Incidence		Deaths	
Breast	2088849	Breast	626679
Colorectum	823303	Lung	576060
Lung	725352	Colorectum	396568
Cervix uteri	569847	Cervix uteri	311365
Thyroid	436344	Stomach	269130
Corpus uteri	382069	Liver	233256
Stomach	349947	Pancreas	205332
Ovary	295414	Ovary	184799
Liver	244506	Oesophagus	151395
Non-Hodgkin lymphoma	224877	Leukaemia	129488
Pancreas	215885	Brain,CNS	105194
Leukaemia	187579	Non-Hodgkin lymphoma	102755
Oesophagus	172335	Gallbladder	94919
Kidney	148755	Corpus uteri	89929
Melanoma of skin	137025	Kidney	61276
Brain,CNS	134317	Lip, oralcavity	57691
Bladder	125311	Bladder	51652
Gallbladder	122024	Multiple myeloma	47280
Lip, oralcavity	108444	Melanoma of skin	25881
Multiple myeloma	70088	Thyroid	25514
Vulva	44235	Nasopharynx	18707
Nasopharynx	35663	Vulva	15222
Hodgkin lymphoma	33431	Larynx	12965
Salivary glands	23543	Hodgkin lymphoma	10397
Larynx	22445	Oropharynx	8889
Oropharynx	18415	Salivary glands	8736
Vagina	17600	Vagina	8062
Kaposi sarcoma	13551	Mesothelioma	7244
Hypopharynx	13112	Kaposi sarcoma	6785
Mesothelioma	8781	Hypopharynx	5569

Total numbers of cases excluding non-melanoma skin cancer
Derived from Globoscan data 2018: http://gco.iarc.fr/today/home

Appendix 4: Answers to self-assessment questions

Chapter 1
1. a, c, g
2. b
3. b, e, g
4. e

Chapter 2
1. b, d, e
2. d
3. b, d, f
4. c, e. g

Chapter 4
1. b, c, g
2. b

Chapter 5
1. c
2. d
3. b, d, e
4. d
5. d
6. c, e, f
7. b, c, f
8. e

Chapter 6
1. a, d, g
2. c
3. b
4. b
5. b, c, f
6. b, c, d
7. c, e, f
8. c
9. d
10. a, c, g
11. e
12. b

Chapter 7
1. a, c, g
2. e
3. d, e, g
4. d
5. b, c, g
6. c
7. a, b, f

Chapter 8
1. d, e, f
2. b
3. a, c, f
4. d
5. e, f, g
6. d
7. b, c, g
8. c

Chapter 9
1. c, d, g
2. b
3. b, c, e
4. a, d, e
5. d
6. c, e, g
7. a
8. a, b, g
9. c
10. b, e, f
11. a, d, g
12. e
13. b, c, e
14. c

Chapter 10
1. c
2. b
3. b, d, g
4. d
5. a, d, e
6. c, f, g
7. e
8. b
9. d
10. e
11. d
12. a, d, g
13. b
14. a

Chapter 11
1. e
2. c
3. a, e, g
4. d
5. e
6. b
7. d
8. a
9. a, d, f
10. c
11. a
12. b
13. c
14. a, b, f

Chapter 12
1. b, c, d
2. d
3. b, e, f
4. b
5. b. d. g
6. b

Chapter 13
1. b, e, g
2. d
3. c, d, f

367

Appendix 4: Answers to self-assessment questions

4. e
5. a
6. a,c,d
7. b
8. a,f,g

Chapter 14

1. c, d, f
2. c
3. a, d, g
4. d

Chapter 15

1. c
2. b
3. b, c, e
4. b
5. e
6. c
7. e, f, g
8. b, d, g

Chapter 16

1. c
2. b
3. a, e, f
4. d
5. e
6. a, b, c
7. c
8. b
9. c, e, g
10. a, b, g

Chapter 17

1. b
2. a, c, f
3. b
4. e
5. b
6. b
7. a, b, g
8. e
9. b
10. d
11. a, d, e
12. b, d, g

Chapter 18

1. a
2. a, b, g
3. d
4. d
5. a, b, d
6. c
7. c
8. a, f, g
9. c
10. d

Chapter 19

1. c
2. a, c, d
3. c, f, g
4. b, e, g
5. a, c, d

6. b, d, f
7. b
8. b, c, d

Chapter 20

1. c, e, g
2. a,b,d

Chapter 21

1. d
2. c, d, e
3. e
4. b, d, f
5. a, c, f
6. c
7. a, d, f
8. b
9. e
10. b, c, d
11. b

Chapter 22

1. b
2. b, d, e
3. a, b, g
4. b
5. d
6. c, e, g
7. d
8. a, c, d
9. e
10. e

Index

Abdominoperineal resection (APR), 148
ABVD, *see* Adriamycin, bleomycin, vinblastine and dacarbazine
Acquired immune deficiency syndrome (AIDS), 7
Acute lymphoblastic leukaemia (ALL), 273, 279; *see also* Leukaemia
   aetiology, 279
   differential diagnosis, 280
   epidemiology, 279
   investigations, 280–281
   natural history, 280
   pathology, 279
   prognosis, 282
   signs, 280
   staging, 281
   staining characteristics of, 280
   symptoms, 280
   treatment, 281–282
   treatment-related complications, 282
   tumour-related complications, 282
Acute myeloid leukaemia, 283; *see also* Leukaemia
   aetiology, 283
   complications, 285
   differential diagnosis, 284
   epidemiology, 283
   investigations, 284
   natural history, 283–284
   pathology, 283
   prognosis, 285
   screening and future prospects, 285
   subtypes of, 283
   treatment, 284–285
Adenoid cystic carcinoma, 227; *see also* Salivary gland tumours
Adenolymphoma, 227; *see also* Salivary gland tumours
Adrenal tumours, 238; *see also* Endocrine tumours
   cortex tumours, 239–240
   phaeochromocytoma, 238–239
Adriamycin, bleomycin, vinblastine and dacarbazine (ABVD), 262
Aflatoxin, 3

AFP, *see* α-Fetoprotein
AIN, *see* Anal intraepithelial neoplasia
ALK, *see* Anaplastic lymphoma kinase
Alkylating agents, 52; *see also* Chemotherapy agents
α-Fetoprotein (AFP), 15, 132, 171, 332
Anal carcinoma, 146; *see also* Gastrointestinal cancer
   aetiology, 146
   anal margin carcinoma, 147
   complications, 149
   differential diagnosis, 147
   epidemiology, 146
   investigations, 147–148
   natural history, 146
   pathology, 146
   prognosis, 149
   pseudomyxoma peritonei, 148
   screening, 149
   staging, 148
   treatment, 148–149
Analgesic ladder, 351; *see also* Palliative care
Anal intraepithelial neoplasia (AIN), 146
Anaplastic lymphoma kinase (ALK), 17
Angiosarcomas, 3
Anorexia, 355; *see also* Palliative care
Anticonvulsants, 354; *see also* Palliative care
Antidepressants, 354; *see also* Palliative care
Anti-emetic drugs in advanced cancer, 356; *see also* Palliative care
Antimetabolites, 51; *see also* Chemotherapy agents
Anxiolytic drugs, 354; *see also* Palliative care
Apoptosis, 1
Aromatase inhibitors, 105
Askin tumour, 250; *see also* Soft-tissue sarcomas
Astrocytoma, 204–206; *see also* Central nervous system tumours
AUC, *see* Area under the serum concentration

Basal cell carcinoma (BCC), 317, 318, 319; *see also* Skin cancer; Squamous cell carcinoma
   aetiology, 317–318
   complications, 322–323

Index

Basal cell carcinoma (*Continued*)
    differential diagnosis, 320
    epidemiology, 317
    investigations, 320
    natural history, 318–319
    pathology, 318
    prognosis, 323
    recurrent, 321
    screening, 323
    staging, 320–321
    treatment, 321–322
BCNU, *see* Bischloroethyl nitrosoureas
BEP, *see* Bleomycin, etoposide and cisplatin
β-human chorionic gonadotropin (HCG), 15, 171, 197, 332
Bevacizumab, 107
Bilateral adrenal metastases, 75
Bilateral breast cancer, 92; *see also* Breast cancer
Bischloroethyl nitrosoureas (BCNU), 52
Bisphosphonates, 109, 354; *see also* Palliative care
Bladder cancer, 165; *see also* Urological cancer
    aetiology, 165–166
    complications, 170
    differential diagnosis, 166
    epidemiology, 165
    investigations, 167
    natural history, 166
    pathology, 166
    prognosis, 170
    rarer tumours, 170
    screening, 170
    staging, 167–168
    treatment, 168–169
Bleomycin, 52
Bleomycin, etoposide and cisplatin (BEP), 191
Bone and soft-tissue tumours, 304; *see also* Paediatric cancer
    rhabdomyosarcoma, 304–306
Bone metastases, 95; *see also* Breast cancer
Bone tumours, 256; *see also* Sarcoma
Brachytherapy, 41–42; *see also* Radiotherapy
Brainstem glioma, 15
Breast cancer, 60–61, 89
    adjuvant systemic therapy, 103–104
    aetiology, 89
    bilateral breast cancer, 92
    breast ultrasound, 96
    chest wall recurrence after mastectomy, 103
    differential diagnosis, 96
    ductal carcinoma *in situ*, 91, 99
    epidemiology, 89
    fine-needle aspiration cytology and needle core biopsy, 97
    hormone therapy in, 61
    inflammatory, 91
    investigations, 96–98
    lobular carcinoma *in situ*, 91
    lytic bone metastases, 94
    male breast cancer, 92
    mammography, 96
    mediastinal lymphadenopathy, 109
    natural history, 92–93
    Paget's disease, 92
    pathology, 90–92
    pericardial effusion, 109
    pleural spread, 96
    prevention, 113
    prognosis, 110–112
    pulmonary lymphangitis, 109
    sclerotic metastasis from, 95
    screening, 112–113
    staging, 98
    treatment, 98–110
Breast self-examination (BSE), 112
Broncho-oesophageal fistula, 120; *see also* Oesophagus carcinoma
Bronchoscopy, 71–72
Buschke–Lowenstein tumour, 175

Cancer pain, 349; *see also* Palliative care
Carcinoembryonic antigen (CEA), 15, 126, 136, 332
Carcinoid tumours, 240; *see also* Endocrine tumours
    aetiology, 240
    complications, 242–243
    differential diagnosis, 241
    epidemiology, 240
    investigations, 241–242
    natural history, 240
    pathology, 240
    prognosis, 243
    staging, 242
    treatment, 242
Carcinoma of unknown primary (CUP), 331
    case history, 335
    differential diagnosis, 332
    investigations, 332–334
    management, 334

Index

prognosis, 334
Carcinomatous meningitis, 213–214; see also Central nervous system tumours
choroidal metastasis, 214
MRI of brain, 214
optic nerve metastases, 214
Case–control studies, 32; see also Clinical trials
Castleman disease, 276
CCNU, see 1-(2-chloroethyl)-3-cyclohexyl-1-nitrosourea
CEA, see Carcinoembryonic antigen
Central nervous system (CNS), 13, 267
Central nervous system tumours, 201, 301; see also Paediatric cancer
    aetiology, 201
    astrocytoma, 204–206
    carcinomatous meningitis, 213–214
    cerebral tumours, 203
    chordoma, 211
    classification of primary, 202
    craniopharyngioma, 208–209
    ependymomas
    ependymomas, 210, 304
    epidemiology, 201
    germ cell tumours, 209
    haemangioblastoma, 211
    high-grade glioma, 202, 205
    lymphoma, 211
    medulloblastoma, 210, 301–304
    meningioma, 206–207
    metastases, 211–213
    multifocal high-grade glioma, 205
    multiple meningeal tumour deposits, 202
    natural history, 202–203
    oligodendroglioma, 206
    pineal tumours, 209
    pituitary tumours, 207–208
    spinal astrocytoma, 206
    spinal tumours, 201, 203
    treatment, 204
Cerebral tumours, 203; see also Central nervous system tumours
Cerebrospinal fluid (CSF), 202, 270
Cervical cancer, 179; see also Gynaecological cancer
    aetiology, 179
    case history, 182–183
    complications, 184
    differential diagnosis, 180
    epidemiology, 179

investigations, 180–181
natural history, 180
patterns of local spread from cervical carcinoma, 180
prognosis, 184
rarer tumours, 185
screening, 184
staging, 181
treatment, 181–184
Cervical intraepithelial neoplasia (CIN), 146, 179
Chemotherapy agents, 4, 51; see also Systemic treatment
    acting on DNA, 51
    acting on mitosis, 52
    alkylating agents, 52
    antimetabolites, 51
    classification, 51
    cytotoxic drugs, 58
    inducing apoptosis, 52
    intercalating agents, 52
    signal transduction inhibitors, 52
    targeting tumour vasculature, 52–53
    topoisomerases inhibitors, 52
1-(2-chloroethyl)-3-cyclohexyl-1-nitrosourea (CCNU), 52
Cholangiocarcinoma, 135; see also Gastrointestinal cancer
    aetiology, 135–136
    complications, 137
    differential diagnosis, 136
    epidemiology, 135
    investigations, 136
    natural history, 136
    pathology, 136
    prognosis, 138
    staging, 137
    treatment, 137
Chondrosarcoma, 256; see also Sarcoma
Chordoma, 211; see also Central nervous system tumours
Choriocarcinoma, 196; see also Gynaecological cancer
    aetiology, 196
    complications, 198
    differential diagnosis, 197
    epidemiology, 196
    investigations, 197
    natural history, 196
    pathology, 196
    prognosis, 198
    screening, 198
    staging, 197
    treatment, 197–198

371

Index

Chronic granulocytic leukaemia (CML), 280
Chronic lymphocytic leukaemia (CLL), 288; *see also* Leukaemia
    aetiology, 288
    complications, 289–290
    differential diagnosis, 289
    epidemiology, 288
    investigations, 289
    natural history, 288
    pathology, 288
    prognosis, 290
    Rai classification for, 289
    staging, 289
    treatment, 289
Chronic myelocytic leukaemia, 285; *see also* Leukaemia
    aetiology, 285
    complications, 287
    differential diagnosis, 286
    investigations, 286–287
    natural history, 286
    pathology, 285–286
    prognosis, 287–288
    treatment, 287
CIN, *see* Cervical intraepithelial neoplasia
Clinical trials, 27; *see also* Treatment policies
    case–control studies, 32
    cohort studies, 32–33
    randomized-controlled trials, 27–32
CLL, *see* Chronic lymphocytic leukaemia
CML, *see* Chronic granulocytic leukaemia
Cohort studies, 32–33; *see also* Clinical trials
Colon and rectum carcinoma, 138; *see also* Gastrointestinal cancer
    aetiology, 139
    epidemiology, 138
    investigations, 141–142
    management, 142–144
    natural history, 140
    pathology, 139–140
    prevention, 146
    prognosis, 144
    screening, 145–146
    staging, 142
Colony-stimulating factors (CSF), 63
Combined surgery and radiotherapy, 35–36; *see also* Surgical oncology
Communication, 24; *see also* Treatment policies

Craniopharyngioma, 208–209; *see also* Central nervous system tumours
CTLA-4, *see* Cytotoxic T-lymphocyte-associated protein 4
Cytomegalovirus (CMV), 261
Cytotoxic T-lymphocyte-associated protein 4 (CTLA-4), 63

Data monitoring committee (DMC), 31
DCIS, *see* Ductal carcinoma *in situ*
Deficient mismatch repair status (dMMR), 144
Denosumab, 109
Diamorphine (Diacetyl morphine), 353; *see also* Palliative care
DIC, *see* Disseminated intravascular coagulation
Diffuse large B-cell lymphoma (DLBCL), 267
Diffusion weighted images (DWI), 158
Disseminated intravascular coagulation (DIC), 127
DLBCL, *see* Diffuse large B-cell lymphoma
dMMR, *see* Deficient mismatch repair status
Drug resistance, 55–56; *see also* Systemic treatment
Ductal carcinoma *in situ* (DCIS), 90, 91, 99; *see also* Breast cancer
Dynamic contrast enhanced (DCE), 158

EBUS, *see* Endobronchial ultrasound-guided node biopsy
ECX, *see* Epirubicin, cisplatin and capecitabine
EGFR, *see* Epidermal growth factor receptor
Endobronchial laser therapy, 80
Endobronchial stent insertion, 80
Endobronchial ultrasound-guided node biopsy (EBUS), 72
Endocrine tumours, 231
    adrenal tumours, 238–240
    carcinoid tumours, 240–243
    multiple endocrine neoplasia, 243
    parathyroid tumour, 238
    thyroid cancer, 231–238
End of life medication, 358; *see also* Palliative care
Endometrial cancer, 61–62, 185; *see also* Gynaecological cancer
    aetiology, 185
    complications, 187
    differential diagnosis, 186
    epidemiology, 185
    investigations, 186
    MR scan, 186
    natural history, 185
    pathology, 185
    prevention, 187

Index

prognosis, 187
staging, 186
treatment, 186–187
Endoscopic retrograde cholepancreaticogram (ERCP), 136
Ependymomas, 210, 304; see also Central nervous system tumours
Epidermal growth factor receptor (EGFR), 17, 52
Epirubicin, cisplatin and capecitabine (ECX), 124
Epstein–Barr virus (EBV), 6, 225, 259
ERCP, see Endoscopic retrograde cholepancreaticogram
Erythrocyte sedimentation rate (ESR), 11
Everolimus, 107
Ewing sarcoma, 254; see also Sarcoma
    aetiology, 254
    complications, 255
    differential diagnosis, 254
    epidemiology, 254
    investigations, 254–255
    natural history, 254
    pathology, 254
    prognosis, 256
    staging, 255
    treatment, 255

FACT, see Functional Assessment of Cancer Therapy
Faecal occult blood testing (FOBT), 145
Familial adenomatous polyposis (FAP), 139
Familial atypical multiple mole melanoma (FAMMM), 126
FCR, see Fludarabine, cyclophosphamide and rituximab
Fentanyl, 352; see also Palliative care
Fibroblast growth factor 3 gene (FGFR3), 166
Fibrosarcoma, 248; see also Soft-tissue sarcomas
FISH, see Fluorescence in situ hybridization
Fludarabine, cyclophosphamide and rituximab (FCR), 289
Fluorescence in situ hybridization (FISH), 15
Fluorodeoxyglucose (FDG), 14, 262
5-Fluorouracil (5FU), 51
5FU, see 5-Fluorouracil

Gallbladder carcinoma, 138; see also Gastrointestinal cancer
γ-glutamyltransferase (GGT), 130
Gastrointestinal cancer, 115
    anal carcinoma of, 146–149
    cholangiocarcinoma, 135–138
    colon and rectal carcinoma, 138–146
    gallbladder carcinoma, 138
    hepatocellular cancer, 131–135

    oesophagal carcinoma, 115–121
    pancreatic carcinoma of, 126–131
    peritoneal tumours, 149–150
    stomach carcinoma, 121–126
Gastrointestinal stromal tumours (GISTs), 8, 125
GC, see Gemcitabine with cisplatin
G-CSF, see Granulocyte colony-stimulating factor
Germ cell tumours, 209, 313; see also Central nervous system tumours; Paediatric cancer
Giant cell tumour, see Osteoclastoma
Glutathione S-transferase (GST), 166
Gonadotrophin-releasing hormone (GnRH), 162
Granulocyte colony-stimulating factor (G-CSF), 63, 342
Granulocytic leukaemia, see Chronic myelocytic leukaemia
Growth factors, 63; see also Systemic treatment
Gynaecological cancer, 179
    cervical cancer, 179
    choriocarcinoma, 196
    endometrial cancer, 185
    ovarian cancer, 188
    vaginal cancer, 192–194
    vulval cancer, 194

Haemangioblastoma, 211; see also Central nervous system tumours
Haematological malignancy, 279
    leukaemia, 279–290
    multiple myeloma, 290–297
Hairy cell leukaemia, 290; see also Leukaemia
Hand–Schüller–Christian disease, 313
HCG, see β-human chorionic gonadotropin
Head and neck cancer, 217
    hypopharynx carcinoma, 224
    larynx carcinoma, 223–224
    nasopharynx carcinoma, 225–226
    oral cavity carcinoma, 217–223
    orbital tumours, 228
    oropharynx carcinoma, 223
    paranasal sinuses carcinoma, 226
    salivary gland tumours, 226–227
Hepatitis B virus (HBV), 6, 135
Hepatocellular cancer, 131; see also Gastrointestinal cancer
    aetiology, 132
    complications, 134–135
    differential diagnosis, 132–133
    epidemiology, 131–132

Hepatocellular cancer (*Continued*)
   investigations, 133
   natural history, 132
   pathology, 132
   prevention, 135
   prognosis, 135
   rare tumours, 135
   screening, 135
   staging, 133–134
   treatment, 134
HER2, *see* Human epidermal growth factor receptor 2
Hereditary non-polyposis colorectal cancer (HNPCC), 139, 166
5-HIAA, *see* 5-Hydroxyindoleacetic acid
Hidradenocarcinoma, 329; *see also* Skin cancer
High-grade glioma, 202, 205; *see also* Central nervous system tumours
HIV, *see* Human immunodeficiency virus
HNPCC, *see* Hereditary non-polyposis colorectal cancer
Hodgkin disease, 306–307
Hodgkin lymphoma, 259; *see also* Lymphoma
   aetiology, 259
   differential diagnosis, 261
   epidemiology, 259
   future prospects, 266
   histological subtypes of classical, 260
   investigations, 261–262
   late effects of radiotherapy, 265
   natural history, 260
   pathology, 259–260
   prognosis, 266
   second malignancies, 265
   staging, 262
   treatment, 262–264
   treatment-related complications, 265
   tumour-related complications, 265
Homovanillylmandelic acid (HVA), 308
Hormone therapy, 60; *see also* Breast cancer; Endometrial cancer; Prostate cancer; Systemic treatment
   mechanisms of androgen release and blockade, 61
Hospital Anxiety and Depression (HAD), 24
HTLV-1, *see* Human T-cell lymphotropic virus type 1
Human epidermal growth factor receptor 2 (HER2), 105
Human herpes virus type 8, 6
Human immunodeficiency virus (HIV), 6
Human papilloma virus (HPV), 6, 179, 217
Human T-cell lymphotropic virus type 1 (HTLV-1), 6, 266

Hydromorphone, 352; *see also* Palliative care
5-Hydroxyindoleacetic acid (5-HIAA), 16, 241
5-Hydroxytryptamine (5-HT), 241
Hypercalcaemia, 337; *see also* Oncological emergencies
   aetiology, 337
   differential diagnosis, 337
   investigations, 337–338
   symptoms, 337
   treatment, 338
Hypopharynx carcinoma, 224; *see also* Head and neck cancer

Ifosfamide, vincristine and actinomycin D (IVA), 305
Immunotherapy, 62–63; *see also* Systemic treatment
Indirect laryngoscopy, 73–74
Inferior vena cava (IVC), 153
Intensity-modulated radiotherapy (IMRT), 43, 129, 161, 221
Intercalating agents, 52; *see also* Chemotherapy agents
Internal isotope therapy, 42; *see also* Radiotherapy
IVA, *see* Ifosfamide, vincristine and actinomycin D
IVC, *see* Inferior vena cava

Kaposi sarcoma, 328; *see also* Skin cancer
Kidneys, ureters and bladder (KUB), 167
Krukenberg tumours, 123; *see also* Stomach carcinoma

Lactate dehydrogenase (LDH), 15, 171
Langerhans' cell histiocytosis, 312–313; *see also* Paediatric cancer
Larynx carcinoma, 223–224; *see also* Head and neck cancer
Leucocyte common antigen (LCA), 268
Leucoplakia, 218; *see also* Oral cavity carcinoma
Leukaemia, 279; *see also* Haematological malignancy; Paediatric cancer
   acute lymphoblastic, 279–282
   acute myeloid, 283–285
   chronic lymphocytic, 288–290
   chronic myelocytic, 285–288
   hairy cell, 290
   paediatric, 301
   prolymphocytic, 290
   rarer forms of, 290
Li–Fraumeni syndrome, 2
Liver Imaging Reporting and Data System (LI-RADS), 133
Lobular carcinoma in situ (LCIS), 90, 91
Loss of heterozygosity (LOH), 311
Low-level microsatellite instability (MSI-L), 140
Lung cancer, 67; *see also* Mesothelioma

aetiology, 67–68
bronchoscopy, 71–72
carcinoid, 82
chemotherapy, 81
complications, 80–81
differential diagnosis, 70
endobronchial laser therapy, 80
endobronchial stent insertion, 80
epidemiology, 67
management, 76
mediastinotomy and/or mediastinoscopy, 72
pancoast tumour, 74
positron emission tomography, 72
prevention, 82
prognosis, 81–82
rare tumours, 82
screening, 82
staging, 74–76
surgery, 81
thymoma, 82
Lymphoma, 211, 259;
   clinical types of, 260
   Hodgkin, 259–266
   non-Hodgkin, 266–276
   paediatric, 306–307
Lytic bone metastases, 94; *see also* Breast cancer

Macrophage colony-stimulating factor (MCSF), 291
Magnetic resonance cholangiopancreatography (MRI/MRCP), 128
Magnetic resonance imaging (MRI), 11, 13–14, 72
Malignancy of undefined primary origin (MUO), 331; *see also* Carcinoma of unknown primary
Malignant histiocytosis, 276
MALT, *see* Mucosal associated lymphoid tissue
MALTomas, *see* Mucosal-associated lymphoid tissue-type lymphomas
Mammography, 96; *see also* Breast cancer
Maximal androgen blockade (MAB), 61, 163
Maximum tolerated dose (MTD), 27
Medulloblastoma, 210–211, 301; *see also* Central nervous system tumours
   aetiology, 301
   complications, 303
   differential diagnosis, 302
   epidemiology, 301
   investigations, 302–303

pathology, 302
prognosis, 304
staging, 303
treatment, 303
Melanoma, 323; *see also* Skin cancer
   aetiology, 323
   complications, 327
   differential diagnosis, 325
   epidemiology, 323
   natural history, 324
   pathology, 323–324
   prognosis, 327
   screening, 327–328
   staging, 326
   treatment, 326–327
MEN, *see* Multiple endocrine neoplasia
Meningioma, 206–207; *see also* Central nervous system tumours
Merkel cell carcinoma, 328; *see also* Skin cancer
Mesothelioma, 83; *see also* Lung cancer
   aetiology, 83
   complications, 86
   CT scan of thorax and abdomen, 85
   differential diagnosis, 84
   epidemiology, 83
   investigations, 84–85
   natural history, 84
   pathology, 83–84
   prognosis, 86
   screening, 86
   staging, 85
   treatment, 85–86
Meta-iodobenzyl guanidine (mIBG), 239, 308
Methotrexate, vinblastine and cisplatin (MVC), 169
MGUS, *see* Monoclonal gammopathy of undetermined significance
mIBG, *see* Meta-iodobenzyl guanidine
Mismatch repair (MMR), 185
Monoclonal gammopathy of undetermined significance (MGUS), 267
Morphine, 351; *see also* Palliative care
   alternatives to, 352
   -resistant pain, 353
Mucosal associated lymphoid tissue (MALT), 126
Multiple endocrine neoplasia (MEN), 231, 243; *see also* Endocrine tumours
   type 1, 131

Index

Multiple myeloma, 290; *see also* Haematological malignancy
   aetiology, 290
   complications, 295
   differential diagnosis, 291
   epidemiology, 290
   investigations, 292
   natural history, 291
   pathology, 290–291
   prognosis, 295
   solitary plasmacytoma, 292
   staging, 292, 294
   treatment, 294–295
MVAC, *see* MVC Adriamycin
MVC, *see* Methotrexate, vinblastine and cisplatin
MVC Adriamycin (MVAC), 169
Mycosis fungoides, 328; *see also* Skin cancer
Myeloblastic leukaemia, *see* Acute myeloid leukaemia

Nasopharyngeal carcinoma, 225–226; *see also* Head and neck cancer
Nephroblastoma, *see* Wilms' tumour
Neuroblastoma, 307; *see also* Paediatric cancer
   aetiology, 307
   complications, 309
   differential diagnosis, 308
   epidemiology, 307
   investigations, 308
   natural history, 307
   pathology, 307
   prognosis, 310
   staging, 308–309
   treatment, 309
Neuron-specific enolase (NSE), 68, 308, 332
Neutropenic sepsis, 342; *see also* Oncological emergencies
   aetiology, 342
   investigations, 342
   signs, 342
   symptoms, 342
   treatment, 342–343
NHL, *see* Non-Hodgkin lymphoma
NLPHL, *see* Nodular lymphocyte-predominant hodgkin lymphoma
Nodular lymphocyte-predominant hodgkin lymphoma (NLPHL), 276
Non-Hodgkin lymphoma (NHL), 266, 306, 328, 332; *see also* Lymphoma
   aetiology, 266–267
   complications, 275
   differential diagnosis, 270–271
   epidemiology, 266
   future prospects, 276
   investigations, 269–270
   natural history, 268
   pathology, 267–268
   prognosis, 275–276
   rare tumours, 276
   staging, 271
   treatment, 271–274
Non-small-cell lung cancer (NSCLC), 68
Non-steroidal anti-inflammatory drug (NSAID), 350–351, 353
NSAID, *see* Non-steroidal anti-inflammatory drug
NSCLC, *see* Non-small-cell lung cancer

OAFs, *see* Osteoclast-activating factors
Oesophagus carcinoma, 115; *see also* Gastrointestinal cancer
   aetiology, 115
   broncho-oesophageal fistula, 120
   case history, 119–120
   complications, 120
   differential diagnosis, 116–117
   epidemiology, 115
   investigations, 117–118
   natural history, 116
   pathology, 115–116
   prognosis, 120
   rare tumours, 121
   screening, 120–121
   signs, 116
   staging, 118
   symptoms, 116
   treatment, 118–119
Oestrogen receptor (ER), 60
Oligodendroglioma, 206; *see also* Central nervous system tumours
Oncological emergencies, 337
   hypercalcaemia, 337–338
   neutropenic sepsis, 342–343
   spinal cord and cauda equina compression, 338–340
   superior vena cava obstruction, 340–342
   toxicities related to immunotherapy agents, 343–345
   tumour lysis syndrome, 343
Oral cavity carcinoma, 217; *see also* Head and neck cancer
   aetiology, 217

Index

complications, 222
differential diagnosis, 219
investigations, 219
leucoplakia, 218
natural history, 218
pathology, 217–218
prognosis, 223
screening, 223
staging, 219–220
treatment, 220–222
Orbital tumours, 228; *see also* Head and neck cancer
   orbital metastasis, 227
Oropharynx carcinoma, 223; *see also* Head and neck cancer
Osteoclast-activating factors (OAFs), 337
Osteoclastoma (Giant cell tumour), 256; *see also* Sarcoma
Osteosarcoma, 250; *see also* Sarcoma
   aetiology, 250
   complications, 253
   differential diagnosis, 252
   epidemiology, 250
   investigations, 252
   natural history, 251
   pathology, 250–251
   prognosis, 253
   rare tumours, 253–254
   staging, 252
   treatment, 252–253
Ovarian cancer, 188; *see also* Gynaecological cancer
   aetiology, 188
   complications, 190–191
   differential diagnosis, 189
   epidemiology, 188
   investigations, 189–190
   natural history, 188
   pathology, 188
   prognosis, 191
   rare tumours, 191–192
   screening, 191
   staging, 190
   treatment, 190
Oxycodone, 352–353; *see also* Palliative care

Paediatric cancer, 301
   bone and soft-tissue tumours, 304–306
   central nervous system tumours, 301–304
   frequency and type of common, 301
   germ cell tumours, 313
   Langerhans' cell histiocytosis, 312–313
   leukaemia, 301
   lymphoma, 306–307
   nephroblastoma, 310–312
   neuroblastoma, 307–310
   retinoblastoma, 313
Paget's disease, 92; *see also* Breast cancer
Palliative care, 349
   acute haemorrhage, 358
   adjuvant analgesics, 353
   agitation and restlessness, 357
   analgesic ladder, 351
   anorexia, 355
   anticonvulsants, 354
   antidepressants, 354
   anti-emetic drugs, 356
   anxiolytic drugs, 354
   bisphosphonates, 354
   confusion, 356–357
   constipation, 356
   cough and dyspnoea, 357
   diamorphine, 353
   end of life medication, 358
   fentanyl, 352
   hydromorphone, 352
   morphine, 351–352
   morphine-resistant pain, 353
   muscle relaxants, 354
   nausea and vomiting, 355–356
   opioids in renal failure, 353
   oxycodone, 352–353
   respiration, 357–358
   resuscitation, 358
   sore mouth, 356
Pancoast tumour, 74
Pancreatic carcinoma, 126; *see also* Gastrointestinal cancer
   aetiology, 126
   complications, 130–131
   differential diagnosis, 127
   epidemiology, 126
   investigations, 127–128
   natural history, 126–127
   pathology, 126
   prognosis, 131
   rare tumours, 131
   staging, 128–129
   treatment, 129–130
Paranasal sinuses carcinoma, 226; *see also* Head and neck cancer

Parathyroid tumour, 238; *see also* Endocrine tumours
PBSC, *see* Peripheral blood stem cell
PCV, *see* Procarbazine, CCNU and vincristine
Penis cancer, 174; *see also* Urological cancer
    aetiology, 174
    complications, 176
    differential diagnosis, 175
    epidemiology, 174
    investigations, 175
    natural history, 174
    pathology, 174
    prognosis, 176
    staging, 175
    treatment, 175–176
Percutaneous endoscopic gastrostomy (PEG), 221
Percutaneous transhepatic cholangiography (PTC), 136
Peripheral blood stem cell (PBSC), 272
Peritoneal tumours, 149–150; *see also* Gastrointestinal cancer
PIN, *see* Prostate intraepithelial neoplasia
Pineal tumours, 209; *see also* Central nervous system tumours
Pituitary tumours, 207–208; *see also* Central nervous system tumours
Pleomorphic adenoma, 226; *see also* Salivary gland tumours
Pleural fluid cytology, 84–85
Plummer–Vinson syndrome, 224
PNET, *see* Primitive neuroectodermal tumours
Primitive neuroectodermal tumours (PNET), 250
Procarbazine, CCNU and vincristine (PCV), 204
Prolymphocytic leukaemia, 290; *see also* Leukaemia
Prophylactic cranial irradiation (PCI), 78
Prostate cancer, 61, 156; *see also* Urological cancer
    aetiology, 156
    differential diagnosis, 158
    epidemiology, 156
    hormone therapy for, 162
    investigations, 158–160
    natural history, 157
    pathology, 156–157
    prognosis, 165
    rarer tumours, 165
    screening and future prospects, 165
    staging, 160
    treatment, 160–164
    treatment-related complications, 164–165
    tumour-related complications, 164
Prostate intraepithelial neoplasia (PIN), 156
Prostate-specific antigen (PSA), 15, 156, 332
Proteosome inhibitors, 52
Pseudomyxoma peritonei, 148; *see also* Anal carcinoma
Psoralens and ultraviolet A exposure (PUVA), 273
Pulmonary lymphangitis, 109; *see also* Breast cancer
PUVA, *see* Psoralens and ultraviolet A exposure

QALY, *see* Quality Adjusted Life Year
Quality Adjusted Life Year (QALY), 30

Radiofrequency ablation (RFA), 134
Radiotherapy, 39; *see also* Surgical oncology
    biological actions of ionizing radiation, 39–40
    brachytherapy, 41–42
    complications, 81
    equipment, 40–42
    external beam, 40–41
    internal isotope therapy, 42
    radiation protection, 47–48
    radiation types, 39
    second malignancies after radiation exposure, 47
    treatment planning, 43–44
    verification, 44
Randomized-controlled trials, 27; *see also* Clinical trials
    end points, 27–30
    ethics of clinical trials, 31–32
    meta-analysis, 32
    placebo-controlled trials, 30
    randomization, 30
    stratification, 30
    trial infrastructure, 31
    trial statistics, 31
Rasburicase, 343
RCHOP, *see* Rituximab, cyclophosphamide, Adriamycin, vincristine and prednisolone
RCVP, *see* Rituximab, cyclophosphamide, vincristine and prednisolone
RECIST, *see* Response evaluation criteria in solid tumors
Renal cell carcinoma, 153; *see also* Urological cancer
    aetiology, 153
    complications, 155
    differential diagnosis, 154
    epidemiology, 153
    investigations, 154
    natural history, 153–154
    pathology, 153
    prognosis, 155
    screening and future prospects, 156

Index

staging, 155
treatment, 155
Response evaluation criteria in solid tumors (RECIST), 28
Retinoblastoma, 313; *see also* Paediatric cancer
RFA, *see* Radiofrequency ablation
Rhabdomyosarcoma, 304
    aetiology, 304
    complications, 306
    differential diagnosis, 305
    epidemiology, 304
    investigations, 305
    natural history, 304
    pathology, 304
    prognosis, 306
    staging, 305
    treatment, 305–306
Risk of Malignancy index (RMI), 189
Rituximab, cyclophosphamide, Adriamycin, vincristine and prednisolone (RCHOP), 274
Rituximab, cyclophosphamide, vincristine and prednisolone (RCVP), 271

SABR, *see* Stereotactic ablative radiotherapy
Salivary gland tumours, 226; *see also* Head and neck cancer
    adenoid cystic carcinoma, 227
    adenolymphoma, 227
    carcinoma, 227
    lymphoma, 227
    pleomorphic adenoma, 226
Sarcoma, 245, 329; *see also* Skin cancer
    bone tumours, 256
    chondrosarcoma, 256
    Ewing, 254–256
    osteoclastoma, 256
    osteosarcoma, 250–254
    soft-tissue, 245–250
    spindle cell, 256
SBRT, *see* Stereotactic body radiotherapy
SIADH, *see* Syndrome of inappropriate antidiuretic hormone secretion
Skin cancer, 317
    hidradenocarcinoma, 329
    Kaposi sarcoma, 328
    melanoma, 323–328
    Merkel cell carcinoma, 328
    metastases, 328
    mycosis fungoides, 328
    non-Hodgkin lymphoma, 328
    rare tumours, 328
    sarcoma, 329
    squamous and basal cell carcinoma, 317–323
Small-cell lung cancer (SCLC), 67
    radical treatment of, 78–79
Soft-tissue sarcomas, 245; *see also* Sarcoma
    aetiology, 245
    classification of, 246
    complications, 249
    differential diagnosis, 246
    epidemiology, 245
    fibrosarcoma, 248
    future developments, 249
    investigations, 246, 248
    natural history, 246
    pathology, 245–246
    prognosis, 249
    rare tumours, 250
    staging, 248
    treatment, 249
Solitary plasmacytoma, 292; *see also* Multiple myeloma
Spinal astrocytoma, 206; *see also* Central nervous system tumours
Spinal cord and cauda equina compression, 338; *see also* Oncological emergencies
    aetiology, 338
    differential diagnosis, 338–339
    investigations, 339
    prognosis, 339–340
    signs, 338
    symptoms, 338
    treatment, 339
Spinal tumours, 201, 203; *see also* Central nervous system tumours
Spindle cell sarcoma, 256; *see also* Sarcoma
Sputum cytology, 71; *see also* Lung cancer
SRS, *see* Stereotactic radiosurgery
Stereotactic ablative radiotherapy (SABR), 77
Stereotactic body radiotherapy (SBRT), 134, 161, 165
Stereotactic radiosurgery (SRS), 204, 211
Stomach carcinoma, 121; *see also* Gastrointestinal cancer
    aetiology, 121
    complications, 124–125
    differential diagnosis, 123
    epidemiology, 121
    investigations, 123
    Krukenberg tumours, 123
    natural history, 122

Index

Stomach carcinoma (*Continued*)
  pathology, 122
  prognosis, 125
  rare tumours, 125–126
  screening, 125
  staging, 123
  treatment, 124
Superior vena cava obstruction (SVCO), 340, 341; *see also* Oncological emergencies
  aetiology, 340
  investigations, 340
  prognosis, 340, 342
  signs, 340
  symptoms, 340
  treatment, 340
Suprasellar teratoma, 209
Surgical oncology, 35
  merits of pre-and post-operative radiotherapy, 36
  palliative surgery, 37
  primary tumour management, 35
  regional lymph node management, 36
  surgery and radiotherapy, 35–36
SVCO, *see* Superior vena cava obstruction
Syndrome of inappropriate antidiuretic hormone secretion (SIADH), 81

TENS, *see* Transcutaneous electrical nerve stimulation
Testis cancer, 170; *see also* Urological cancer
  aetiology, 170
  complications, 173–174
  differential diagnosis, 171
  epidemiology, 170
  investigations, 171
  natural history, 171
  pathology, 170–171
  prognosis, 174
  rarer tumours, 174
  screening, 174
  staging, 171–173
  treatment, 173
TGFβ, *see* Transforming growth factor β
Thymoma, 82
Thyroid cancer, 231; *see also* Endocrine tumours
  aetiology, 231
  anaplastic, 236
  complications, 236–237
  differential diagnosis, 232
  epidemiology, 231
  investigations, 232–234
  medullary carcinoma, 233
  natural history, 232
  palliative treatment, 236
  pathology, 231–232
  prognosis, 237
  rare tumours, 237–238
  screening, 237
  staging, 234
  treatment, 234
Thyroid-stimulating hormone (TSH), 7, 234
Topoisomerases inhibitors, 52; *see also* Chemotherapy agents
Total mesorectal excision (TME), 143
Transarterial chemo-embolization (TACE), 134
Transcutaneous electrical nerve stimulation (TENS), 355
Transforming growth factor β (TGFβ), 337
Transurethral resection of bladder tumour (TURBT), 167
Transurethral resection of the prostate (TURP), 160
Trastuzumab, 110
TSH, *see* Thyroid-stimulating hormone
Tumour necrosis factor (TNF), 291
Tyrosine kinase inhibitors (TKIs), 80, 155

Urological cancer, 153
  bladder cancer, 165–170
  penis cancer, 174–176
  prostate cancer, 156–165
  renal cell carcinoma, 153–156
  testis cancer, 170–174

VA, *see* Vincristine and actinomycin D
VAC, *see* Vincristine, actinomycin D and cyclophosphamide
Vaginal cancer, 192; *see also* Gynaecological cancer
  aetiology, 192
  complications, 193
  differential diagnosis, 193
  epidemiology, 192
  investigations, 193
  natural history, 192
  pathology, 192
  prognosis, 194
  rarer tumours, 194
  screening, 194
  staging, 193
  treatment, 193
Vaginal intraepithelial neoplasia (VAIN), 192
Vascular disrupting agents (VDAs), 51
Vascular endothelial growth factor (VEGF), 52, 107, 153

Index

Vasoactive intestinal peptide (VIP), 308, 309
VIA, *see* Vincristine, ifosfamide and actinomycin D
VIDE, *see* Vincristine, ifosfamide, doxorubicin and etoposide
Vinca alkaloids, 52
Vincristine, actinomycin D and cyclophosphamide (VAC), 191, 255
Vincristine and actinomycin D (VA), 305
Vincristine, ifosfamide and actinomycin D (VIA), 255
Vincristine, ifosfamide, doxorubicin and etoposide (VIDE), 255
Von Hippel–Lindau (VHL), 153
Vulval cancer, 194; *see also* Gynaecological cancer
    aetiology, 194
    complications, 196
    differential diagnosis, 195
    epidemiology, 194
    investigations, 195
    natural history, 194
    pathology, 194
    prognosis, 196
    rare tumours, 196
    staging, 195
    treatment, 195

Waldenström macroglobulinaemia, 276
Whole brain radiotherapy (WBRT), 204, 213
Wilms' tumour (WT), 310; *see also* Paediatric cancer
    aetiology, 310
    complications, 312
    CT scan, 311
    differential diagnosis, 311
    epidemiology, 310
    investigations, 311
    natural history, 310
    pathology, 310
    prognosis, 312
    rare tumours, 312
    staging, 311
    treatment, 311–312

Xeroderma pigmentosum, 4

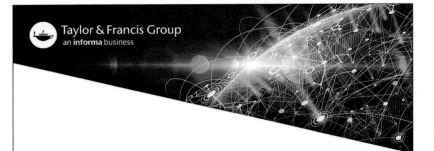